Population Policy & Women's Rights

Population Policy & Women's Rights

Transforming Reproductive Choice

Ruth Dixon-Mueller

PRAEGER

Westport, Connecticut
London

Library of Congress Cataloging-in-Publication Data

Dixon-Mueller, Ruth.
   Population policy and women's rights : transforming reproductive
choice / Ruth Dixon-Mueller.
     p. cm.
   Includes bibliographical references (p.   ) and index.
   ISBN 0–275–94504–9 (Permanent Paper).—ISBN 0–275–94611–8 (alk.: pb.)
   1. Population policy.   2. Birth control.   3. Women's rights.
4. Feminism.   I. Title.
HQ766.7.D58   1993
304.6—dc20   92–28547

British Library Cataloguing in Publication Data is available.

Library of Congress Catalog Card Number: 92–28547
ISBN: 0–275–94504–9 (hb)
      0–275–94611–8 (pb)

First published in 1993

Praeger Publishers, 88 Post Road West, Westport, CT 06881
An imprint of Greenwood Publishing Group, Inc.

Printed in the United States of America

The paper used in this book complies with the Permanent
Paper Standard issued by the National Information Standards
Organization (Z39.48—1984).

10 9 8 7 6 5 4 3 2 1

Copyright Acknowledgments

The author and publisher wish to acknowledge the following for permission to include their
material in this volume:
   Extracts from "Abortion Policy and Women's Health in Developing Countries," by Ruth
Dixon-Mueller, in *International Journal of Health Services*, Vol. 20(2), 1990, pp. 297–314,
published by the Baywood Publishing Co., Inc.
   Extracts from "U.S. International Population Policy and the Woman Question," by Ruth
Dixon-Mueller, in *Journal of International Law & Politics*, Vol. 20(1), Fall 1987, pp. 143–
167, by permission of the Journal of International Law & Politics.
   Extracts from "Psychosocial Consequences to Women of Contraceptive Use and
Controlled Fertility," by Ruth Dixon-Mueller, in *Contraceptive Use and Controlled Fertility*,
1989, published by National Academy Press, Washington, D.C., reprinted with permission.
   An earlier version of chapter 4, "Population Policy and Women's Political Action in Three
Developing Countries" appears in *The Politics of Family Planning in the Third World*,
edited by Jason L. Finkle and Alison McIntosh, published as a supplement to *Population
and Development Review*, Volume 19 (© The Population Council, 1993).

CONTENTS

PREFACE

This book has evolved over a period of 25 years. My interest in domestic and international population policies was first stimulated by Kingsley Davis, Judith Blake, William Petersen, and Calvin Goldscheider during graduate studies in sociology and demography at the University of California, Berkeley in the late 1960s. In 1972 I took a year's leave from the University of California at Davis to work with the Section on the Status of Women at the United Nations in New York. Energized by the emerging feminist movement and eager to put the tools of social demography to good use, I prepared a report on *The Status of Women and Family Planning* for the celebration of World Population Year in 1974 and International Women's Year in 1975. The study illuminated the connections between women's reproductive and productive lives in ways that have defined virtually all of my subsequent work on women's employment, marriage and childbearing, and the impact of development on women.

The international conferences on women sponsored by the United Nations in Mexico City in 1975, Copenhagen in 1980, and Nairobi in 1985, along with their associated nongovernmental forums, inspired women throughout the world to work for the elimination of oppressive gender ideologies and practices and for the equitable development of their own societies. The U.N. Convention on the Elimination of All Forms of Discrimination Against Women (1979) is particularly important as an international standard-bearer for women's rights as broadly defined. In addition, the population conferences held by the United Nations in Bucharest in 1974 and Mexico City in 1984, together with their nongovernmental forums, pulled together policymakers, social scientists, and other activists in a broad-ranging effort to focus attention on problems of population growth and distribution as experienced in diverse national settings. Because these documents and events have reflected and shaped much of the thinking in the international arena about women's rights and population processes, they form a logical framework for this book.

Many people share responsibility for the ideas and motivation that have resulted in this book. Collectively, they include friends and colleagues at the United Nations, the Department of Sociology at the University of California at Davis, the Departments of Sociology and of Demography at the University of California at Berkeley, the Committee on Population of the National Research Council, the Association for Women in Development, the Population Council, and the International Women's Health Coalition in New York. Individually, for their valued friendship over the years, their inspired intellect, and their commitment to "the cause," I am deeply indebted to Judith Bruce, Joan Dunlop, Karen Paige Ericksen, Judith Helzner, Rounaq Jahan, Judith Justice, Kristin Luker, Judith V. May, Emily C. Moore, Hanna Papanek, Harriet B. Presser, Judith Stacey, Judith Tendler, Irene Tinker, and Norma J. Wikler. I couldn't have done it without them. Others who should be listed here are excluded only for reasons of space. A special note of appreciation goes to Adrienne Germain of the International Women's Health Coalition, coauthor of chapter 4, for persuading me to work with the Coalition's international programs on behalf of women's reproductive rights and health and for contributing many of the ideas in this book. By a long and gradual process of osmosis, I have come to think of them as my own.

INTRODUCTION

One of the major questions addressing the world today is whether the growth of the global population will slow down sufficiently over the next two decades to preserve a sustainable standard of living for all people without resorting to coercive measures of population control. On the one hand, the urgency of the global environmental crisis is eliciting new calls for decisive action on the "population front" in the most populous southern[1] countries, excluding China, along with charges that the world will soon be forced to reckon with the consequences of years of population policy neglect (e.g., Ehrlich and Ehrlich 1990; Brown et al. 1991; "Priority Statement on Population" 1991). On the other hand, feminists and women's health advocates in both southern and northern countries are increasingly outspoken in their criticisms of population control rhetoric that blames Third World women for their "excess fertility" and leads to overzealous recruitment of family planning "acceptors" and other program abuses (e.g., Hartmann 1987; Sen and Grown 1987; Karkal and Pandey 1989). These are not new arguments. They first burst into public consciousness in the 1960s as the U.S. government began its large-scale funding of contraceptive research and domestic and international family planning programs. The arguments are becoming increasingly powerful, however, as calls for stronger antinatalist measures intensify on one side and resistance to the rhetoric hardens on the other. At the same time, rising waves of religious fundamentalism, ethnic nationalism, and an organized international "right-to-life" movement threaten to undermine much of what has been achieved in the fields of family planning, women's rights, and reproductive freedom over the past three decades.

Feminists in many countries have been caught between the antinatalist ideologies of the "controlistas" and the pronatalist ideologies of nationalist and fundamentalist forces, both of which lay claim to the control of women's bodies and women's lives. The controlista ideologies have tended to elicit greater resistance from feminists, however, in large part because they are seen as First World programs aimed at limiting the growth of Third World populations by forcing women to use imported and imposed birth control technologies under unsafe conditions. As a consequence, some radical feminist groups insist that family planning programs in most southern countries are by definition coercive and that all artificial methods of fertility control should be rejected. This is an extreme position, of course, but it illustrates the extent to which opposition can go. Indeed, the most radical feminist position on birth control has come dangerously full circle to join that of some anti-choice "right-to-life" organizations. There is also a tendency among some feminist groups to deny the existence of a global population problem. By focusing on pervasive social injustice and inequalities in the distribution of resources across and within nations they do a great service to our understanding of the root causes of poverty. Unfortunately, however, the analysis often leads to the conclusion that family planning programs are unnecessary, or that they must be rejected under certain political circumstances, or that the fundamental problems of poverty and injustice must be solved first. Where does this leave those women who are desperately trying to preserve their health and regulate their fertility by spacing their pregnancies and resorting to unsafe abortion? How does one justify withholding from poor women in southern countries those methods of fertility control that wealthy women in the south and the north take for granted? In what way is the principle of distributive justice or equity—or, indeed, of "sisterhood"—served by these restrictions?

There is an urgent need for a gathering of feminist forces that will (1) recognize that population growth at the global level is a problem that must be solved; (2) articulate a set of feminist principles on which a responsive population (reproductive) policy could be based; (3) build alliances with human rights advocates, development specialists, government planners, legislators, and the population/family planning community in the policy-making process; and (4) work to extend to all women the full range of sexual and reproductive health and rights to which they are, in principle, entitled.

At the same time, population policymakers, researchers, and family planning providers must learn to listen closely to what women's health advocates and women of all social classes have to say about their fears, concerns, and needs. Population researchers and planners are dealing in fundamental ways with women's bodies and lives, yet the language of their discourse reveals little awareness of this basic fact. Preoccupations with the mathematical modeling of population processes, the biotechnology of contraceptive development, and the demographic effectiveness and efficiency of various program interventions have taken precedence. Moreover, the rhetoric of population control that has tainted contraceptive service delivery in so many countries does a disservice to the cause of empowering women to take control over their own lives. It also devalues women's concerns about their reproductive health and their children's survival and security.

How can this chasm be bridged? Through dialogue, through cooperation, through reformulating the goals and methodologies of population policies and programs. It is time for a sea change in our thinking, for a return to the ideas of some of the early feminist crusaders about the liberating capacity of birth control in the context of broader social transformation. The purpose of this book is to take one step in that direction.

The essays presented here, several of which have been published previously in different form, present a particular point of view. They represent the perspective of a feminist demographer (if this is not a contradiction in terms) who is passionately committed to the idea that a woman's ability to decide whether, when, if, and with whom to have sex and have children is a fundamental component of her rights as a woman and of her human dignity. The perspective is undoubtedly a western one in its emphasis on an intellectual tradition that values individual freedom and personal choice. It is liberal in its pragmatic approach and its willingness to work within existing institutions to bring about change. It is radical in its condemnation of male power and privilege and the universal oppression of girls and women. It is optimistic in its hope that reason and good intentions will prevail, and pessimistic in its fears that they will not. Above all, it is an appeal to listen to the voices of the world's women, in all their diversity, of which only a barest hint can be presented here.

The book is organized in four parts. The first part, "Women's Rights as Human Rights," lays the groundwork for the discussion of women's rights and population policies throughout the book. It addresses several broad issues relating to the evolution of concepts of human rights in western thought and the progressive identification of women's rights and, more recently, of sexual and reproductive rights as legitimate human rights concerns. Many of these ideas are reflected in United Nations documents such as the Universal Declaration of Human Rights and the Convention on the Elimination of All Forms of Discrimination Against Women, both of which set international standards for the exercise of individual freedoms and social entitlements.

Part Two includes three chapters about the politics of feminism and birth control/population control as social movements. The intent here is to tell a story about how feminists and advocates of population control have come to have such contradictory views about the nature of women's reproductive capacities and needs. It is a story of misunderstandings, ideological differences, and divergent political agendas. Part Three, "Women's Rights, Women's Lives," looks more closely at the conditions of women's lives and their sexual and reproductive choices. These chapters draw on findings from surveys and ethnographic research in southern countries, with some comparisons with the north. Part Four, "Toward a Feminist Population Policy," lays out a policy agenda: a set of propositions defining a woman-centered reproductive policy and program based on the concepts of sexual and reproductive health and women's rights. Recognizing that women around the world define and interpret many of their needs quite differently, this chapter draws on a set of minimal but essential components of a feminist perspective. These include building on women's shared and diverse social experiences in program design, and recognizing that girls and women everywhere are subject—although in different ways and degrees—to oppression under patriarchy. Policies and programs must incorporate systematic means of recognizing the risks women face and strengthening alternative bases of survival, security, and empowerment.

The thesis of this book is that the exercise of women's reproductive rights depends in fundamental ways on the exercise of women's rights in other spheres. Policies to reduce fertility can accomplish their objectives by eliminating the "coercive pronatalism" inherent in patriarchal institutions and gender inequalities in the family and society without introducing an equally coercive antinatalist agenda. Indeed, population control policies and programs would probably be unnecessary if women could exercise their basic economic, political, and social rights and genuine reproductive choice. In addition, programs need to address the widespread unmet need in many countries for reproductive health services that would enable women to regulate the timing of their childbearing and, in particular, help women to avoid unwanted and mistimed pregnancies and unsafe abortion.

The "population problem" and its possible solutions need to be redefined. Women's rights advocates throughout the world are increasingly united in their commitment to the protection of women's sexual and reproductive rights, if not in their analysis of the major threats to these rights or in their political agendas. At the same time, population policymakers are increasingly concerned about the sluggish pace of fertility decline in some countries and the tremendous growth projected for the global population before numbers can be stabilized. Past efforts at population control have triggered resistance from many quarters based on charges of cultural insensitivity, program abuses, and even genocide. The premise of this book is that a policy approach that places the entitlement to high quality, comprehensive reproductive health services at the center of a focused program for promoting women's economic, social, and political rights could help to (1) legitimize efforts at population regulation; (2) promote their effectiveness, efficiency, and equity; and (3) win the support of advocates of human rights, women's rights, and reproductive freedom, who should be natural allies in a common endeavor.

Note

1. The terms "southern" and "northern" are used in this book as synonyms for "developing" and "industrialized" or "less developed" and "more developed." The line between north and south is drawn along the southern border of the United States and Europe, the former Soviet Union and Japan, and then dips down to include Australia and New Zealand. The more neutral geographical terms are intended to avoid the assumptions that all "developing" countries are indeed developing, or that all "industrialized" countries are industrialized.

Part One

WOMEN'S RIGHTS AS HUMAN RIGHTS

1

HUMAN RIGHTS, WOMEN'S RIGHTS, AND REPRODUCTIVE FREEDOM: THE EVOLUTION OF IDEAS

Two streams of thought with somewhat parallel histories shape the arguments in this book. In an oversimplified fashion they can be summarized as follows:

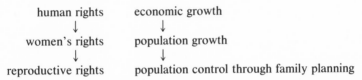

The first stream of thought originates in concepts of human rights expressed in seventeenth- and eighteenth-century theories about the "natural" or inalienable rights of man. Ideas about individual liberties underlying the French and American revolutions—that is, about civil and political rights—created a fertile ground for later ideas about economic and social rights, or entitlements. In the nineteenth century, a few liberal reformers and radical utopians proposed the startling idea that the rights of man might properly extend to women, too. Thus was born the first movement for female emancipation which, in its second wave in the mid-twentieth century, became a movement for women's liberation. Ultimately, ideas about reproductive rights and freedoms emerged from both sets of principles. The idea that family planning was a human right—that is, that couples should be free to decide the number and spacing of their children—was first recognized at the 1968 U.N. International Conference on Human Rights in Teheran, Iran. Feminists since the nineteenth century have elaborated on the idea of reproductive rights by articulating the principle of a woman's right to "control her own body." This idea transcends the narrower U.N. formulations to encompass a broader range of sexual and reproductive rights and freedoms.

The second stream of thought flows through a sequence of theories about the relationship between population size and growth rates and the "wealth of nations." These ideas can be traced from the seventeenth- and eighteenth-century European mercantilists who stressed the economic and political advantages of large and growing populations, to the English and French utopians who believed that social reforms and modern science could provide for any size population, to Malthusian thinkers who—taking prevailing social institutions as fixed—believed that unrestrained population growth would perpetuate poverty and quickly outstrip the means of subsistence. The stream flows through a series of post-Malthusian theories of classical and neo-classical economists, socialists and Marxists, demographic transitionists, modern-day Malthusians, and free marketeers, each with their own notions of how population growth affects economic growth and of their policy implications (United Nations 1973b:33–63). Out of Malthus was born the nineteenth-century movement for birth control in Europe and North America. And out of the birth control movement was born the twentieth-century movement for family planning and population control in developing countries.

The two streams of thought incorporate somewhat contradictory ideas. But there are also commonalities in their origins and evolution, how the ideas are represented in laws and policies, what their adherents and opponents believe, and how they are played out in everyday life. Relationships among these ideas and social movements are explored in this book with a special emphasis on women's rights and population policies. This connection can be understood only within the framework of the other linkages, however. How are reproductive rights related to human rights, for example, and to what extent do population policies, laws, and programs infringe on rights that are considered universal (see the discussion in this chapter)? Are family planning programs more properly seen as the means of controlling population growth or the means of enabling women and men to exercise their reproductive rights (chapters 2 to 4)? How are reproductive rights related to the exercise of women's rights in other spheres such as education, employment, the family, and the community (see chapter 5)? How does fertility regulation affect the physical and emotional health of women in diverse circumstances, as women themselves perceive it (chapter 6)? Does the right to family planning articulated in U.N. declarations include a right to abortion as well (chapter 7)? Finally, how can the principles of human rights, women's rights, and reproductive rights be integrated in population policies that effectively *define* the sexual and reproductive rights of women and *protect* them from violations by agents of the family, the community, and the state (chapter 8)?

This chapter introduces the major themes of the book. It begins with the concept of *human rights*—of individual freedoms and social entitlements—as it has developed historically and is embodied in the Universal Declaration of Human Rights of the United Nations. *Gender inequality* is introduced as a human rights issue in the discussion of the natural and social rights of women and their violation by customary beliefs and practices. The concept of *reproductive rights* draws on human rights principles of freedom and entitlement. It also draws on the feminist principle of a woman's right to control her own body, that is, her right not to be alienated from her sexual and reproductive capacity, and her right to the integrity of her physical person.

The discussion then turns to concepts of population and family planning. As a formal statement by a government of perceived demographic problems and desired policy goals and objectives, a *population policy* generally attempts to alter levels of fertility, mortality, and/or migration in order to bring demographic processes in balance with national development goals. Fertility policies may attempt to raise or lower birth rates, using direct or indirect means, targeting everyone or specific population subgroups. The role of *family planning* programs is to provide individuals and couples with the means to regulate their fertility more safely or effectively than indigenous methods may allow. It is not a means of lowering the birth rate per se, but of enabling people to achieve their own childbearing intentions.

Do population policies that attempt to raise or lower birth rates violate human rights? The discussion of how pronatalist and antinatalist policy interventions by governments may impinge on the exercise of human rights is followed by an analysis of the role of family and community institutions and interest groups that mediate between the individual and the state. These institutions can have powerful pronatalist agendas that may be reflected in, or counteracted by, government policies. Both public policies and kinship/community claims are potential violators of the rights of individuals. This double threat is especially compelling in the case of girls and women. The argument is made that the most fundamental threats to women's rights to sexual and reproductive self-determination can be found within the patriarchal family system. Patriarchal institutions are built on power hierarchies of age and gender in which girls and women have little control over their sexual and marital lives, the number and spacing of their children, and the allocation of and returns to their labor. The chapter concludes that the goal of a "rights-conscious" antinatalist population policy should be twofold: (1) to challenge patriarchal family

and community controls that limit women's freedom; and (2) to extend
to all women those social and economic entitlements and reproductive
health services that are preconditions for genuine reproductive choice.

EVOLVING CONCEPTS OF HUMAN RIGHTS

The Universal Declaration of Human Rights adopted by the United
Nations in 1948 incorporates two ideas about the nature of human rights.
The first is the theory that certain individual rights are "natural" or "inalienable." The evolution of this notion in seventeenth- and eighteenth-
century western thought is embodied in the English Bill of Rights of 1689,
the American Bill of Rights of 1789, and the Declaration of the Rights of
Man and of the Citizen adopted by the French National Assembly in 1789.
These and subsequent documents set forth a concept of *individual liberty*
in which the primary role of the state is to ensure freedom of the citizenry
from abuses of power (e.g., from governments not freely elected, from
arbitrary arrest and detention). The newly defined rights to "life, liberty,
and the pursuit of happiness" encompassed rights to own property and
to compete freely in a market economy, along with other civil and political
rights such as freedom of assembly, religion, and speech. The Universal
Declaration of Human Rights continues this tradition by affirming the
right of all people to life, liberty, and security of person; to recognition
before the law; to freedom of movement within each state; to property
ownership; to free choice of employment; to freedom of thought, conscience, and religion; to freedom of peaceful assembly and association;
and to self-governance by freely chosen representatives, among other
provisions (United Nations 1973a:1–3).

The second concept of human rights is one of *social entitlement,* that
is, the responsibility of society and the state to guarantee not only freedom
of *opportunity* to its citizens but also achievement of *results*. Although
the earlier concept of individual liberty was universal in theory, in practice
it applied primarily or solely to adult males (and, in the United States, to
white males), often only to those who owned property. The new concept,
which evolved in large part from nineteenth- and twentieth-century socialist thought, affirmed that *all persons* were to be assured of certain
entitlements. These entitlements are often called economic and social
rights, or "welfare rights," as distinct from the civil and political rights
articulated in earlier theories. As set forth in the Universal Declaration,
they include the right to an adequate standard of living, to education, to
work, to just and favorable conditions of work, and to protection against
unemployment. These rights and freedoms are intended to apply to everyone "without distinction of any kind, such as race, colour, sex, language,
religion, political or other opinion, national or social origin, property,
birth or other status" and without regard to the "political, jurisdictional

or international status of the country or territory to which a person belongs'' (United Nations 1973a:1).

With the extension of the concept of human rights to include social entitlements as well as personal freedoms, governments are charged not only with protecting individual liberty but also with ensuring social well-being. Furthermore, if everyone has the right to such personal freedoms and social entitlements, then no person or institution can deny another person or group the exercise of these rights. The state must thus protect its citizens not only from the tyranny of government—that is, from itself—but also from the tyranny of their fellow citizens.

The transition from individual liberty to social entitlement carries new *obligations* for the citizen as well. For instance, the "right" to an education becomes a moral obligation for parents (and a legal requirement in many countries) to send all children of a certain age to school. Similarly, the right to health becomes an obligation to vaccinate one's children against certain infectious diseases; the right to decide "freely" on the number and spacing of one's children becomes an obligation to decide "responsibly" as well. (The constitution of China, for example, makes family planning not only an individual right but also a duty.) As Simone Veil, France's former minister of health, remarks, "We have therefore arrived at a curious reversal of things: out of liberty is born obligation, and the exercise of a right is rendered essentially compulsory" (Veil 1978:314).

Countries differ considerably in the precedence they ascribe to civil and political rights (freedoms) compared with economic and social rights (entitlements) as well as in their interpretation of the origin and meaning of these rights. In general, governments of northern countries have stressed the primacy of political and civil liberties in their domestic policies and in international discourse. Southern countries and communist or socialist regimes have more often stressed the primacy of economic and social rights (Johnson 1988). The southern perspective has also been more sharply critical of north-south inequalities in the distribution of resources (Ferrero 1986) and more insistent on the rights of national sovereignty in setting their own policies (Callahan 1981). Crosscutting these distinctions, regimes differ in the importance they attach to the individual relative to the community as a locus of social identity and human rights; the importance of duties relative to rights (that is, obligations on the part of the individual *to* the community or the state); and on the extent to which socioeconomic inequalities are correctable or inevitable (Johnson 1988).

Proclamations of human rights by the United Nations have multiplied since 1948 in the form of declarations and resolutions, which are not binding, and in the form of convenants and conventions which, in theory, bind ratifying member states to translate principles into action. (Unless they are embodied in national laws, however, such proclamations have no legal applicability to specific persons or situations.) International standards have been issued on the right of self-determination, the elimination of racial discrimination, prevention of genocide, abolition of forced labor, the political rights of women, rights of nationality and of refugees, freedom of information, freedom of association, consent to marriage and minimum age for marriage, children's rights, and social progress and development, among others (United Nations 1973a). Most significant for our purposes is the Convention on the Elimination of All Forms of Discrimination Against Women (reproduced in part in Appendix A), which was adopted by the General Assembly in 1979 and ratified or acceded to by over 100 countries by 1991.

GENDER INEQUALITY AS A HUMAN RIGHTS ISSUE

Gender forms a basis in all societies for the division of labor and the social allocation of rights and responsibilities. Interwoven with hierarchies of age, race, ethnicity, religion, lineage, caste, and class, among other distinctions, inequalities based on gender pervade every aspect of social life and affect girls' and women's chances for survival and security in fundamental ways. The nature and degree of inequality between the sexes derive from a complex set of conditions within each society that determines the relative access of women and men to valued resources, that is, to material goods and to personal freedoms and entitlements. Although individual women may outrank individual men, men as a group invariably wield more power and acquire more prestige than women do. According to one sociologist, the power differential ranges across societies "from near equality to full-blown male tyranny" (van den Berghe 1973:60).

One of the earliest treatises on the idea of equality between the sexes appeared in 1792 amidst the highly charged atmosphere of debate over the ideologies of the French and American revolutions. Writing as a liberal reformer in passionate defense of civil liberties and a rational and just social order, British feminist Mary Wollstonecraft in *Vindication of the Rights of Woman* challenged the attitudes of liberal and conservative thinkers alike in their advocacy of the rights *of man* (literally interpreted) and their denigration of women's capabilities (Wollstonecraft [1792] 1982). John Stuart Mill followed three-quarters of a century later with his treatise on *The Subjection of Women* (1869). Perhaps best described as a "liberal feminist" in his advocacy of equal opportunities for women to prove themselves in public life, Mill presented what some have called a *radical critique* of the economic and social causes of women's oppression together with *reformist proposals* for their elimination (Tulloch 1989:67). Both Wollstonecraft and Mill were in the classical liberal tradition of deploring discriminatory beliefs and practices that prevented women from achieving their full potential in a competitive market economy (Eisenstein 1986). Both had radical and utopian sympathies, visualizing a better world in which social justice and personal liberty would prevail. These ideas were to form the foundation of the nineteenth- and early twentieth-century crusade for the recognition of women's rights as *human rights* among feminists and social reformers in Europe, North America, and in some Asian and Latin American countries as well.

The Convention on the Elimination of All Forms of Discrimination Against Women represents a culmination of this line of thought. It says little about reproductive rights except to confirm women's rights to family planning information, counseling, and services and to have equal rights with men to decide on the number and spacing of their children. Despite this gap, the convention is a remarkable document in several respects. First, it elaborates on the Universal Declaration of Human Rights in affirming "on a basis of equality of men and women" woman's right to individual freedoms such as voting and free choice of a profession, and to social entitlements such as schooling and employment. State parties to the convention agree to "pursue by all appropriate means and without delay a policy of eliminating discrimination against women" in all fields of human endeavor. Second, the convention introduces rights specific to women, such as prohibitions on dismissal from employment on grounds of pregnancy and the right to maternity leave and child-care benefits, that are intended to *prevent* discrimination and ensure women's effective (i.e., nondiscriminatory in outcome) right to work. Third, the convention acknowledges the need in some cases for "temporary special measures aimed at accelerating *de facto* equality between men and women." These affirmative action measures are not considered discriminatory as long as they are discontinued "when the objectives of equality of opportunity *and treatment* have been achieved" (Appendix A, Article 4, Part I, emphasis added).

Fourth, and perhaps most important, the convention stresses the obligation of states to modify discriminatory social and cultural patterns of conduct "with a view to achieving the elimination of prejudices and *customary and all other practices* which are based on the idea of the inferiority or the superiority of either of the sexes or on stereotyped roles for men and women" (emphasis added). Rooted in systems of social stratification in which each person acquires at birth certain entitlements and obligations according to his or her position in the social hierarchy, the concept of customary rights exerts a powerful influence on the exercise of human rights in most societies. *Customary rights based on social differentiation are the antithesis of universal rights.* It was those customary beliefs in male privilege and female inferiority that Wollstonecraft and Mill attacked as inherently irrational and unfair.

The convention thus addresses three concepts of rights: *natural rights* deriving from theories of individual liberties, *social rights* deriving from theories of state responsibility, and *customary rights* deriving from traditional beliefs and practices. It recognizes that the achievement of equal rights of women and men sometimes requires special gender-specific policies and programs. It stresses the need to eliminate those customary attitudes and practices that are responsible for the persistent gap—or chasm—between the law as it is written and the law as it is enacted in everyday life. Although many nations have not ratified or acceded to the convention, the document symbolizes a commitment to the ideal of women's rights in the international political arena and serves as an organizing tool for feminist activists throughout the industrialized and developing world (Cook 1989c). It also serves as a standard against which prevailing gender inequalities can be assessed.

MEASURES OF GENDER INEQUALITY

To what extent are women able to exercise the range of human rights— of individual freedoms and social guarantees—to which they are, in theory, entitled? This is a classic case of examining the gap between law and practice. The more than 100 governments that have ratified or acceded to the convention (the United States has not yet done so) technically commit themselves to bringing national laws and policies into conformity with its provisions. They include virtually all European, Latin American and Caribbean countries and about one-third of North African and Middle Eastern nations, one-half in Asia, and two-thirds in sub-Saharan Africa. Almost 100 countries (but again, not the United States) have incorporated equal rights provisions into their constitutions (see Appendix D). It is unrealistic to expect a close correspondence between what is said and what is done, however, because discriminatory institutions and behaviors are remarkably resilient. In some Middle Eastern and South Asian countries that have signed the convention, for example, discrimination against women in law and in practice is intense and pervasive. That is why systematic assessments are needed of what progress has been made in the advancement of women's rights.

One of the many accomplishments of the U.N. Decade for Women has been the proliferation of publications documenting international trends and variations in the social and economic condition of girls and women compared with boys and men (e.g., Boulding et al. 1976; Sivard 1985; Population Crisis Committee 1988; United Nations 1984, 1988c, 1991). Organizations such as the International Women's Rights Action Watch (IWRAW, based in Minneapolis) and the U.N. Committee on the Elimination of Discrimination Against Women (CEDAW) monitor progress within each of the convention's substantive areas. These include eliminating gender discrimination in political and public life, rights of nationality, access to and conditions of education and employment, health care, marriage and family life, and social and economic security, and eliminating the sexual exploitation of women in prostitution (International Women's Rights Action Watch 1988).

Compilations of indicators of inequality at the national level are limited in what they can do, however. Inequality has both objective and subjective aspects, the latter of which are not captured in standard statistical measures. Inequalities in one sphere of activity, such as sexuality or childrearing, are linked with inequalities in other spheres such as economic and political life in systematic ways (Dixon 1976). Moreover, the many facets of gender inequality take on different form and meaning in different contexts, varying across nations and by class, caste, and other bases of social rank (Mason 1986). Forces of change inevitably affect individuals and groups differently. In rural areas of many developing countries, for example, women's traditional rights to resources such as land, livestock, food crops, or indigenous forms of income-generating employment have been eroded both by planned development and by forces of commercialization, economic diversification, labor migration, land fragmentation, and social change (Boserup 1970; Benería 1982; Overholt et al. 1984; Tinker 1990). Yet, although girls and women have frequently lost ground in absolute or relative terms, they have sometimes gained in important areas such as schooling, better health, or new wage-earning opportunities. In some cases gender inequality is exacerbated by economic, social, and demographic change; in others it is diminished.

Reviewing the global situation, one study representing 92 percent of the world's female population used 20 indicators of health, education, employment, marriage and childbearing, and equality under the law to rank 99 countries on a scale of women's *overall status* and on the size of the *gender gap* (Population Crisis Committee 1988). Gender inequalities in the exercise of basic human rights according to this analysis are least pronounced in Finland, Sweden, Norway, the former Soviet Union, and the United States, and most pronounced in Bangladesh, Saudi Arabia, Egypt, Syria, and Nigeria. International trends in marriage and divorce, contraceptive use and childbearing, and school enrollment and employment reveal improvements in women's rights and reductions in gender inequality in many countries. The gains women have made differ markedly by world region, economic class, and between rural and urban areas. They have been undercut in some countries by deteriorating national economies and requirements of structural adjustment policies (United Nations 1991). Moreover, women's voices are scarcely heard in the top policy-making positions in most countries. In the late 1980s, women held only 10 percent of the seats in national legislatures worldwide and 3.5

percent of the cabinet posts. *In almost 100 countries, women held no positions at the cabinet level.* Yet, it is at these levels that policy decisions are made that can affect women's lives in fundamental ways.

THE IDEA OF REPRODUCTIVE RIGHTS AND FREEDOMS

The idea of reproductive rights and freedoms cannot be considered apart from the exercise of other basic human rights. Reproductive freedom lies at the core of individual self-determination. The principle of "voluntary motherhood" was central to the movement for female emancipation among nineteenth-century liberal feminists, for example (see chapter 2), whereas birth control for socialist and radical feminists was more often a means to sexual and social liberation. One of the earliest international documents on family planning (the 1966 Declaration on Population by World Leaders) reflected the liberal tradition by defining family planning as a means of "assuring greater opportunity to each person" and of "free[ing] man to attain his individual dignity and reach his full potential" (United Nations 1975:9).

At least three types of reproductive rights can be distinguished: (1) the freedom to decide how many children to have and when (or whether) to have them; (2) the right to have the information and means to regulate one's fertility; (3) the right to "control one's own body." The first two concepts have been formalized in various U.N. declarations since the mid-1960s while the third has emerged primarily from feminist discourse. What do these rights imply for the individual, the family, the state?

Reproductive freedom refers in most U.N. documents to the freedom of all persons of "full age" to marry or not, to choose one's spouse, to have children or not, and to decide when to have them and how many to have. The concept has gone through an evolutionary process that is not yet complete. The "right to decide freely . . . the number and spacing of children" was vested initially in "each individual family" (a General Assembly resolution in 1966), then in "parents," then "couples," and finally (although perhaps unintentionally) in "couples *and individuals*" (plans of action of the 1974 and 1984 world population conferences) (van de Kaa 1988:183; see also United Nations 1990b:56–60). By implication, this right cannot be infringed by other individuals, by the community, or by governments: it is a *civil liberty.* One cannot be forced to marry or have children against one's will, nor can one be prevented from doing so. It is not an *entitlement,* however, for an individual cannot lay claim to be married or to have children in the face of a partner's opposition (van de Kaa 1988), nor is the state obliged to provide. Nor, as yet, is there a recognized "basic right" of individuals or couples to terminate an unhappy marriage through divorce even though this principle is consistent with the right not to be married against one's will and has been recognized in the laws of most member states.

The freedom to choose among alternative courses of action may be considered a fundamental human right from which all other human rights derive. But the freedom to choose is not absolute, for it may conflict with other rights and freedoms and thus conveys certain responsibilities. The United Nations declares that individuals and couples have a basic right to decide freely *and responsibly* on the number and spacing of their children, taking into account "the needs of their living and future children and their responsibilities towards the community." These responsibilities are to be "assumed freely and without coercion," however, which poses a tension between the protection of individual freedoms and the common good.

Freedom to choose is also contingent upon the state's fulfilment of certain social and economic rights (entitlements) that make genuine choice possible. It is here that feminists and leftist social critics, in particular, have identified the range and intensity of discriminatory practices based on class, ethnicity, age, and gender that limit freedom of choice across and within nations, communities, and families. "The critical issue for feminists is not so much the content of women's choices," writes historian Rosalind Petchesky, "or even the [abstract] 'right to choose,' as it is the ... conditions under which choices are made. *The 'right to choose' means little when women are powerless*" (Petchesky 1984:11; emphasis added).

The second element of reproductive rights and freedoms is the right *to be able* to regulate one's fertility, that is, the right to obtain family planning information and services. From its tentative origins in U.N. documents as a right "to adequate education and information" permitting couples to regulate their fertility, the concept was broadened to include the right to the "information, education *and means* to do so." This right is an entitlement in theory if not in fact: if people are to exercise their reproductive freedom, they are entitled to have the means to do so safely and effectively.

In one sense, of course, everyone *does* have the means to regulate their own fertility. Throughout history, individuals and couples have used a variety of methods such as prolonged celibacy, periodic abstinence, coitus interruptus, or herbal potions and mechanical devices to avoid or terminate an unwanted pregnancy. The right to family planning thus presumably involves a right to *use* rather than to have access to these methods, along with the right to learn about, obtain, *and use* "modern" methods within the ordinary limitations that states may impose to protect consumers' health or welfare (van de Kaa 1988). According to this formulation, governments cannot intervene to prevent people from obtaining or using a contraceptive method (people have a "right to privacy" in this regard, according to U.S. Supreme Court interpretations) nor can one individual or group stand in the way of another. Religious values and social norms designed to limit the right to use any or all methods of fertility regulation such as artificial contraception or abortion may be freely accepted by individuals but cannot be imposed on those who choose not to accept such values and norms. The principle of tolerance is intended to prevail.

The third element of reproductive rights and freedoms is the more comprehensive *right to control one's own body*. Articulated as a feminist principle, this formulation recognizes the potential for conflict inherent in male-female relationships and includes sexual as well as reproductive rights.

The idea of a right to determine the uses of one's own body is not new. It can be found in liberal, neo-Marxist, and radical philosophical traditions, none of which originally carried a feminist connotation. Emerging in seventeenth-century liberal thought in England, the idea of "property in one's own person" paralleled a "natural right" to property in goods. It included a right not to be detained without due cause, not to be alienated from one's labor (e.g., in slavery or other forms of economic bondage), and not to be bound in marriage against one's will (Petchesky 1984:3). Marxist and socialist thought also considered the alienation of labor as a violation of individual integrity and workers' rights. More radical interpretations of the right to control one's body have celebrated the ideal of sensual self-expression as an elementary form of personal development and social participation (ibid.:4).

The extension of these ideas to feminist analysis is natural. The right to control one's body—that is, to determine what one does with it and who has access to it—can apply to a woman's right *not to be alienated from her sexual and reproductive capacity* (e.g., through coerced sex or marriage, prostitution, female "circumcision," denial of access to birth control, sterilization without informed consent, prohibitions on homosexuality), and to her right to the *integrity of her physical person* (e.g., freedom from sexual violence, from false imprisonment in the home, from unsafe contraceptive methods, from unwanted pregnancies or coerced childbearing, from unwanted medical interventions). Radical feminists emphasize women's rights to full sensual expression and sexual pleasure as an aspect of sexual and reproductive freedom. Whereas many of the reproductive rights claimed by feminists deriving from the liberal tradition have been established at least indirectly in international standards (with the exception of the right to terminate an unwanted pregnancy), these more radical assertions of sexual rights, which impinge directly on patriarchal ideologies, clearly have not.

All of the elements of reproductive rights and freedom mentioned here incorporate the principles of individual liberty and social entitlement within a broad human rights framework. The *individual liberty* elements consist of the freedom to choose among alternative sexual and reproductive behaviors without coercion from governments or from individuals or social institutions. In turn, individual behavior is to be governed by a sense of social responsibility. The exercise of certain freedoms is also circumscribed by the obligation not to deny—or, more positively, by the obligation to tolerate and support—the rights and freedoms of others (Macklin 1989). The *social entitlement* elements consist of the obligation of the state, or of "society," to ensure that everyone can exercise the full range of economic, social, political, and civil rights that infuse reproductive choice with real meaning.

POPULATION POLICIES AND THE ROLE OF FAMILY PLANNING

The role of governments, ideally, is to balance in practice the sometimes contradictory demands of individual freedom and social entitlement as abstractly defined. The dilemma of how to reconcile these rights in a sociopolitical context of contradictory customary beliefs and practices (some of which are embodied in powerful religious institutions) is confronted head-on in the design and implementation of population policies. While the protection of individual liberty implies a hands-off, minimalist governmental role, the provision of social guarantees requires hands-on intervention. Too little state intervention can make it impossible for people to decide freely on the number and spacing of their children, for example, because they lack the economic resources, information, and services to do so or because their rights are violated by other individuals or groups. Too much intervention can infringe on individual choice in the name of collective security or the common good.

A *population policy* as narrowly defined is a formal statement by a government of perceived national demographic problems, solutions, and desired goals and objectives, together with a systematic organizational plan of implementation (Godwin 1975; Roberts 1990). Policies generally originate from technical analyses that reveal serious current or projected imbalances between demographic conditions such as population size, growth, or distribution and the attainment of national development goals or values. Broadly speaking, the role of a population policy is to modify the demographic behavior of a given population in a desired direction.

Population policies can be grouped into three categories: (1) *reproductive policies* (or fertility policies) whose objective is to raise or lower the birth rate, either universally or selectively, in order to affect population size, growth, or composition; (2) *health policies* whose objective is to reduce mortality and morbidity; and (3) *migration and urbanization policies* whose objective is to achieve a more rational spatial distribution of the population or to alter its size or composition (e.g., through selective immigration). A fourth category is *family and welfare policies* whose objective is to enhance the well-being of individuals and families in areas such as marriage and divorce, child care, maternity benefits, and old-age security (van de Walle 1990:10). Family and welfare policies can have a significant effect on reproductive behavior. This category is probably best excluded from a consideration of population policies, however, unless its primary purpose is to influence the birth rate—for example, by making it easier for women to raise children—in which case it could be treated as a policy of the first type.

A population policy may attempt to influence demographic processes *directly* by such means as raising the legal minimum age of marriage, targeting high-fertility groups for intensive birth control propaganda, creating a package of economic incentives to reward (or penalize) couples with small (or large) families, launching massive disease-prevention programs, or inducing or restricting internal or international migration of certain types. Alternatively, or in addition, a policy may try to alter the economic, political, or sociocultural environment in which people make demographic decisions in order to affect these behaviors *indirectly*. Policy measures of this type include family allowances, subsidized child care or paid maternity leaves, the expansion of primary or secondary education, and increases in female employment, among other possibilities. Social and economic policies designed with other purposes in mind are not "population" policies per se, even though they may affect demographic behavior.

The boundaries of a population policy are unclear, for they blend easily and inevitably into more comprehensive social, economic, and political policies. Although a population policy may set specific demographic targets, its implementation almost always depends on an interlocking set of sectoral programs relating to employment, education, health, housing, family welfare, urban planning, and agricultural and industrial growth. Each sectoral program has its own goals that may complement or counteract the intent of a demographic policy. The policy of granting more family control over agricultural production in China, for example, while achieving the desired result of raising farm output and rural incomes, has encouraged rural couples to have more children despite the official one-child demographic policy. And in Europe, pronatalist family policies in some countries have been diluted or negated by other social and economic policies such as those supporting the aged.

Where does family planning fit in this scheme of things? In the early years of public concern with runaway rates of population growth in developing countries, demographer Kingsley Davis (1967) emphasized that "population policies" and "population control" are not synonymous with "birth control" and "family planning." First, fertility is only one factor in population growth: health and migration policies are also "population policies." Second, population control refers to state efforts to regulate population growth at the aggregate level, whereas birth control refers to the practices of individuals and couples who are trying to regulate their own fertility. Third, a program of voluntary family planning is not a population policy unless it is accompanied by additional measures intended to influence desired family size. A policy that simply enables each couple to have the number of children they want, when they want them—what Davis calls the "doctrine of family planning"—will not slow down population growth if couples are not motivated to space or limit their births. A family planning program offers people the *opportunity* to regulate their fertility more safely and effectively than some indigenous methods allow. In policy terms, however, it is a means to an end and not an end in itself. When demographers and policymakers discuss the need for fertility policies that go "beyond family planning," then, they are referring to measures intended to alter the socioeconomic or political environment of reproductive decision making *with a specific demographic objective in mind* (Davis 1967; Berelson 1969).

The public provision of family planning services nevertheless lies at the heart of most antinatalist population policies, as well as at the heart of health and welfare policies of many countries with no antinatalist agenda. A strong *antinatalist* policy will include (1) comprehensive national contraception, abortion, and sterilization services (a family planning *service* strategy); a weaker one, some family planning integrated with health services, or governmental support for private sector initiatives (Godwin 1975:53). Beyond this core, governments may add (2) a national effort to persuade couples to have fewer children (an antinatalist *communications* strategy); (3) a comprehensive national system of direct payments for not having children, plus a system of indirect incentives through public programs (an *incentives* strategy); (4) a formal, top-level, codified commitment to achieve specific fertility and population growth targets within a given time frame (a *leadership* strategy); and (5) a total integration of fertility policy-making into the national planning process, including a broad program of research, coordination, supervision, and support (a *coordination* strategy) (ibid.:53–59). Of course, governments may invest in some but not all of these antinatalist strategies, or commit at a lower level to each one, or have no specific policy at all, or promote a pronatalist policy (e.g., prohibitions on most forms of birth control, public exhortations to have large families, direct payments to couples with many children, a coordinated pronatalist program) with the opposite demographic intent.

POLICY RESPONSES TO HIGH AND LOW FERTILITY: DO THEY VIOLATE HUMAN RIGHTS?

Despite rapid fertility declines in many developing countries, birth rates in the developing world remain substantially above those of industrialized countries on the whole. Total fertility rates (TFRs) in the late 1980s ranged from about 5.3 children per woman on average in Southern Africa to 6.7 in Western Africa, from 2.3 in East Asia to 5.6 in the Middle East, and from 3.2 in the Caribbean to 4.4 in Central America (Appendix B). Whereas women were bearing seven or more children on average in almost 20 countries in Africa and the Middle East, they were bearing two children or fewer in Mauritius, Singapore, Taiwan, South Korea, Hong Kong, and Cuba. The low birth rates in East Asia and the Caribbean fall well within the range typical of industrialized countries. Holding steady at about 2.0 children per woman since the mid 1970s, TFRs in more developed regions range from a low of 1.6 in Western Europe, to 2.0 in Eastern Europe and North America, to 2.3 in the former Soviet Union.

Dramatically declining infant mortality in many areas of the developing world in the face of slower declines in fertility (or even rising birth rates in some African countries) has intensified the interest of many governments in fertility reduction policies (Appendix D). As of the late 1980s, 55 of 131 developing countries considered that some form of intervention to *lower their birth rates* was appropriate: 21 in Africa, 19 in Asia and the Pacific, and 15 in Latin America and the Caribbean (United Nations 1988d:106). An additional 13 governments, while believing their birth rates were too high, did not consider intervention appropriate. At the same time, the governments of 21 developing countries believed in interventions to *maintain or raise their current fertility levels,* along with 18 of 39 industrialized countries. Among those wanting to maintain their current levels are such diverse countries as Singapore, with a TFR of 2.0 children per woman, and Iraq, with a TFR of 7.3 (one of the highest in the world). Among those wanting to reverse the decline of fertility are virtually all of the Eastern European countries and the former Soviet Union, along with some Western European countries such as Greece, Belgium, and France.

The policy responses of governments that are attempting to speed up, slow down, or reverse the declining birth rates in their countries (or to slow down or reverse migration flows from the countryside to the cities or across international borders) have elicited a great deal of interest among ethicists concerned with potential human rights violations. To what extent have specific population policies in industrialized and developing countries served to restrict rather than facilitate the exercise of basic human rights? How have the constraints or inducements of population policies and programs been distributed among population subgroups, and between women and men? Who benefits, and who suffers?

Policies aimed at maintaining or raising fertility levels in Europe generally include paid parental leaves and child allowances, the expansion of child-care services, and other family welfare benefits intended to ease the difficulties of childrearing, especially for employed women. Promoted *in part* with a demographic intent, family welfare policies such as these have historically attempted to raise the birth rate through expanded social and economic entitlements without denying anyone's personal freedom to practice birth control (Winter 1989). Some countries have deliberately restricted access to contraception or abortion in order to raise the birth rate, however (e.g., Romania in the 1970s and 1980s), which constitutes a clear violation of people's right to the means of family planning and hits hardest those who cannot obtain private illegal services. Other governments have introduced economic incentives or special privileges to promote childbearing among particular subpopulations. For example, Singapore's policy of selecting women with higher education for pronatalist incentives has triggered charges of ethical violations because similar benefits are not available for women with less schooling.

Among antinatalists, the Chinese policy is clearly the most restrictive with its top-down, multi-layered, and multi-faceted scheme for rewarding one-child families, penalizing most couples with more children, and imposing fertility targets at the state, district, community, neighborhood, workplace, and household levels (Hardee-Cleaveland and Banister 1988). Justified on the grounds that personal freedoms must be subordinated to collective needs if the population's long-term welfare is to be assured in the face of limited economic and natural resources, the Chinese policy has stimulated international debate on ethical grounds (Crane and Finkle 1989). It has also elicited considerable domestic resistance from rural couples who refuse to abide by its provisions. Antinatalist programs combining intensive persuasion, widespread family planning services, and in some cases small-scale incentive schemes are also found in countries such as Indonesia, Thailand, Sri Lanka, Bangladesh, the Republic of Korea, Colombia, Mexico, Tunisia, and India, among others (Mauldin and Lapham 1987). These, too, have raised some charges of violations of the rights of individuals who are persuaded, tricked, or coerced into accepting contraception or sterilization by over-zealous family planning promoters in the absence of truly informed consent (e.g., Warwick 1982; Hartmann 1987).

Resolutions adopted over the years by the United Nations have repeatedly affirmed the sovereign right of governments to formulate their own population policies in accordance with their development goals. Yet, population policies touch inevitably on human rights that are deemed universal. Some experts insist that certain freedoms are so fundamental that any state interference with them would be intolerable, while others argue that it is impossible to take a categorical position without considering historical circumstances or compelling state needs (World Population Conference 1974:31). Governments might appropriately offer economic or social incentives to couples to have fewer (or more) children, for example, as long as such incentives do not result in discrimination on grounds of race, sex, language, religion, property, or income. Advocates of this position contend that some degree of coercion is implied in any law, such as that requiring compulsory education, setting a minimum age at marriage, or limiting the number of spouses a person can have. However, critics point out that people's perceptions and compliance are determined by their socioeconomic resources and the nature of the measures and means of enforcement (Isaacs and Cook 1984:130–134; David 1987). Incentive or disincentive schemes intended by governments to raise or lower birth rates are inevitably discriminatory in societies characterized by unequal distribution of resources because they appear coercive to some individuals or groups but trivial or beneficial to others.

It is important to emphasize that program incentives may *expand* the range of options for some individuals and groups. For example, antinatalist incentive schemes and propaganda can help to counteract what Judith Blake (1972) calls the "coercive pronatalism" of family and gender ideologies and of other social and economic institutions. In turn, pronatalist incentives such as child allowances offered in Canada and some European countries may help to counteract the antinatalist pressures of high costs of living or maternal employment (Demeny 1986), thus broadening individual choice.

Perceptions and outcomes of incentive and disincentive schemes and other population policy components need to be analyzed among population subgroups in each national setting in order to understand their impact on the exercise of human rights. Most experts agree that population policies must form part of a broader strategy of development and implementation of human rights in a democratically responsive regime if they are to be considered legitimate (e.g., World Population Conference 1974; United Nations 1990b). This point has a fundamental bearing on the question of women's rights and population policies. From an ethical standpoint, the process by which a population policy is formulated and implemented can be as important as the substance of the policy itself (Berelson and Lieberson 1979). Process is especially relevant where the "objects" of population policies believe that the policies are not in their own best interests, or that they have been unfairly singled out as policy targets. The first component of an ethical appraisal is thus the *procedural* question of how policies are formulated and implemented, including the participation of persons and groups who will be most fundamentally affected. The second is the *substantive* question of what sorts of ethical considerations a particular policy embodies. The participation of women in policy-making and the extent to which women's sexual and reproductive behavior are singled out for policy intervention are clearly crucial to an ethical appraisal of this type.

THE INDIVIDUAL, THE STATE, AND THE ROLE OF
MEDIATING INSTITUTIONS

Posing the dynamics of population policy-making as inevitably pitting the state against the individual, which is conventional in many ethical treatments of the subject, is undoubtedly too simplistic. First, it assumes a conflict of interest that may not exist. In many cases, the motivations of individuals—to defer marriage, say, or to space and limit births—may be congruent with state policies. Second, the "individual versus the state" model masks the complexity of the institutional setting in which demographic decisions are made, both at the policy-making level and at the level of individuals and families. Indeed, the institutional layers between the state and individual may be so thick as to filter out the substance of state policies almost beyond recognition, particularly where the state apparatus is weak and where resistant social institutions are deeply entrenched (Greenhalgh 1990).

Analysts have noted that policy-making in developing countries generally has a state-centric character in which decisions are made by a (male) policy elite of cabinet ministers and chief executives (Thomas and Grindle 1990). Antinatalist policies are often advocated by foreign donors and expatriate advisors in conjunction with like-minded national professional or political elites. Political leaders may have more to lose than to gain domestically by taking a strong antinatalist stance, however, especially where societies are fragmented and socially heterogeneous, where pronatalist values permeate a wide range of institutions, or where the leaders themselves are of tenuous legitimacy or tenure (Anglim 1975:185). (Bureaucrats, in contrast, may have more latitude to make unpopular policy choices because they are less concerned with the quest for legitimacy.) From this "soft" domestic policy commitment, observers contend, flows only a weak commitment to effective policy implementation (Thomas and Grindle 1990).

The articulation of mass-based interest groups within the population that might exert pressure on policy questions is, according to this analysis, often weak. But policymakers can be influenced by the *perceived* power of constituencies that have a stake in policy outcomes, such as ethnic or religious groups or trade unions with a mass base or outspoken leadership, opposition political parties, the military, business and professional associations, industrial leaders, women's organizations, and the popular press, whether or not such groups are highly mobilized in fact (ibid.). Interest groups such as these are unlikely to *demand* a reproductive policy from the state, except perhaps in the case of demanding or opposing family planning services, but they may actively *oppose* any efforts at restricting fertility as a threat to group security, wealth, privilege, or national power, or as an affront to public morality and national values. Thus, policy elites may try to co-opt potential opposition by including powerful interest group leaders in a consultative process because the costs of making a mistake are high. Or, they may try to win popular support by avoiding the issue and turning to other, more appealing programs, even if they are not indifferent to the logic of fertility control (Anglim 1975:185).

Exceptionally difficult to implement in any case because of the breadth of coordination and depth of commitment required at all levels, population policies—like policies of women's rights—may have little if any relation to actual practice. A report of a seminar on population and health policy in sub-Saharan Africa, for example, noted with simple eloquence that "The policies have changed, but the system remained fundamentally the same" (van de Walle 1990:12). Attempts at implementation of unpopular policies can meet with polite indifference or with hostility and rebellion on the part of affected groups (Kokole and Mazrui 1990; Panandiker and Umashankar 1990). Governments may compromise by announcing an official antinatalist stance while failing to offer specific programs to achieve this end, or by justifying support for family planning on health, human rights, or family welfare grounds but not on demographic grounds, or by declaring a laissez-faire or pronatalist stance while tolerating or actively supporting private sector family planning initiatives, among other possibilities. Each of these processes mediates between the state and the individual. Protecting individual liberties *from* infringements by the state, each intervening layer also leaves individual liberties vulnerable *to* infringement by the mediating institutions themselves.

Institutionalized ideologies and practices within families and communities can have significant demographic consequences, some of which complement state efforts and some of which countermand them. Individuals are not reached directly by population policies but through the filters of overlapping group membership. Population policies that are uniform on their surface affect each population subgroup in different ways.

The notion of group rights, which is sometimes expressed as the rights of the *community* to self-determination, has gained some currency in recent years (Callahan 1981:316). A "group" in this context may be created by religious, racial, linguistic, ethnic, or other traditional identities that define the nature of social collectivities within national boundaries. Interposed between the individual and the state, a community may represent itself as an interest group in the politics of national policy-making. It also imposes expectations on the behavior of group members, some of which are likely to violate members' basic human rights. Such expectations are often pronatalist both in intent and outcome, in part because they are so often fired by religious injunctions or ethnic rivalries. Proscriptions against certain forms of sexual expression or birth control, expectations of early and universal marriage for girls, restrictions on the physical movement and social roles of girls and women, economic discrimination resulting in female dependency, prohibitions on divorce or the encouragement of polygyny, strong social incentives for the birth of children, especially sons, and so on, all create conditions favoring if not requiring high fertility. Cultural prescriptions such as these can be as coercive as official population policies—or even more so—in limiting the range of individual choice. The struggle to establish individual rights thus confronts both group and national claims.

Individual rights are also determined by the claims of smaller units within the boundaries of larger communities, that is, of households, families, and lineages. These units form additional layers between the individual and the state that governments may feel compelled to protect. The Declaration on the Elimination of Discrimination Against Women adopted by the U.N. General Assembly in 1967, for example (the predecessor of the current convention), included a qualification that women's "equal" civil rights were to be exercised "without prejudice to the safeguarding of the unity and the harmony of the family, which remains the basic unit of any society" (United Nations 1973a:39). This symbolic deference to what is sometimes called "the sanctity of the family unit," which was added as a compromise during debate in the General Assembly and renders the notion of equal rights meaningless, serves as a reminder of the pervasiveness of patriarchal ideologies in both international and national discourse on population policy and women's rights. Family harmony, unity, and strength have been consistently identified in both northern and southern countries with the authority of the father and husband, and female emancipation with the disintegration of the family and the loss of male privilege (Michele 1960).

WOMEN IN THE FAMILY: THE PATRIARCHAL BASES OF SOCIAL CONTROL

Perhaps the most fundamental threat to women's right to self determination is the patriarchal family system. Patriarchal institutions are systems of social relations by which the old dominate the young, men dominate women, and those at the center of male descent lines dominate "outsiders" who marry or are adopted into the lineage. To varying degrees in different settings, patriarchal family and community systems impose the collective wills of their older and more powerful members on girls and women (as well as on boys and young men). Social institutions are structured in ways that perpetuate the gender- and class- or caste-based division of labor, reinforce beliefs in female inferiority, and impose behavioral rules that curtail women's abilities to exercise those basic human rights to which they are, in principle, entitled (Mies 1986).

Generational hierarchies, gender hierarchies, and lineage hierarchies are the building blocks of patriarchal family (and community) systems.

The absolute and relative strengths of age, sex, and blood ties as organizing principles vary across social settings. In joint family systems characterized by patrilineal descent and patrilocal residence typical of much of South Asia, the Middle East, and Africa, for example, all three ideological building blocks are firmly in place even if they are not always cemented by the necessary material resources. In-marrying women who have achieved seniority in the family reap some of the benefits of patriarchy by acquiring authority over adult daughters, daughters-in-law, or younger co-wives and their children. Senior women rarely achieve the level of control over family resources that senior men do, however, and exhortations to reproductive conformity by the patriarch's wife to her sons and daughters-in law are "nearly always [made] within the moral framework approved by her husband" (Caldwell 1982:172).

Conjugal family systems tend to weaken the authority of elders and of the male lineage, although filial obligations remain strong in the patriarchal regimes of China, Korea, and Japan even when they are not reinforced by joint residence. Patriarchal ideology in Latin America has tended to emphasize male dominance and female subordination rather than the rule of elders, especially as institutionalized in the form of somewhat unstable conjugal unions (legal or consensual). Elements of patriarchy, particularly assumptions of male privilege, pervade European and North American societies as well, of course, in addition to those of Southeast Asia and the Pacific where family structures and ideologies are generally more egalitarian.

Patriarchy has both a material base and an ideological justification. The material base involves, to varying degrees, control by elder male heads of a lineage, extended family, and/or household, or by the male in a couple, over the means of production and reproduction, that is, over valued property (especially land, livestock, capital) and its uses; over family (especially female) labor and its returns; and over the circumstances under which family (especially female) members enter and leave sexual unions and have children. The ideological justification consists of assertions in various forms of the "natural" or "divine" origins of filial obligation, male dominance, and female subordination, and their expression in legal and moral codes of behavior. Patriarchal ideologies can wield considerable influence independent of a material base, for instance by mandating female seclusion as a symbol of family honor even among resource-poor households, or by convincing girls and women that their paid or unpaid work has little value even if it contributes significantly to family and community welfare.

Depending on the ideologies of political elites, a government may *reinforce* community claims and patriarchal controls as a way of maintaining its own power base, or it may try to *undermine* them for the same reason (Agarwal 1988:1–28). The first situation is illustrated most vividly by political regimes founded on the principles of religious fundamentalism where religious doctrines relating to marriage, divorce, birth control, inheritance, property rights, freedom of movement, and other behaviors are encoded in legal statutes and enforced by state authorities. Multiple layers of patriarchal enforcement (the state, the community, the household or family head) pose a triple threat to the exercise of women's rights to self-determination. More moderately, a socially heterogeneous and divided state may recognize the legitimacy of separate family laws for distinct religious communities (e.g., a Hindu code, Muslim code, Christian code, etc.), or perhaps even distinct ethnic groups (e.g., customary tribal law), while imposing secular law on all who are not group members. Even in so-called secular states, laws and policies are likely to incorporate patriarchal elements, however; indeed, the persistence of discriminatory gender ideologies in law and in practice forms the raison d'être of the convention on discrimination against women. Consider, as a simple example, the requirement in some legal codes or family planning programs that a woman must obtain her husband's permission for contraception, abortion, or sterilization, or that an unmarried woman cannot obtain services (Cooke and Maine 1987). In contrast, governments may specifically attempt to destroy patriarchal relations by imposing non-discriminatory laws and policies and punishing violations, even to the extent of punishing such outward forms of deference to religious and patriarchal (rather than state) authority as the wearing of the veil in Islamic societies, as was the case historically in Turkey and Soviet Central Asia (Massell 1974; Jayawardena 1986; Kandiyoti 1991).

The essence of patriarchy is that girls and women have little control over the circumstances under which they work, the returns for their labor, their sexuality, and the timing and number of their children. But patriarchal institutions interact with institutions of caste, class, and ethnicity within historically specific settings to produce diverse patterns of productive and reproductive behavior (Cain 1984; Dixon-Mueller 1989). The control of men and elders over women's labor, for example, can result in the visible deployment of female labor outside the home in agriculture and marketing, as in much of sub-Saharan Africa, or in the invisible confinement of female labor to the home or compound, as in parts of North Africa, the Middle East, and South Asia. Patterns vary in important ways by social rank and according to the woman's age and sexual/reproductive status. Patriarchal control over reproduction can produce very early arranged marriages (sub-Saharan Africa, South Asia) or later marriages (East Asia) depending on the benefits flowing to elders from each pattern. It can produce high or low rates of divorce and female remarriage (Muslim and Catholic or Hindu countries, respectively), monogyny or polygyny, pregnancies closely or widely spaced. And it can produce not only high birth rates and low levels of contraceptive use, but also more controlled birth rates and higher levels of contraceptive use. Among the Chinese in Southeast and East Asia, for example, the interests of powerful kin lie in investing more heavily in fewer children, especially sons, for the family's social advancement (Greenhalgh 1985).

The demographic aspects of patriarchal control over female labor, sexuality, and reproduction can be understood as reflecting more general strategies by which individuals (or households, families, lineages) in each society attempt to secure a minimal standard of living or (depending on their class position) to accumulate status or resources and to transmit them intergenerationally (Mason and Palan 1981:570). As members of a corporate unit such as a household, family, or lineage, individuals face certain joint risks and rise and fall together in the social hierarchy (Cain 1981). But within the corporate unit, each member invents distinct survival, security, or mobility strategies that are shaped by opportunities and risks both within and outside the family that are not necessarily shared by other members. A woman's personal reproductive strategy, for example, may coincide or conflict with the policies of the state or of her community, her powerful kin, or her male partner. The degree of convergence depends on how thoroughly she has internalized particular ideologies and on the social and material resources she has at her disposal as insurance against marital, reproductive, or economic "failure" (Cain 1986).

Girls and women in every society have devised means, subtle or otherwise, to try to influence the outcome of decisions that concern them or to circumvent the authority of men and elders while appearing to acquiesce (e.g., Bledsoe 1980; Benería and Roldán 1987; Mandelbaum 1988). Moreover, patriarchal institutions are subject to numerous internal contradictions and shifting alliances among group members that can provide girls and women with some leverage. As Petchesky emphasizes (1984:10), "Social divisions, based on differing relationships to power and resources, mediate the institutional and cultural arrangements through which biology, sexuality, and reproduction among human beings are expressed, and *such relations are essentially antagonistic and complex*" (emphasis added). The potential antagonism between opposing interests inherent in patriarchal family and community systems (between younger men and their elders, for example, or between mothers and daughters-in-law, husbands and wives) can create tensions that trigger important social changes or indicate the direction that such change is likely to take (Caldwell 1982:160).

Awareness of these potential (or actual) antagonisms—that is, of the stress points of patriarchal structures and ideologies—is critical to our understanding of the potential for women's reproductive self-determination in a policy context. For many girls and women, the most severe violations of their human rights are rooted deeply within the family system, bolstered by community norms of male privilege and frequently justified by religious doctrines or appeals to custom or tradition. These hidden injuries of gender are rarely addressed in public policies and international assemblies because they threaten collective beliefs in the "sanctity, harmony, and stability" of the family unit. Laws and policies can be directed toward undermining these patriarchal controls and advancing the equal rights of women and men. The challenge of a reproductive policy is to ensure that the abstract principle of reproductive rights becomes a reality in women's lives.

Part Two

THE POLITICS OF FEMINISM AND BIRTH CONTROL/ POPULATION CONTROL

2

"POPULATION CONTROLLERS" AND THE FEMINIST CRITIQUE

Feminism, women's rights, birth control, population control: they are all social movements engaged in political action to promote specific policy agendas. Connected in complex and sometimes combative ways with one another, they are also involved in collaborative or antagonistic relationships with other social/political movements: with liberalism, radicalism, and socialism, for example, and with ethnic and state nationalism and religious fundamentalism. The ideas of these and other movements compete in a clash of contradictory ideologies backed by interest groups with varying degrees of power. Competing claims often incorporate the control of women's bodies and women's lives as symbols of group power. In the midst of antinatalist and pronatalist agendas, feminists claim the right to control their own bodies and their own lives.

The three chapters of this section analyze the politics of the women's movement and the birth control/population control movements from different vantage points. This opening chapter tells the story of feminist reactions to the campaigns for birth control in Europe and North America in the latter part of the nineteenth century and for population control in the latter part of the twentieth. It examines the roots of the contradiction between early liberal-reformist feminism and the birth control movement that raise questions of relevance today. Are artificial methods of contraception truly liberating for women or do they simply make it easy for men to have unlimited sexual access without having to engage in "cooperative self-denial" (for example, by practicing coitus interruptus or periodic abstinence to avoid unwanted pregnancy)? The early feminists were passionately committed to the idea of "voluntary motherhood," but on their own terms. It was not until the beginning of the twentieth century, with the rise of socialist agitation and radical feminism, that birth control was defined by activists such as Margaret Sanger and Emma Goldman as vital to the class struggle and to women's sexual liberation. The first clinics opened their doors in a spirit of open defiance of legal and social conventions. The subsequent evolution of the family planning "establishment" took quite another turn, however. Increasingly professionalized, medicalized, and respectable, it lost its feminist fervor in the decades following the 1920s. "Responsible parenthood," not women's liberation, was the primary goal.

The renewal of feminist activism in the late 1960s in the United States involved, among many other issues, a protracted struggle for the recognition of reproductive rights and the legalization of abortion. But feminist health advocates have been increasingly critical of many of the developments in family planning programming and contraceptive development. The growth of a powerful movement for population control has attracted strong opposition. Although feminists insist that every woman has a right to birth control information and services, they have challenged population control policies and programs because the latter's political agendas seemed to exclude a fundamental concern with empowering women. "The major difference . . . between the feminist agenda and most population agencies is that feminists see the use of family planning within the context of sexual power dynamics that subordinate women, and *they place the highest priority on helping women change these dynamics*" (Helzner and Shepard 1990, p. 153; emphasis added). Programs that do not recognize these priorities do women a disservice, feminists contend, by perpetuating male power and privilege.

The perspective of the population establishment is addressed in chapter 3, which tells a story about the shifting position of the United States government on population and family planning at home and abroad. The government's position evolved from a tentative interest in supporting family planning research and programs in the 1950s, to enthusiastic endorsement of international population control efforts in the 1960s and 1970s, to revisionism in the 1980s when U.S. policy fell under the sway of conservative economic ideologies and organized attacks on family planning by fundamentalist religious groups. Because most policymakers revealed little awareness of (or interest in) the implications of their policies for women's lives, the "woman question" remained peripheral to most of the domestic and international policy debates. Planners and researchers were more interested in macro-level analyses of the effects of population growth on economic development, environmental deterioriation, food supplies, and political security. These were the "hard" questions. Except for some expressed concern with women's and children's health and family welfare, the "soft" questions remained largely unexamined. Advocates of women's rights along with other critics of the ethics and practices of the population controllers were alienated from the policy process. Only recently have they mobilized around the issues of improving the quality of care in family planning programs and protecting women's health and rights in domestic and international programs.

The dilemma of women's health advocates in developing countries who are caught between the ideologies of population controllers (generally reflecting U.S. policy) and of nationalist and religious pronatalist movements is described in chapter 4. Womens' organizations in Brazil, Nigeria, and the Philippines have tried in various ways, some successful and some not, to influence or challenge the population policies of their countries as democratization in the 1980s has opened up new avenues of political engagement. The possibilities of extending comprehensive reproductive health services to women as a basic entitlement have been tempered by the harsh realities of economic austerity as well as by political resistance from conservative sources. Feminists in these and other southern countries are struggling to identify key issues and programs that will reflect their *own* sense of priorities rather than those of national political parties and elites, powerful religious institutions, and the international population establishment. They are also developing a unique feminist identity which, on some political issues, sets them apart from or even in opposition to many feminists in the north. Histories of colonialism, imperialism, racism, and economic exploitation that have produced glaring international disparities in power, privilege, and wealth are far too powerful to be ignored. A major challenge to the global women's movement is to transcend these geopolitical divides in the defense of women's reproductive health and rights.

The women's movement in both northern and southern countries has been caught in a double bind on the birth control question, largely because the feminist concept of fertility control as an individual, autonomous act of empowerment has been eclipsed by the political concept of population control as a public policy imposed by governmental authorities or other ruling elites. The feminist response has been a sharp and vocal critique of "controlista" ideologies and practices launched from outside the major population institutions, a persistent attempt at reform by feminists (both male and female) from within, and an unanticipated and potentially devastating co-optation of feminist criticisms by anti-feminist, "right-to-life" organizations.

The feminist critique has shaped the dynamics of the relationship between women's groups and the population/family planning establishment in fundamental ways. Unfortunately, it has also contributed to a situation in which groups that in principle should be natural allies in the defense of reproductive rights often work at cross purposes in an atmosphere of mutual distrust. Some radical feminist groups attack virtually all new contraceptive technology on political grounds without engaging in the kind of scientific fact-finding that might make their arguments more persuasive and their conclusions more nuanced. Some insist that virtually all family planning programs are imperialist or racist by definition and thus should be rejected. In short, they are too prone to throw out the baby with the bathwater. At the same time, population planners and contraceptive researchers tend to dismiss feminist complaints as uninformed, emotional, and representing a minority view. Preoccupied with achieving their own political and scientific goals, they fail to take seriously the legitimate concerns that feminists raise about women's health and rights. The contradictions embedded in these issues, which have divided the women's movement from the birth control/population movements and the women's movement within itself, can be traced to the first organized campaign for birth control in England over a century ago.

THE ROOTS OF CONTRADICTION: FEMINISTS AND NEO-MALTHUSIANS IN THE NINETEENTH CENTURY

The deep ambivalence of many contemporary feminists about the promotion of artificial methods of contraception has its roots in the reactions of first-wave feminists to the rise of the neo-Malthusian birth control movement in England in the latter part of the nineteenth century.

Birth rates were falling throughout the nineteenth century in England and in some northern and western European countries, beginning earliest in France (and the United States). Delayed marriage, nonmarriage, and the practice of coitus interruptus within marriage were primarily responsible. By the late nineteenth century, birth control information and technology, originally the preserve of the propertied middle classes, permeated the "popular" or working classes (Fryer 1965; Shorter 1973). In Germany, for example, entrepreneurs were producing rubber and chemical products such as condoms, diaphragms, douches, and vaginal suppositories advertised "for the Malthusian," while professional and indigenous health-care practitioners offered abortion and sterilization services (Woycke 1988:4). Pharmacies in England displayed a variety of contraceptive wares. The sensational trial of birth control crusaders Annie Besant and Charles Bradlaugh in 1877 on charges of obscenity for publishing a book on contraception (Charles Knowlton's *Fruits of Philosophy,* first published in the United States in 1832) had sparked enormous interest in birth control among the general public. A Dutch physician opened the first office to dispense contraceptives (primarily the diaphragm) to women in 1882. At the same time, the ideology of female emancipation was politicizing women in England and throughout Europe among the bourgeoisie and the intellectual classes. The rise of a European liberal-reformist feminist movement protesting women's unequal opportunities was reflected in the rapid growth of local, national, and international women's associations concerned with female suffrage and other aspects of women's social, economic, and political rights (Riemer and Fout 1980:59–62).

Based largely on the theories of Thomas Malthus in the multiple versions of his *Essays on the Principle of Population* (first published in 1798), the Malthusian League for the promotion of birth control was started in England in 1877. Meetings of neo-Malthusians were held throughout Europe in the 1880s and 1890s. Organizations were formed in Holland, Germany, and France, and an International Neo-Malthusian Federation started in 1900 (Pierpoint 1922; Glass 1940). Attracting a variety of freethinkers, liberal reformers, and utopians, the movement adopted Malthusian economic arguments but departed from Malthus's own views in crusading for the adoption of birth control *within* marriage. Malthus had preached "moral restraint" rather than contraception as the check against excessive childbearing among the poor. Men and women were to abstain from marriage and from illicit sexual relations until they could properly afford through their hard work and frugality to marry and raise a family. In no case was "promiscuous intercourse" to be countenanced, by which Malthus meant "that which employed improper arts" to prevent the birth of children, because it would "weaken the best affections of the heart, and in a very marked manner . . . degrade the female character" (Malthus [1817] 1963:266). In contrast, the neo-Malthusians promoted birth control both for its economic advantages and as a means of avoiding "the evils of abstinence" for men or their resort to prostitution (Banks and Banks 1964:118).

Neo-Malthusian propaganda aroused a storm of protest from some quarters, especially as expounded by the Malthusian League and its precursors in their "crusade against poverty" (Fryer 1965:89–189). The British labor movement challenged the League's economic argument that surplus labor was the root cause of low wages and poverty. Public figures in the medical profession claimed artificial contraception to be unnatural and unhealthy. The greatest resistance came from religious moralists who believed that birth control would encourage licentiousness both within and outside marriage by making possible the enjoyment of sexual pleasure while preventing procreation (Banks and Banks 1964:120). In this sense the moralists shared Malthus's view that intercourse without the consequence of childbirth was wrong.

Ironically, bourgeois Victorian feminists appear to have acquiesced in the moralists' view, although from a different perspective. According to historians J. A. and Olive Banks (1964), "Far from believing family limitation by means of contraception to be a further step towards their emancipation, they appear to have seen it as yet another instance of their *subordination to man's sexual desires*" (emphasis added). Expressed in this way, their reactions have a certain radical bent. It was not that British feminists were oblivious to the problems of excessive childbearing; far from it. Nor were they oblivious to the advantages that female-controlled contraceptive methods such as douching, vaginal suppositories, cervical caps, or vaginal sponges might bring in comparison with male-controlled methods such as condoms or withdrawal (coitus interruptus). Indeed, a number of them undoubtedly used such methods themselves. But, in their public stance, feminists were concerned that artificial contraception would weaken whatever control women may have gained over their own persons by undermining their ability to regulate sexual access on the grounds of avoiding unwanted pregnancy. Women also feared that contraception would encourage philandering on the part of their husbands, who could take other women at will without fear of pregnancy. Sexual and reproductive autonomy were closely linked in this view: a woman's control over childbearing would be achieved primarily through her control over marital sexual relations. A husband should respect his wife's wishes by practicing withdrawal or abstinence—that is, through *cooperative self-denial*.

The theme of sexual autonomy—of women achieving control over the couple's sexual relations—also appears among early liberal feminists in the United States. The Grimké sisters, Elizabeth Cady Stanton, Charlotte Perkins Gilman, and Elizabeth Blackwell all attested to the healthy nature of women's sexuality. Indeed, women's sex drives could equal or exceed men's, they noted, were it not for the pervasive social efforts to suppress it and for the "ignorance and selfishness of men in the sexual act" (Degler 1980:265–268). Nevertheless, in uneasy partnership with social purists who preached against excessive sexual indulgence, early American feminists also advocated sexual limitation within marriage as a means of granting women greater sexual autonomy. Elizabeth Cady Stanton, for example, asserted in 1853 that "Man in his lust has regulated long enough this whole question of sexual intercourse." One of the Grimké sisters insisted on woman's right "to decide when she shall become a mother, how often, and under what circumstances" (ibid.:272). In other words, feminists argued for a wife's unilateral right to refuse her husband's sexual demands. This was a revolutionary concept at a time when a wife was considered the private property of her husband in law and practice.

The hopes of reformers that husbands would cooperate in a regimen of self-imposed or female-controlled periodic celibacy appear to us now as idealized and fundamentally class-based. Even upper middle-class women lacked access to potentially empowering resources beyond those of moral persuasion. Working class women struggling to survive economically could not possibly have identified with (or been mobilized by) the principle of "sexual limitation." Nevertheless, the concept of women having ultimate control over their sexual and reproductive capacity—that is, the principle of voluntary motherhood—was a powerful component of the early feminist agenda for female emancipation and women's rights (Gordon 1976). Women would gain this control either within marriage or, at the extremes, by rejecting marriage altogether through singlehood or divorce.

Nineteenth-century bourgeois feminists remained suspicious of those advocates of artificial contraception who, it seemed, were men concerned primarily with their own sexual pleasures. Feminism was not a causal factor in the advent of family planning in Victorian England (Banks and Banks 1964:129). Rather, it was the neo-Malthusian crusade combined with socioeconomic changes, especially in the middle classes, that appeared to be primarily responsible for the spreading practice of family limitation in that country (Banks 1954). In the United States, the birth control movement was fueled in the first half of the twentieth century by liberal lay persons (both women and men) concerned with issues of family health and welfare who increasingly won the medical professionals over to their cause (Fryer 1965:215). There was little feminist activism within the movement, with the notable exceptions of Emma Goldman and Margaret Sanger.

BIRTH CONTROL AND SOCIALIST/RADICAL FEMINISM IN THE EARLY TWENTIETH CENTURY

The movement for socialist feminism which arose in Europe and North America in the latter part of the nineteenth century and flourished in the first two decades of the twentieth century was inspired in part by August Bebel's feminist tract, *Women Under Socialism*. Published in 1879, the book went through 55 editions by 1930 and was translated into 20 languages (Winter 1989:123). Socialist feminists were demanding the same economic and political rights as men and equality within the family, which included the right to divorce and to limit the number of births (Quataert 1979; Riemer and Fout 1980).

The demand for birth control divided the socialist movement, however, particularly in Europe where many socialists adhered to an orthodox line (Petersen 1989; Winter 1989). Some birth control opponents spoke from a position of ideological purity: family limitation was reformist, they argued; moreover, it sacrificed the collective and revolutionary interests of the working classes to the personal interests of the individual. Excessive individualism was causing dangerous declines in birth rates which threatened the future of socialism. Other opponents disassociated themselves from the economic theories and reformist politics of the neo-Malthusians and from the anarchists, whose advocacy of birth control—rooted in hostility to the state and the bourgeois family—carried a strong (and not at all respectable) element of sexual liberation. Still other socialist critics spoke against the movement from a position of compromise. With a relatively small base of electoral support in most European countries, they contended, socialist parties should build coalitions with middle-class constituencies by emphasizing family and nation-building as common values (Winter 1989:134).

The idea of separating sex from reproduction was becoming generally accepted in the United States by the second decade of the twentieth century. Women, especially working-class women, were entering the labor force in large numbers. The birth control movement that began in the United States in 1914 was, according to historian Linda Gordon (1976:207), " . . . part of a general explosion of resistance to economic and social exploitation." Its radical proponents (both socialist and anarchist) argued that birth control was not an incrementalist reform but a revolutionary change that would transform society toward free sexual expression, reproductive self-determination, and human rights.

Self-proclaimed freethinkers and "militant feminists" Emma Goldman and Margaret Sanger, both of whom published pamphlets on contraceptive techniques among their many other writings and speeches, crusaded for birth control as a means of opposing male tyranny and liberating female sexuality (a radical feminist position). Their crusade had a socialist and pacifist justification as well: birth control among the poor and working classes would serve as a weapon in the class struggle against capitalist exploitation, which relied on a reserve army of workers to keep wages down, and against militarism, which relied on mass mobilization (Gordon 1976:212–219; Kennedy 1970:127–135; Fryer 1965:201–219).

In Goldman's view, birth control was "the most dominant issue of modern times" which "cannot be driven back by persecution, imprisonment or a conspiracy of silence" (Goldman 1916:471). The federal Comstock law, which was passed in 1873 and not repealed until 1971, forbade the importation or distribution through the mails of so-called obscene materials such as birth control information or supplies. In 1914 Sanger launched a short-lived monthly publication called *The Woman Rebel* which had two purposes: first, to test the Comstock law; second, "to rally friends and supporters to the cause of militant feminism in general, contraception in particular" (Fryer 1965:204). The first issue included an extract from Goldman's essay on love and marriage urging women not to have children if they did not want to. Sanger, in turn, asserted women's right to have children without being married, as well as their firm duty "to look the whole world in the face with a go-to-hell look in the eyes; to have an ideal; to speak and act in defiance of convention" (ibid.). The expression "birth control" was printed for the first time in the fourth issue of *The Woman Rebel* in June 1914 (Fryer 1965:205). Sanger and her friends had searched for a name that would convey the "social and personal significance" of the movement. Having rejected a number of alternatives, they finally agreed on birth control as the perfect name for the cause.

In 1914 Sanger also published the first edition of *Family Limitation,* a widely distributed birth control pamphlet that ran eventually to ten editions. *Family Limitation* described in graphic terms how a woman could prevent pregnancy with douches, condoms, pessaries, sponges, and vaginal suppositories, while condemning the use of coitus interruptus because it was unreliable and could have a "degrading" and "injurious" effect on women (Jensen 1981:559). The journal *Birth Control Review* inaugurated by Sanger in 1917 continued publication until 1940.

Despite anti-obscenity laws and harassment from moralists, in 1916 Margaret Sanger opened the first birth control clinic in the United States in an impoverished working class neighborhood of Brooklyn. With several colleagues she distributed leaflets printed in Yiddish, Italian, and English throughout the neighborhood. Hundreds of women showed up for services the first day. The movement spread: women in other locations quickly followed by opening clinics (usually for fitting vaginal diaphragms) in defiance of the law. The resulting arrests and trials brought much publicity and support for the cause. The first public centers for family planning service delivery in the United States were thus created in the spirit of a strong feminist ideology as a direct challenge to oppressive legal and social institutions that denied women their rights to reproductive self-determination. Birth control formed the basis of a large and radical movement involving not only educated but also working-class women in participatory and defiant social action (Gordon 1976:229).

Similiar events followed in England a few years later. In a working class community in 1921, feminist author Marie Stopes and birth control crusader Humphrey Verdon Roe opened what they claimed was the first contraceptive clinic in the British Empire (Fryer 1965:228). Like Sanger, Stopes was also subjected to years of legal harassment as well as to attack by the medical profession, church representatives, and other defenders of public morality. The Malthusian League opened its first clinic a few months later. The number of clinics grew rapidly in Britain following these beginnings, primarily under the aegis of the Society for the Provision of Birth Control Clinics formed in 1924. By the late 1920s at least 300 birth control centers were to be found in Great Britain, Germany, Austria, and the United States (Robinson 1930). In the Soviet Union, a law was passed in 1920 under the administration of feminist Alexandra Kollontay, Commissariat of Public Health, entitling any woman with less than three months' pregnancy to procure an abortion from a qualified physician, and to rest and care after the operation at the expense of the state. Leftist feminists in Czechoslovakia, Germany, Austria, and Great Britain, were agitating for similar rights (Pierpoint 1922:42).

The influence of these early feminist crusaders was to be felt in many parts of the world, not only in North America and Europe but in southern countries as well. In Yucatán in Southeast Mexico, for example, Sanger's book *Family Limitation* was published and disseminated widely following the first Feminist Congress held there in 1916 which was chaired by the governor of the state. In 1925, during a strongly anti-clerical political regime, the book was distributed freely throughout Mexico (Cabrera 1990). In 1922, Margaret Sanger reported to the Fifth International Neo-Malthusian and Birth Control Conference held in London on her triumphal tour of Japan, China, and Korea. Sanger's American Birth Control League had affiliates in Mexico, Hawaii, Japan, and China, and an Indian Birth Control Society had been started under her influence.

The 1920s marked a turning point in the birth control movement. The Report of the Fifth International Neo-Malthusian and Birth Control Conference in 1922 had a crusading ring to it, but the movement was determined to appear respectable in its promotion of "decency and sexual purity;" in its economic and medical justifications for birth control; and, increasingly, in its eugenic arguments on the scientific improvement of the human race (Pierpoint 1922). The voice of women's liberation was dimming. Speaking as a member of "a very small minority" in the movement, British feminist and communist Stella Browne told the audience that "In my opinion . . . the fundamental importance and value of Birth Control lies in its widening the scope of human freedom and choice, its *self-determining* significance for women. For make no mistake about this: Birth Control . . . means freedom for women, social and sexual freedom, and that is why it is so intensely feared and disliked in many influential quarters today" (ibid.:40; emphasis in the original). Wondering aloud why scientists could not invent better contraceptive methods that would "prevent conception without injuring health or impairing natural pleasure," Browne announced in conclusion her profound conviction that abortion is a "woman's primary right" (ibid.:42).

PROFESSIONALIZING PLANNED PARENTHOOD

As socialist and feminist agitation faded following the First World War, the birth control movement in the United States became increasingly professionalized, institutionalized, and national in scale (Gordon 1976: 249–300; Piotrow 1973:7–19). As early as 1915, a variety of birth control leagues had been organized by middle-class, reformist women (Hodgson 1991:15). Although some socialist women remained committed to the cause, many abandoned and some attacked the fight for women's sexual and reproductive rights after 1920 to focus on union organizing, a class-based action considered less divisive to the socialist cause. Meanwhile, sharing with other political groups a widespread concern over declining birth rates and prospects of impending "depopulation" in Europe (especially in France, Belgium, and Germany), European socialists were favoring pronatalist family protection policies over women's rights and the fight for birth control (Winter 1989).

The evolution of Margaret Sanger's career embodies the transformation of the birth control movement from its feminist and radical phase to one of social reformism and medical respectability. In the 1920s and even later, many physicians were still publicly opposed to contraception, which, with the exception of periodic abstinence (taught incorrectly in ignorance of the true fertile period), most believed to be injurious. Physicians were also worried about the association between contraception and adultery, premarital sex, radical feminism, and medical quackery (Hodgson 1991:14). By the 1930s birth control was becoming a legitimate medical issue under Sanger's leadership. It was not until 1937, however, that Sanger's efforts to win over the medical establishment resulted in the American Medical Association's endorsement of contraception as a therapeutic health measure (Kennedy 1970:172–217). Even then, many physicians in the United States as well as in England and Canada hoped to disassociate themselves from a movement influenced by lay persons (e.g., Sanger herself) and from a subject they considered "distasteful" (Field 1983:226–230).

From the 1920s on, Margaret Sanger directed her attentions not only to winning medical respectability for birth control within the United States but also, increasingly, to winning scientific and political support internationally. Her efforts began in earnest in 1922 with her highly publicized visits to China, Korea, and Japan. A world conference which she organized in New York in 1925 resulted in the formation of the International Federation of Birth Control Leagues (ibid.:219). In 1927 she organized the first World Population Conference in Geneva. Sanger's sponsorship apparently caused the assembled scientists some discomfort, however: not only did they refuse to acknowledge her role officially, but they also barred the topic of contraception from the agenda (Piotrow 1973:8). Meeting privately in Paris the following year, the scientists organized the International Union for the Scientific Study of Population (IUSSP). At a 1948 conference Sanger helped to form the International Committee on Planned Parenthood which in 1952 became the International Planned Parenthood Federation (IPPF) with Sanger and Lady Rama Rao of India as joint honorary presidents. Although the scientific community was never at ease with her activism, Sanger had muted much of her early feminism and grass-roots orientation in her quest for scientific acceptance of the cause.

The American movement's change of name from Birth Control to Planned Parenthood was symbolic. The movement would now enable married couples to "plan their families." The concepts "planned parenthood" and "family planning" reflected an ideological shift toward *strengthening the family as a unit* rather than *freeing women,* married or unmarried, to accept or reject sexual relationships and motherhood on their own terms. In 1938, rival organizations such as the American Birth Control League (Sanger's organization) and the Voluntary Parenthood League joined to form the Birth Control Federation of America, which in 1942 changed its name to the Planned Parenthood Federation of America (PPFA) in order to shed the "negative" image of birth control (Gordon 1976:341). Planned parenthood represented the triumph of experts—of scientists, physicians, economists, statisticians—over grass roots activists, not only obliterating the movement's radical and feminist flavor but also attracting eugenicists who were specifically anti-feminist in their fears of family breakdown and race suicide.

The eugenics attraction was not new. The possibilities of selective birth control had drawn believers in racial improvement from the start, both in Europe and North America. Writers in the United States in the 1890s spread fears of "racial degeneration" from the profligate breeding of the genetically unfit, including the Southern European "races" (Hodgson 1991). The movement gained momentum with the passage of discriminatory immigration laws setting national origins quotas in the early 1920s. Proponents advocated both "positive" and "negative" eugenics: the former to encourage higher birth rates among the white, educated, and native-born; the latter to discourage births among "inferior" people. Reaching its height in the 1930s, the eugenics movement subsequently fell from favor as a result of Nazi atrocities. Few experts were entirely immune from the appeal of "scientific breeding" in the early years, however. Having insisted on very clear differences between birth control and eugenics movements in 1919, for example, Margaret Sanger argued in 1926 that the national origins quota acts did not go far enough in controlling the quality of the population. Measures were needed, she said, to "cut down the rapid multiplication of the unfit and undesirable at home" (quoted in Hodgson 1991:15).

Paralleling the trend toward professionalism in the United States, the Malthusian League in England dissolved itself at the end of 1927 on the grounds that the principle of birth control was now widely accepted (Fryer 1965:250–253). In 1930, the National Birth Control Council was established to coordinate the work of existing societies and promote scientific contraception. With the amalgamation of several other societies in 1939, the British organization adopted a new name: the Family Planning Association, which corresponded more closely to the Association's activities.

By the 1930s, writes Linda Gordon, "the birth controllers had virtually ceased expressing any concern with the women's rights aspects of birth control" (Gordon 1976:310; see also Berkman 1979:32). It appears that a reformist women's movement had also abandoned the partnership. In

Great Britain, Canada, and the United States, laws regulating contraception that had been adopted on obscenity grounds were gradually being overturned. Women's organizations rarely took the lead in efforts to secure policy change, however (Field 1983). Although English women's groups at the Labour Women's Conference in 1925 and the Women's National Liberal Federation in 1927 passed resolutions supporting the provision of birth control advice at public maternity centers, in the United States neither the National Woman's Party nor the League of Women Voters were willing to risk association with the issue. Meanwhile, France and Belgium had passed restrictive laws forbidding the sale of contraceptives in an attempt to counter their declining birth rates, while Italy and Germany were increasingly advancing pronatalist measures under fascist regimes. Although the predominantly liberal legislation in Scandinavia remained intact, Stalinism was to threaten contraception and abortion rights in the Soviet Union.

During the 1940s and 1950s, birth control services in the United States were mainstreamed under the organizational umbrella of the Planned Parenthood Federation of America. Family planning was not accepted everywhere, however. In Louisiana, for example, there were no public or private birth control clinics in the early 1960s and the state criminal code made it a felony for physicians or others to disseminate information about any contraceptive method (Ward 1986:3). But, in general, although a number of state legal codes still blocked access to information and services, and although the Roman Catholic church remained firmly opposed, contraception for married couples as a means to responsible parenthood and even to sexual happiness had become respectable (Piotrow 1973:23–29).

Important new contraceptive methods also made their appearance. The progesterone pill, developed in 1953 after extensive earlier experimentation, was tested on a large scale in Puerto Rico in 1956 and approved for commercial distribution by the U.S. Food and Drug Administration in 1960. By 1965, 4 million American women were using oral contraceptives and, in the late 1960s, perhaps 12 to 15 million women worldwide (Seaman 1969:12). The intra-uterine device (IUD), different forms of which had been invented earlier in Germany and Japan, appeared in a new guise in the 1950s and was about to be incorporated into national family planning programs of Taiwan, Republic of Korea, Hong Kong, Singapore, India, and Pakistan (Piotrow 1973:97). Techniques of male and female sterilization as well as of identifying a woman's fertile period for practicing the rhythm method were improving. In combination with other attitudinal and demographic changes, the widespread acceptability and use of contraception undoubtedly contributed to the resurgence of feminism in the late 1960s and to the articulation of the movement's demands (Gordon 1976; Davis and van den Oever 1982).

SECOND WAVE FEMINISTS: NEW ISSUES, NEW CONTROVERSIES

The second wave of feminism swept North America and Western Europe in the late 1960s and 1970s, stimulated in part by Simone de Beauvoir's book *The Second Sex* (1949) and Betty Friedan's *The Feminine Mystique* (1963). Both books—among many others to follow—offered critical (although very different) analyses of women's subordination.

In the United States, the movement for "women's liberation" took three forms (Hole and Levine 1971). First, feminists founded the National Organization for Women (NOW) in 1966, a predominantly liberal-reformist organization of women and men supporting a broad range of women's rights. Similar organizations and caucuses were soon to follow within academic institutions, bureaucracies, and professional associations. Second, hundreds of small, independent, leaderless groups of radical feminists burst into bloom throughout the country to engage in personal consciousness raising and "guerilla" political activism. Third, women's caucuses emerged from new left, civil rights, and anti-war groups to challenge male leadership and debate gender-based as well as class- and race-based sources of oppression. The demands of the women's liberation movement ranged from economic and political rights to sexual and reproductive rights; from the transformation of intimate interpersonal and family relationships to institutional structures to national and international public policies.

The intensifying abortion controversy in the 1960s galvanized this second wave of American feminists around the issue of establishing and protecting women's reproductive rights, just as the struggle for liberal abortion and divorce laws was to unite European feminists of otherwise diverse views during the 1970s in countries such as England, Italy, and France (Bassnett 1986; Duchen 1986). The 1960s witnessed two additional developments in the domestic and international birth control movements that mobilized some feminists. The first was the rapid spread of new contraceptive techniques such as female hormonal methods and the IUD. Women's health advocates concerned with contraceptive safety disliked the direction the new technology was taking. Although the effective new methods offered more choice to some women, they carried the seeds of coercion and harm for others. The second development was the U.S. government's new enthusiasm for family planning as an anti-poverty measure at home and abroad, backed by a strong contingent of "population controllers" in the family planning organizations, foundations, academia, and federal and state legislatures. Feminists found themselves torn between their advocacy of reproductive control for all women and their distaste for the anti-feminist methods and neo-Malthusian motives of the population control movement.

THE STRUGGLE FOR ABORTION RIGHTS

Widespread legal prohibitions on abortion were largely a feature of laws and statutes adopted in Europe and North America throughout the nineteenth century (Field 1983:62–67). Abortion apparently raised little official concern before that, and the first definitive Papal condemnation did not occur until 1869. Nineteenth-century bourgeois feminists were not ardent supporters of abortion rights: they saw abortion and contraception "as symptoms of women's sexual exploitation rather than means toward the 'right to choose' motherhood" (Petchesky 1984:76). Sanger herself was ambivalent. Distressed with the dangers of clandestine abortion, she chose to advance legal contraception as an alternative rather than to promote safe abortion as a right. In this she departed from the demands of other radical and socialist feminists who insisted that women had a fundamental right to free abortion on demand.

With the exception of the Soviet Union, movements for liberalization emerged first in Scandinavia and Iceland during the 1930s and 1940s. Almost all Eastern European countries liberalized their abortion laws in the 1950s. In 1960, Spain, Italy, France, Ireland, Canada, and most of the United States retained the most restrictive laws, permitting abortion only to save a woman's life. At the other end of the spectrum, several Eastern European countries and the Soviet Union granted abortion on request or for broad social or health reasons (Field 1983: 25–26). Legislation in other European countries allowed abortion under more narrowly defined conditions. Abortion (and divorce) laws were liberalized under the impetus of various special interest reform groups in many countries during the 1960s and 1970s, including the United States.

In 1962, the American Law Institute proposed a model code that would provide for abortion on certain health, eugenic, and ethical grounds as approved by a physician (Luker 1984:66–91). The intent was to "rationalize" and standardize abortion laws across the states. (Similar efforts were addressed to divorce laws and other civil and criminal codes.) Initiated by legal reformers, the movement for abortion law reform was supported by liberal legislators, physicians, public health professionals, the family planning establishment, and many civic and church groups. Organized women's groups played little part in the early years, although some radical feminists had been working underground to help women who needed an illegal abortion.

In the heady atmosphere of social protest that was developing in the 1960s, abortion rights soon became a feminist issue (Hole and Levine 1971:278–302; Petchesky 1984:125–132). Reformers, fearing that radical feminist rhetoric might jeopardize their cause, were not overjoyed (Faux 1988:209). It was not *reform* feminists wanted, but *total repeal* of all laws regulating abortion. "Abortion, they said, should be of concern only to the woman herself; physicians and other 'authorities' had no right to intervene.... [Feminists] wanted to redefine how abortion decisions should be made and who should make them; they wanted, in fact, to redefine the ground rules on abortion that had held sway for centuries" (Luker 1984:95). Reflecting the earlier arguments of radical and socialist feminists, the women's movement defined abortion as a woman's unconditional *right* requiring no legal, social, or medical justification. The right to freely obtained abortion, they argued, was essential to individual freedom, sexual liberation, and gender equality.

By 1970, recommendations for repeal of restrictive abortion laws were sweeping the country. Supporters of liberalization or repeal included NOW, Planned Parenthood, the Young Women's Christian Association (YWCA), the League of Women Voters, the American Civil Liberties Union (ACLU), the newly formed National Association to Repeal Abortion Laws (NARAL), the Unitarian Church, and the American Baptist Convention, among other organizations (Field 1983:81; Faux 1988). Twelve states reformed their abortion laws between 1967 and 1973, with four permitting abortion virtually on request. In response, a nascent right-to-life movement mobilized coalitions of political conservatives and religious fundamentalists opposed to reform or repeal, and the bitter fight that preceded (and followed) the Supreme Court's 1973 decision in Roe v. Wade was fully launched (Piotrow 1973:190–198).

In Roe v. Wade, which decriminalized abortion throughout the United States, the court found that a *right of privacy* inherent in the concept of personal liberty could be logically extended from a married couple's decision to use contraceptives (established in Griswold v. Connecticut, 1961) to a woman's decision to terminate a pregnancy. But the right was not unqualified. Although the state could not intervene during the first trimester of pregnancy, it had a "compelling interest" in later stages in protecting the woman's health and a "potential life" (Faux 1988:298–299). The responsibility rested with the physician. Roe v. Wade did not establish a woman's right *not* to bear a child against her will, nor did it remove the element of legal-medical control (Petchesky 1984:289–294).

The right to abortion in the United States under specified conditions was established (however precariously) as an individual *freedom,* not an entitlement. It carried no corresponding obligation on the part of a physician or hospital to perform one. In 1982, only 16 percent of all public hospitals in the United States performed abortions at all, and only 26 percent of non-Catholic general hospitals. Nor was the state obliged to pay. In the same year as Roe v. Wade, the U.S. Congress passed the Helms Amendment to the Foreign Assistance Act prohibiting the direct use of U.S. foreign aid funds for abortion services in recipient nations (Fox 1986:641–643). Similar prohibitions were attached to the federal funding of abortions in the United States. Many state legislatures followed suit; as a result, impoverished women in most states could not obtain subsidized services. The years since 1973 have been marked by continued legislative and legal assaults on abortion rights in the states, in Congress, and in the Supreme Court (NARAL Foundation 1991).

The battle over abortion in the United States and other Western countries has made feminists uneasy with their dependence on legal and legislative initiatives for rights they consider fundamental. Major legal decisions on access to contraception and abortion have been based largely on non-feminist grounds. Liberal policies and statutes are vulnerable to erosion or reversal as the political winds change direction. Although by the late 1980s women could obtain abortions on broad health or social grounds or on request in all but two countries in North America and Europe (Henshaw and Morrow 1990), the "legalistic bias" of these achievements made them seem fragile in the face of political opposition and weak or nonexistent support for the principle of safe and legal abortion at the international level. "The contradiction," feminists noted, "lies in being forced into the uneasy position of appealing to an unsympathetic government to create and protect our 'legal' rights" (Clark and Wolfson 1984:116).

Many feminists have also been uneasy with the single-issue politics of the abortion movement, insisting that greater attention must be paid to winning grass roots support for a full range of reproductive (and economic and social) rights and freedoms (e.g., Fried 1990). Socialist feminists charged the liberal women's movement in the United States with insensitivity to the concerns of poor and working-class women and women of color, both at home and abroad (Davis 1981:202–221; Clark and Wolfson 1984). "Birth control—individual choice, safe contraceptive methods, as well as abortions when necessary—is a fundamental prerequisite for the emancipation of women," writes Angela Davis in *Women, Race and Class*. The inability of middle-class feminists to unite women of different social backgrounds around this issue has resulted from their failure to popularize the genuine concerns of working-class women, and from the historical record of the birth control movement which "leaves much to be desired in the realm of challenges to racism and class exploitation" (Davis 1981:202–203).

RESISTING THE MEDICALIZATION OF CONTRACEPTIVE TECHNOLOGY AND SERVICES

The feminist critique of medicalization has focused on two related issues: the health risks and neglect of women's interests in the development of new birth control technology, and the appropriation of technology and service delivery by physicians. An emerging women's health movement in the late 1960s and 1970s, represented in the United States by the National Women's Health Movement, contributed early critiques. Since then, a growing network of domestic and international women's health advocates has continued to confront established institutions on these and other concerns, including groups such as the Women's Global Network on Reproductive Rights (based in Amsterdam) and the International Women's Health Coalition (based in New York).

The *contraceptive safety* issue raises several related points. First, feminists charge that women's health advocates have had no say in the development of fertility regulating methods such as hormonal pills, IUDs, female sterilization—and, more recently, hormonal injections and implants—or in designing and staffing the experimental tests and delivery systems for these methods. Decisions have been made by the drug industry and by scientists and doctors in the population and biomedical professions who are promoting their own interests. Women as a political constituency are simply not considered (Seaman 1969; Jaquette and Staudt 1985). Second, feminists charge that most research has been done on female methods because male scientists are reluctant to pursue technologies that put men at any risk of side effects or that might be perceived as interfering with male sexuality (Frankfort 1972:22; Gray 1974:171–173). Research on acceptability pays no attention to female sexuality and little attention to certain side effects which, although not life-threatening, can cause women great anxiety. Third, both research and service delivery are dominated by an "inoculation mentality" in which the best method for most women (especially the poor) is viewed as a single anti-pregnancy "shot" such as an IUD insertion, injection, implant, or tubectomy (Joffe 1986:24–26). The reproductive concerns of women themselves are largely neglected in the scientists' quest for the perfectly effective, provider-controlled method.

Fourth, the effectiveness of hormonal and surgical methods has been purchased at the cost of significant dangers to the health or even the life of some users, feminists charge, especially in the early years of high-dose estrogen pills and injections and unsafe IUDs. Yet, medical professionals insist that the risks of preventing a birth must be weighed against the even higher risks to poor women—especially those in developing countries—of unsafe childbirth and clandestine abortion. Women's health advocates find this comparison insulting and unfair (Holmes 1979:4–5; Hartmann 1987:168–175), particularly in view of the limited resources devoted to primary health care in most countries (Germain 1987). Researchers and service providers should place more emphasis on mechanical and chemical barrier methods such as diaphragms and spermicidal foams, they contend, and on traditional methods such as withdrawal and periodic abstinence. Although less effective, these methods are generally without side effects (Bruce and Shearer 1979; Bruce 1987). Safe, legal abortion must be available as a backup for contraceptive failure and as a basic right.

Fifth, feminists have objected to the conditions under which many field tests of new contraceptives have been performed in both industrialized and developing countries. Of critical importance is the lack of genuinely informed consent and the apparent overrepresentation of vulnerable groups (the poor, the uneducated, racial or ethnic minorities) among experimental "subjects" (Ruzek 1978:36–47; Hartmann 1987). Sixth, new contraceptive methods requiring considerable skills and surveillance on the part of service providers are often introduced into settings with inadequate health infrastructures, thus exposing women to unnecessary risks of side effects and unwanted pregnancies (WHO 1991).

In the same vein, feminists have accused clinic-based family planning programs of pushing female methods at the expense of condoms or vasectomy. Although some women undoubtedly benefit from achieving greater reproductive autonomy, they also assume the sole responsibility for, and health risks of, fertility regulation. Sanger had pronounced this outcome inevitable. "In an ideal society," she wrote, " . . . birth control would become the concern of the man as well as the woman. The hard, inescapable fact which we encounter to-day is that man has not only refused any such responsibility, but has individually and collectively sought to prevent woman from obtaining knowledge by which she could assume this responsibility for herself" (Sanger 1920:93). Modern-day feminists found that husbands and lovers seemed eager to shift the responsibility for birth control to women while at the same time benefiting from greater sexual access. Some insist with their nineteenth-century counterparts that only natural family planning (periodic abstinence) is safe and acceptable. Others, although committed to furthering research on male methods so that men can share the responsibility for birth control and sexually transmitted disease prevention more equitably, are reluctant to depend on their male partners and want to maintain this control for themselves.

The *medical-hierarchical model of service delivery* constitutes a second theme of the critique. Sanger's efforts to win over the medical establishment undoubtedly helped to legitimize artificial methods of birth control on health grounds and to broaden women's access to services, but at a cost. Feminists have objected to the medicalization of contraceptive service delivery because it signifies a loss of female control and feminist consciousness, just as they have objected to the medicalization of childbirth in Europe and North America and to medical control over abortion and women's reproductive health in general (Ruzek 1978; Rothman 1982). When Marie Stopes opened her British clinic in 1921, for instance, the medical profession challenged her failure to have a qualified gynecologist in attendance all day (cervical caps were fitted by nurses) and even her right to use the word "clinic" (Fryer 1965: 229). Doctors have long insisted on their professional perogative to control service delivery even when female paramedical personnel could do the job as well or better. The campaign by physicians' associations to penalize paramedical or lay providers of medical services continues almost everywhere: in most countries only licensed doctors can prescribe pills, sterilize clients, or perform abortions.

Women's health activists in the United States, in other industrialized countries, and in some developing countries have experimented with alternative models of health care delivery (Ruzek 1978; Jones, Toss, and Scottish Health Education Group 1987). "Alternative" in this sense generally refers to women-controlled, non-hierarchically organized health centers that include abortion and birthing services, feminist therapy, and rape crisis counseling in the context of meeting women's needs for a broad range of sexual and reproductive information, support, and advocacy (Simmons, Kay and Regan 1984:624). The concept of self-help, promoted through the publication of books such as *Our Bodies, Ourselves* by the Boston Women's Health Book Collective (1973, 1984) and translated into many languages, is intended to circumvent the *traditional-authoritarian* model of service delivery in which "patients" are passive recipients of "expert" advice with which they are expected to "comply." Two feminist models are offered in its place (Ruzek 1978:104–112). In the *traditional-feminist* model, female para-professionals provide much of the reproductive health care to clients in an atmosphere of mutual respect and egalitarianism, thus reducing the potential for (usually male) physician control. In the *radical-feminist* model, women are encouraged to assume major responsibility for their own care with the assistance of lay women facilitators who are usually members of a health care collective. Feminists have also attempted to transform service delivery in *traditional-authoritian* family planning clinics in the United States (Joffe 1986; Ward 1986) and in some developing countries by introducing sexuality counseling by the woman's peers, sensitivity training of male and female staff, and woman-to-woman community outreach, among other reforms.

Professionalized, mystified, elitist, hierarchical, male-dominated, and often profit-oriented, medicalization is a top-down approach that—in the views of feminist health advocates—tends to *displace* paramedical personnel and traditional health practitioners such as midwives; *denigrate* women's knowledge about their own bodies, their own lives, and their own needs; and *deny* the reality of women's experience. This is not to romanticize women's traditional knowledge and skills, for some indigenous reproductive health practices are extremely harmful and others are harmless but ineffective (e.g., Hull 1979; Newman 1985). The feminist critique nevertheless raises a critical point about the locus of decisions regarding women's reproductive lives and, quite literally, about the control of medical professionals over women's bodies.

CHALLENGING THE DEMOGRAPHIC IMPERATIVE

The third development that caused feminists in North America and Europe as well as in southern countries considerable alarm from the 1960s onward was the growing preoccupation of many birth control supporters with the cause of population control. Drawing in part on nineteenth-century Malthusian theories, concerns about the rapid growth of population as a cause of poverty on the individual and family level and of economic underdevelopment on the national level burgeoned in the United States and internationally in the 1960s and 1970s (see chapter 3). In the United States, subsidized family planning was to become a centerpiece of President Lyndon Johnson's domestic War on Poverty in the mid 1960s. Although a number of scientific and political leaders and domestic organizations such as Zero Population Growth (ZPG) advocated birth rate reductions within the United States, the demographic imperative was most pronounced as a basis for U.S. foreign aid to developing countries. The Office of Population of the U.S. Agency for International Development (USAID) was soon to launch its "inundation strategy" to make contraceptives and sterilization available to all couples who wanted them (and some who did not) in developing countries. The U.S. delegation to the United Nations World Population Conference in Bucharest in 1974 argued strongly for an international policy setting demographic targets for reductions in population growth.

Once again, feminists were caught in a dilemma. On the one hand, subsidized services for low-income women at home and USAID's inundation approach abroad benefited women by broadening the range and accessibility of birth control information and services. Governments and non-governmental organizations (NGOs) created infrastructures for delivering family planning and, in the best programs, other reproductive health services to previously unserved populations, especially in rural areas. In the United States, the "great experiment" in subsidized family planning had developed by the early 1970s into a major system for the delivery of preventive health care to women of low or marginal incomes (Ward 1986:74). In many developing countries the numbers of women claiming to know of at least one "modern" method of family planning soared while contraceptive prevalence rates rose steadily. The emphasis on reaching large numbers of acceptors helped to undermine physicians' control over contraception by extending services through networks of health and family planning clinics, paramedical personnel, and community motivators, many of whom were women. Services were also increasingly delivered through commercial and community channels. The demographic imperative helped to mobilize medical science to develop more effective contraceptives and simpler techniques of abortion (e.g., vacuum aspiration by hand-held syringe, hormonal pills) and male and female sterilization (e.g., female minilaparascopy) that could be performed by paramedics.

From a feminist perspective, however, the demographic bias of the expanded birth control movement was damaging to women's interests. Women of childbearing age—especially if they were poor—were targeted as "at risk reproducers" with little if any understanding of, or concern for, their social and economic survival and security (Jaquette and Staudt 1985). Few population experts appeared to recognize that a reduction in fertility in the absence of other social changes could actually worsen, rather than improve, women's position in societies where childbearing is their main source of satisfaction and exclusive claim to social consideration as an adult woman (Tangri 1976:902; see also chapter 6). Moreover, some authoritarian governments seemed eager to promote population control in the absence of any genuine social, economic, or political reform; in this sense, the political context rather than the services themselves were unacceptable.

Within most family planning programs, the *quality* of reproductive health services was sacrificed to the *quantity* of family planning acceptors, the safety of contraceptive methods sacrificed to efficiency and technical effectiveness (Seaman 1969). Quantitative goals in service delivery were measured in numbers of acceptors, contraceptive prevalence rates, couple-years of protection, and—at the bottom line—numbers of "births averted." Governments and service providers appeared preoccupied with limiting family size ("stop at two" campaigns, for example) rather than with meeting women's traditional interest in child spacing or their fears of subfecundity or sterility. Excesses among overenthusiastic governments and overzealous community motivators eager to reach their targeted numbers of IUD or sterilization acceptors were common (Warwick 1982; Hartmann 1987). Providers often promoted long-lasting methods such as the IUD, injectables, or sterilization over methods that a woman could easily stop or switch on her own. Some providers believed that nonliterate women could not use other methods correctly; others were receiving incentive payments for persuading clients to accept IUDs or sterilization. Providers often failed to advise clients about possible side effects or contra-indications for fear that this would discourage them from adopting a method. At the same time, the rapidly expanding market for contraception in southern countries (much of it supplied by USAID or its grantees), combined with heightened concerns about liability litigation in the United States, encouraged some cases of corporate dumping overseas of contraceptives that were no longer in use (or never approved for use) in the U.S. domestic market, such as high estrogen orals, the Dalkon Shield IUD, and injectable Depo-Provera (Ehrenreich, Dowie and Minkin 1979).

More generally, feminists charged that the world view of population planners focused too narrowly on women's "excess fertility" without paying sufficient attention to the entire pronatalist and discriminatory system within which women live. Even those demographers who were aware of the pronatalist implications of gender inequality (e.g., Davis 1967) often proposed policy solutions that would intensify rather than reduce the conflicts most women experienced between their productive and reproductive roles. At the same time, the single-minded preoccupation of the population controllers with averting births neglected women's other vital health concerns (Germain and Ordway 1989). The concept of birth control as potentially liberating for women and for the poor, which was so central to radical and socialist feminism in the early part of the century, had been submerged.

Ultimately, the feminist critique of the demographic imperative rests on the conviction that women have a right to make their own decisions and to "own and control" their own bodies without governmental intervention. Women will make rational choices if they have the information and resources. Feminists have spoken out against program abuses and against the underlying ideologies of population control. As described more fully in the next chapter, however, women's views and concerns were scarcely represented in the bureaucracies of the population controllers— in the research centers, the corporations producing the contraceptive technologies, the medical establishments, the foundations, the legislatures, the governmental and nongovernmental agencies. It seemed that women had lost control over their own bodies to these outside agents at the same time that they were finally able to plan whether and when to bear children.

3

THE ELUSIVE "WOMAN QUESTION" IN UNITED STATES INTERNATIONAL POPULATION POLICY

Feminist commentary dominated the analysis in the previous chapter of the relationship between the movements for women's rights and for birth control/population control. In this chapter, women's voices are conspicuously absent. As a counterpart to the previous chapter, this one tells an "official story" about population and family planning policies in the United States. The story involves a search for rationales that would justify U.S. government support for family planning programs in developing countries and, to a lesser extent, domestically as well. The details are important because they have shaped much of the international environment of population funding and research.

Whereas feminists insist that a woman's right to control her own body entitles her to high quality reproductive health services, including safe and affordable contraception and abortion, neither the presumed right nor the entitlement have entered the official discourse in the United States. As the decade-by-decade review in this chapter will show, the closest approximation to a recognition of women's rights can be found in three contexts. The first is the congressional hearings on domestic and international population issues held in 1965 in which a number of expert witnesses urged the government to support family planning on grounds of personal freedom and civil liberties, that is, as a human right. The second is the justification for federal funding (Title X) of domestic family planning programs in 1970 on the grounds that poor women were entitled to have access to family planning assistance as a matter of social justice. The third is the 1972 recommendation of a presidentially appointed Commis-

sion on Population Growth and the American Future that women should
be free to determine their own fertility, which included a right to legal
abortion. These are scattered examples; perhaps more could be found.
By and large, however, public debates on population and family planning
policy have been concerned with "more important" issues.

Population policy and research in the United States have drawn heavily
on Malthusian fears of overpopulation fueled since the 1950s by unprecedented rates of global population growth. United States international
population policy in the 1960s and 1970s was driven by perceptions of
demographic crisis. Policymakers defined rapid population growth in developing countries as a critical problem with potentially disastrous social,
economic, political, and environmental consequences. The United States
urged governments in developing countries to set population growth reduction targets; foreign aid was mobilized in support of comprehensive
family planning programs as the major component of international population assistance.

The debate on U.S. international population policy during the past
several decades has been dominated by three major issues. The first is
the nature of the relationship between population growth and social, economic, political, and environmental conditions in developing countries.
Points of controversy include the extent to which rapid population growth
hinders improvements in per capita incomes, food consumption, health,
education, and general welfare; exacerbates social unrest and inequalities
in income distribution within and among nations; and accelerates environmental deterioration and resource depletion (e.g., National Academy
of Sciences 1971; Meadows et al. 1972; Easterlin 1980; Simon 1981; National Research Council 1986; Johnson and Lee 1987). Answers to these
questions would determine whether the U.S. government has a strategic
interest in reducing population growth in southern countries, and on what
grounds.

The second issue is the demographic effectiveness of different strategies
for reducing birth rates in developing countries, given the many possible
rationales for doing so (Berelson 1969). Proponents of family planning
programs as a population control strategy argue that improving access to
modern methods of birth control and raising the quality of service delivery
can have a substantial impact on population growth in most countries
(Mauldin and Berelson 1978; Mauldin and Lapham 1987; Jain 1989; Bongaarts, Mauldin and Phillips 1990). Others insist that stronger and more
direct measures are necessary in many countries, such as institutional
reforms to provide alternatives to childbearing or incentive schemes to
reward couples with fewer children or penalize those with more (Davis
1967; Ehrlich 1968; Ridker 1976). Still others contend that agrarian reform
and other structural changes to reduce class inequalities are necessary to
create conditions favorable to lower fertility (Kocher 1973; Rich 1973;

Hernandez 1984). The outcome of this debate determines the manner in which U.S. aid funds should be invested if they are to achieve a significant demographic impact. It also raises the ethical question of how far any government should go in its efforts to alter the reproductive behavior of all or part of its population (Berelson and Lieberson 1979; Callahan 1981). Are government-imposed incentive schemes for motivating couples to accept family planning or to "stop at two" children inherently coercive, for example? Where is the line to be drawn between coercion and free choice?

A third component of the policy debate concerns what role the U.S. government should play in the actual delivery of birth control information and services, at home or abroad. Quite apart from its possible demographic consequences, U.S. support for family planning has been justified as a means of enhancing the freedom of individuals and promoting family welfare. But U.S. support for family planning has also been challenged as interventionist and immoral. Points of controversy include the nature of sexual and reproductive rights and the "right of privacy"; the role of the family in society and of patriarchal authority within the family; and the moral and health aspects of specific means of family planning such as intrusive artificial contraception, sterilization, and abortion (Jaffe 1981; Luker 1984; Roberts 1990). Should the U.S. government be in the business of providing people with birth control information and services, either directly or through other agencies? Should American taxpayers have to pay for it?

Important questions of women's rights are raised implicitly or explicitly in each of these policy debates. With few exceptions, however, the "woman question" has remained peripheral throughout the evolution of the U.S. policy position. For example, the question of whether gender inequalities in access to schooling, employment, or health care are intensified by rapid population growth has been ignored. Population policy-makers have tended to view women of childbearing age as "targets" for specific program interventions in their attempts to achieve demographic objectives such as a specific percentage-point decline in the birth rate or a particular number of family planning "acceptors." What women in diverse circumstances might actually *want*, or how they might define their own needs and aspirations, has not been considered. The idea that a woman could exercise her basic human rights more effectively by gaining control over her own body—that is, over her own sexuality and reproductive capacity—is only occasionally acknowledged. And while the human rights justification for providing family planning has focused on freedom of information and services, there has been little awareness of the ways in which patriarchal attitudes and practices in different social contexts prevent girls and women from exercising the rights to which they are entitled.

This chapter describes the evolution of U.S. international population policy over four decades. Beginning in the cautious years of the 1950s, the story moves through the period of enthusiastic endorsement of population control and international family planning in the 1960s and 1970s. It culminates with the revisionist policy stance of the 1980s in which the guiding rationales were thrown into considerable disarray. On the one hand, official policy backed off on the economic rationale to focus on health and welfare concerns in the context of maintaining "respect for family values." On the other hand, a resurgence of pressure for stronger efforts to reduce global population growth marked a return to the "controlista" mentality of earlier years. The chapter concludes that both of these ideologies—the preservation of family values and population control—threaten to undermine the movement for expanded sexual and reproductive rights for women and the provision of a full array of reproductive health services.

THE 1950S: NO POLICY IS THE BEST POLICY

At the international level, family planning organizations in Europe and North America had been holding meetings since 1880. Much of the early enthusiasm for birth control (especially in nineteenth-century England) can be attributed to anxieties about excessive population growth. However, the fears expressed by many European governments between the two world wars of incipient population *decline* overrode such Malthusian concerns. In the years following World War II, rapid population growth in some developing countries combined with a recovery of fertility in Europe and North America triggered a new interest in birth control policies. Sweden took the initiative by sponsoring an international meeting that led to the establishment of the International Planned Parenthood Federation (IPPF) in 1952. Sweden was also the first country to extend international technical assistance for family planning, to Sri Lanka (then Ceylon) in 1958 (Field 1983:61).

Although some American researchers were showing considerable interest in international population questions, the official U.S. position in the 1950s on population growth and family planning was characterized by nervous caution on all fronts. Neither "the woman question" nor human rights issues had been explicitly raised at the domestic or international level in connection with family planning. The primary concern at the time was whether the U.S. government should become involved at all in the population problems of developing countries or in the distribution of family planning services at home.

Reliable demographic statistics on the world's population situation were lacking in the early postwar years. According to the best estimates, the world's population had reached 2.5 billion by 1950, a 32 percent increase since 1920 (United Nations 1973b:526). Growing at an annual rate of about 1.2 percent throughout the preceding three decades, the population of Asia, Africa, and Latin America was 1.6 billion in 1950, up from 1.2 billion in 1920. Population growth was declining rapidly in Europe, North America, Oceania, and the Soviet Union, however, dropping from 1.1 percent annually during the 1920s to 0.3 percent in the 1940s. The decade of the 1950s showed a sharp upsurge in growth rates. By 1960, the world's population had reached 3.0 billion. A postwar surge of marriages and births raised the annual rate of increase in industrialized countries to 1.3 percent, but the populations of developing countries were now growing twice as fast as they had in the 1920s, at 2.0 percent per year.

As early as 1946, the newly formed United Nations had established a Population Commission, primarily at the instigation of the United States and Great Britain (Symonds and Carder 1973:41–43). In 1950, a U.N. report supported by the United States declared that high birth rates *could* pose obstacles to more rapid economic growth in some countries. The report encouraged governments of developing countries to consider adopting policies to curb population growth (ibid.:69–71). Even this careful recommendation elicited opposition, however. Representatives of some pronatalist western European Catholic countries where birth control was still illegal, and of some eastern European socialist countries where birth control had been liberalized, attacked the "neo-Malthusian pessimism" of the report. Proponents of the proposal, in order to avoid controversy, dropped the issue. Meanwhile, expressions of concern about the potential consequences of overpopulation were appearing in the late 1940s and early 1950s in the U.N. specialized agencies: UNESCO, the Food and Agriculture Organization (FAO), the International Labour Office (ILO), and the World Health Organization (WHO) (Johnson 1987).

Within the United States, momentum for a policy change in the domestic arena had been building. Advocates of legal and medical liberalization of contraception had made great strides (Piotrow 1973:7–11). Margaret Sanger had waged an unrelenting battle to eliminate legal barriers blocking access to birth control services and to focus medical attention on the issue. Progressive lawyers and physicians united in urging the removal of arbitrary, outmoded restrictions on the prescription of contraceptives. While the Roman Catholic church hierarchy remained adamantly opposed to artificial birth control, Protestant churches were breaking away from their traditional prohibitions. The idea of contraception for married couples was generally accepted for health and social reasons (Symonds and Carder 1973:89–95; Piotrow 1973:23–29). Public opinion polls showed that, by 1959, about 80 percent of white men and women of reproductive age agreed that birth control information should be publicly available even though its dissemination was still illegal in some places. Among the remaining 20 percent were many who claimed no opinion on the subject (Blake 1969:522–523).

By 1958, Massachusetts and Connecticut were the only states with laws prohibiting contraceptive use. But some interest groups were still trying to promote such legislation. In 1958, for example, a Roman Catholic group in New York tried to prevent doctors from giving contraceptive advice to patients of municipal hospitals (Symonds and Carder 1973:95). Having failed to uphold restrictive legislation on moral grounds, the group argued that it was inappropriate for the government to pay for contraceptive information and services with taxpayers' money. This theme was to reappear later in the domestic and international abortion policy debates.

Responding to the rising interest in family planning as means of reducing rapid population growth in southern countries and even among rapidly growing subgroups in the United States, a group of Catholic bishops in Washington D.C. in November 1959 unambiguously declared that "United States Catholics believe that the promotion of artificial birth control is a morally, humanly, psychologically, and politically disastrous approach to the population problem. They will not support any public assistance, either at home or abroad, to promote artificial birth prevention, abortion or sterilization, whether through direct aid or by means of international organizations" (quoted in Piotrow 1973:43). The church's opposition to government-supported family planning services both in the United States and in the developing world may have derived only partly from its historical condemnation of the so-called artificial means of fertility control, however. According to some analysts, the church's opposition also drew from its desire to maintain church authority regarding the sanctity of the traditional (i.e., patriarchal) family against the inroads of secularism and women's emancipation, as well as with avoiding drastic declines in birth rates among its constituents (Donaldson 1990:12–14).

Meanwhile, private foundations such as The Population Council, The Ford Foundation, and The Pathfinder Fund had initiated research in human reproduction that included contraceptive development, and, to a limited extent, support for family planning programs in developing countries such as Pakistan and India (Bachrach and Bergman 1973). Their efforts were aided by important technological advances in birth control such as the hormonal pill and the IUD.

In 1959, the President's Committee to Study the U.S. Military Assistance Program (also known as the Draper Committee) issued a report that addressed the "population question" by recommending that "in order to meet more effectively the problem of economic development, the United States [should] assist . . . countries . . . on request in the formulation of . . . plans designed to deal with the problem of rapid population growth" (Symonds and Carder 1973:94; see also Piotrow 1973:40). As the first advisory body to address the problem in detail and to recommend specific action, the committee was also concerned with possible threats to U.S. national security posed by widening income disparities between rich and poor nations.

Apparently nervous about the political implications of the proposal, President Dwight D. Eisenhower passed the report on to the Senate Foreign Relations Committee without commenting on this section. The senate committee, agreeing with the report, recommended that the U.S. government *should* provide assistance in contraceptive development to developing countries (Symonds and Carder 1973:94). A horrified President Eisenhower responded that "I cannot imagine anything more emphatically a subject that is not a proper political or governmental activity or function or responsibility.... As long as I am here," he insisted, "this government will not have a positive political doctrine on birth control" (*New York Times*, 3 Dec. 1959:1, 18; see also Piotrow 1973:45–48 for additional comment).

Although Eisenhower subsequently supported U.S. family planning assistance to developing countries and acknowledged that his earlier concerns about violating the religious convictions of large groups of taxpayers were probably "taken too far," his 1959 statement was interpreted as a policy banning the use of foreign aid funds for family planning. At the end of the decade, officials of the International Cooperation Administration (predecessor of the Agency for International Development) assured Congress that "Not one penny of foreign aid funds has ever been used for dissemination of birth control information *and there are no plans to do so*" (quoted in Piotrow 1973:51; emphasis added).

THE 1960s: ENCOURAGEMENT AND ASSISTANCE

The U.S. government took its first steps in providing direct international economic aid by passing the Foreign Assistance Act of 1961. In 1963, Congress authorized research on problems of population control and technical assistance, including the provision of family planning information for couples who requested it. Funds dispersed by the U.S. Agency for International Development (USAID) could not be spent on contraceptive supplies, however, which had been on the prohibited list for commodity assistance since 1948 (Piotrow 1973:83). Although the rationale offered for the prohibition was that developing countries could manufacture their own contraceptives, nervousness over the Roman Catholic vote at home seemed more responsible. Indeed, in 1964 the United States stated its position at the United Nations as being "opposed to the United Nations undertaking any activity involving the supply of specific birth control devices to member states, since *such devices were repugnant to many people*" (Symonds and Carder 1973:140, emphasis added). (This theme resurfaces in the U.S. international abortion statement in 1984.) Nevertheless, in a small but significant step forward, the United States did approve assistance in providing contraceptive information.

By the early 1960s the population of the developing world was growing faster than in the early 1950s because death rates were dropping. The populations of developing regions were growing by almost 2.4 percent annually compared with 1.1 percent in developed regions, reflecting a total fertility rate of about six children per woman. Although President John F. Kennedy recognized that rapid population growth posed special problems in underdeveloped countries and was willing to provide assistance if requested, it was President Lyndon B. Johnson who took action. In his 1965 State of the Union message, Johnson declared that he would "seek new ways to use our knowledge to help deal with the explosion in world population and the growing scarcity in world resources" (*New York Times*, 5 Jan. 1965:16). By June of that year he had moved even further. At the twentieth anniversary of the founding of the United Nations in San Francisco, Johnson overenthusiastically proclaimed, "Let us act on the fact that less than five dollars invested in population control is worth a hundred dollars invested in economic growth" (quoted in Piotrow 1973:90).

Census results revealed that the population of most developing countries had been growing at a considerably higher rate than was commonly assumed. Unable to deny the existence of a "population explosion," the U.S. government adopted a plan of "direct attack" to reduce the birth rates of developing countries through its War on Hunger, primarily through investment in family planning programs. The *demographic imperative* was born, a child of the so-called population coalition of intellectuals and professionals who formed an influential, interlocking network of politicians and experts ("a men's club," according to some commentators) in the foundations, universities, legislatures, and government agencies (Bachrach and Bergman 1973; see also Donaldson 1990:53–74). Key congressional supporters included Senators Ernest Gruening, George Bush, and Joseph Clark, backed by President Johnson and, subsequently, President Richard M. Nixon as well (Field 1983:22).

The year 1965 marked the modest beginning of USAID's support for family planning in foreign assistance (USAID 1974). In the same year, Senator Gruening launched a series of congressional hearings on domestic and international population issues that attracted a great deal of attention during the next two years (Piotrow 1973:103–111). A stream of expert witnesses recommended the expansion of contraceptive services at home and abroad for reasons such as personal and family health and welfare, abortion prevention, environmental protection, and the amelioration of poverty and malnutrition. Concerns about population growth in developing countries were linked with concerns about population growth in

the United States. According to one observer, however, "it was the freedom of information, civil libertarian, personal-freedom-of-choice argument that received the greatest emphasis" with respect to justifying the
government's policy (ibid.:107). If this interpretation was valid, the U.S.
government would be hard pressed to justify withholding birth control
information and services from people who wanted and needed them. The
issue was no longer based solely on demographic concerns: out of the
congressional hearings emerged an implied personal "right" to family
planning.

The right to family planning was soon formally recognized on the international level as well. In 1966, the U.N. General Assembly passed a
resolution pushed by Sweden, the United States, India, Pakistan, and
Ceylon calling upon the Population Commission, the Economic and Social
Council (ECOSOC), and the U.N. regional commissions and specialized
agencies to strengthen training, research, and advisory services in the
field of population and family planning (Johnson 1987:33). The specialized
agencies such as WHO, FAO, UNESCO, ILO, and UNICEF were increasingly active, as was the World Bank, whose president, Robert
McNamara, announced a major commitment to population assistance in
1968 (ibid.:34–41). The 1968 U.N. Teheran Declaration on human rights
declared that couples have a basic human right to decide freely and responsibly on the number and spacing of their children. The initiative for
the Teheran declaration on family planning had come largely from the
U.N. Commission on the Status of Women and from IPPF, which has
official U.N. status as a non-governmental organization (Symonds and
Carder 1973:178–179). The 1968 meetings of ECOSOC also raised the
crucial issue of the link between population and the status of women. The
Commission on the Status of Women invited the United Nations and its
member states to undertake surveys and case studies on the Status of
Women and Family Planning, with special reference to the protection of
human rights, and, in particular, the rights of women (Johnson 1987:33).
The United Nations published the results of this effort in 1975.

POPULATION ACTIVISTS AND THEIR CRITICS

The second half of the 1960s witnessed a surge of public interest within
the United States in the global population crisis. Popular books warned
of massive starvation and environmental disaster unless runaway world
population growth rates were checked by immediate and drastic means
(e.g., Day and Day 1964; Paddock and Paddock 1967; Ehrlich 1968). As
public concerns grew, population supporters such as Senator J. William
Fulbright claimed that USAID was not giving the population problem the
high priority it deserved (Piotrow 1973:133). In 1967, Fulbright introduced
legislation authorizing $35 million to support voluntary family planning

programs overseas. The funds would be distributed primarily through
agencies already providing family planning services abroad, such as IPPF,
The Population Council, and The Pathfinder Fund; through grants to U.S.
institutions for demographic and contraceptive research; through direct
bilateral assistance to governments requesting it; and through the United
Nations Fund for Population Activities (UNFPA), which, beginning operations in 1969, was the major coordinating agency for multilateral governmental assistance.

In 1966, Congress had amended the Food for Peace Act in order to
grant USAID the authority to use foreign currencies to manufacture or
distribute "medical" supplies such as contraceptives (Piotrow 1973:118).
The enthusiastic new director of the population office at USAID was
eager to remove all obstacles to direct grants of contraceptives to developing countries with U.S. currency and soon did so. USAID was now
firmly committed to population control in developing countries, primarily
through a strategy of family planning program assistance. Domestic critics
of U.S. policy were quick to respond (Clinton 1973; Glassheim, Cargille
and Hoffman 1978). Leftists accused the U.S. "population establishment"
of promoting the interests of the capitalist ruling class through population
control in the Third World. At the same time, black militants were charging
the U.S. government with genocidal birth control policies at home and
abroad (e.g., see Littlewood 1977; Stycos 1977).

The domestic charges of genocide were aimed at federally subsidized
programs of family planning for the poor that had been instituted in President Johnson's War on Poverty. In 1964, only 13 states had rudimentary
state-funded family planning programs; by 1966, 40 states had services,
although none statewide (Ward 1986:39). Amendments to the Social Security Act of 1965 required state health departments to extend health
services, including family planning, to all areas within 10 years. Federal
grants were available for services in isolated rural areas and among the
urban poor. According to one analyst, "Family planning became synonymous with the civil rights of poor women to medical care" (ibid.:xiii).

Economic Opportunity Program funds were channeled primarily
through affiliates of the Planned Parenthood Federation of America. In
the final month of the decade, Congress passed the Family Planning Services and Population Research Act of 1970 (otherwise known as Title X
of the Public Health Services Act), the major enabling legislation for
subsidized family planning services in the United States. Title X established a program of categorical funding of federal grants—up to $382
million for the next two years—for family planning services through public
and private providers. Rationales for the family planning initiative included the concerns of environmental groups about the negative consequences of population growth in the United States, and the liberal
economic assumptions driving the War on Poverty (Aries 1987:1471).

Foremost among the rationales was the belief that low-income women were *entitled* to public services. "It is my view that no American woman should be denied access to family planning assistance because of her economic condition," declared President Nixon in announcing the program. "I believe, therefore, that we should establish as a national goal the provision of adequate family planning services within the next five years to all those who want them but cannot afford them" (quoted in Ward 1986:68). Most states lacked the commitment and necessary infrastructure to respond effectively, however.

The domestic family planning program raised some of the same outcry as the program overseas. Critics favoring a national population policy challenged the assumption that federal family planning programs would result in smaller families or help to alleviate poverty, even if they *were* justifiable on individual grounds (Blake 1969). More radical social reforms were needed—particularly in women's roles—if the reproductive motivations of American couples were to be transformed. Defenders argued that the national family planning program was not intended as a *population* policy because it included no fertility reduction goals; rather, it was a *public health* and *civil rights* policy for poor women (Ward 1986:69). The fact that Title X emphasized birth control over other health services, and that blacks and other minorities were disproportionately represented among America's poor, elicited charges of genocidal conspiracy from black militants, however, who aimed their protests at federally funded birth control clinics in poor or black neighborhoods (ibid.:92). Hurled in an atmosphere of intense political mobilization as the decade of the sixties drew to a close, these charges divided the family planning movement as well as the black community. Many black women found themselves torn between their loyalties to the cause of black nationalism and their insistence on fertility regulation and reproductive health services as a woman's right.

THE 1970s: ENTHUSIASM AND ADVOCACY

In the late 1960s and early 1970s, the United States experienced an unprecedented surge of social and political activism. As noted in chapter 2, the movement for women's liberation emerged in part from the experiences of women activists in the civil rights movement, the students' movement, socialist-leftist groups, and the movement against the war in Vietnam. Demands for economic and political rights competed with demands for reproductive and sexual rights as the new wave of feminists campaigned for the repeal of all restrictive abortion laws so that women could "control their own bodies." Perceiving the illegality of abortion as tantamount to compulsive pregnancy or coercive childbearing, advocates of legalized abortion insisted that the government should not intervene in this personal decision. At the same time, anti-abortion activists lobbied to repeal the new, liberalized abortion laws passed by a few states.

In 1969, President Nixon had appointed a Commission on Population Growth and the American Future to formulate a domestic policy that would reflect "the pervasive impact of population growth on every facet of American life" (U.S. Commission . . . 1972:preface). Chaired by John D. Rockefeller 3rd, the Commission considered a broad range of domestic trends and policies relating to population growth and distribution, employment and economic growth, resources and the environment, government and public policy, immigration and internal migration, education and research, and, tellingly, "the status of children and women." In its final report of 1972, the commission recommended among many other policies setting a target of zero population growth for the United States and instituting a policy of comprehensive family planning services, including contraception for all regardless of age or marital status, and legalized abortion. "Women should be free to determine their own fertility," the report proclaimed (ibid.:103). The commission noted that pervasive pronatalist institutions and practices in American society were channeling women into childbearing while restricting their access to rewarding alternatives (Blake 1972). To counter these social forces, the commission recommended congressional and state approval of the Equal Rights Amendment to the U.S. Constitution. Nixon's response to the report was hostile. Singling out the recommendations on legal abortion and on contraception for teenagers for public attack, he effectively repudiated the entire report and condemned it to inaction.

In 1973, the same year that abortion was legalized in the United States in the Supreme Court decision of Roe v. Wade, Congress passed the Helms Amendment to the Foreign Assistance Act of 1961 prohibiting the direct use of U.S. foreign aid funds for abortion services or for abortifacient devices or drugs in recipient nations. This event marked the beginning of an increasingly restrictive U.S. policy in which organized right-to-life groups turned their attention to blocking international aid for abortion and family planning. The Office of Population of USAID stopped funding its "highest priority" research to develop a safe, post-conceptive, once-a-month substance "which, when self-administered on a single occasion, would ensure the nonpregnant state at completion of a monthly cycle" (USAID 1974:14). The Office of Population had also been distributing vacuum aspiration kits for early abortion ("menstrual regulation" or MR) to family planning providers in a number of countries. This all came to an end.

Congress had repeatedly rejected an even more restrictive draft of the Helms Amendment which would also have barred funding for biomedical research on abortion. (The latter was added to the FAA in 1981.) The Helms amendment thus denied support to women in developing countries for the full range of birth control options now available to American women. The newly won right to abortion in the United States came under immediate attack, however. Several legislators proposed amendments to the U.S. Constitution that would authorize the states to regulate abortion, or, more fundamentally, bestow the rights of full "personhood" on the fetus. In addition, 188 anti-abortion bills were introduced in 41 states within six months of the Roe v. Wade decision (Faux 1988:318–319).

Despite these conservative tendencies, several liberal policy changes were introduced the same year. In accordance with the Nixon-Ford Administration's New Directions strategy in international assistance, the foreign aid program was now mandated to emphasize basic human needs and "growth with equity" (Staudt 1985:30–32; Fox 1986:618–619). This strategy attempted to reach the poor majority in developing nations more directly through smaller, community-based projects. Population program assistance was to stress "low-cost integrated delivery systems for health, nutrition, and family planning" and to incorporate an awareness of the relationship between population growth and "improvements in the status and employment of women," among other factors. Also in 1973, responding to pressure from U.S. women's groups, Congress added the Percy Amendment to the Foreign Assistance Act which provided that relevant sections of the act be administered "so as to give particular attention to those programs, projects, and activities which tend to integrate women into the national economies of developing countries, thus improving their status and assisting the total development effort."

These provisions marked the first public policy recognition in U.S. international aid of a connection between population and development processes and the status of women. To some extent, they reflected the findings of the Commission on Population Growth and the American Future that gender discrimination created pronatalist pressures by preventing women from exercising greater reproductive choice. Feminists successfully lobbied national delegations, including U.S. representatives, for similar language at the U.N. World Population Conference at Bucharest in August of the following year. But the debate in Bucharest was to concentrate almost totally on the question of whether population growth was a contributing cause of underdevelopment (Mauldin et al. 1974).

THE 1974 WORLD POPULATION CONFERENCE AT BUCHAREST AND ITS AFTERMATH

The Bucharest conference was a landmark in the movement for official recognition of population issues at the international level. World Population Conferences held in Rome in 1955 and Belgrade in 1965 had involved scientists in their personal capacity, but the 1974 meeting in Bucharest was the first to include government representatives in their official capacity. The U.N. Population Commission and the Population Division prepared a draft World Population Plan of Action following intensive consultation with member states and reviews of the findings of pre-conference symposia on population and development; population and the family; population, resources, and the environment; and population and human rights.

At the meeting itself, the U.S. delegation strongly recommended setting national goals for reductions in population growth together with a world goal of replacement level fertility by the year 2000. The population of the developing world had reached 2.6 billion by 1970—almost one billion more than in 1950—and was growing faster than ever before at over 2.4 percent annually despite a slight drop in the total fertility rate. The global population had reached 3.6 billion and was projected to reach somewhere between 5.9 and 6.7 billion by the year 2000 (Frejka 1973). The U.S. delegation stressed not only the urgency of making subsidized information, education, and the means of family planning available to all people as a basic human right, but also the importance of increasing funds for bilateral and multilateral health and population programs in developing countries (United States 1974:2, 4–5). USAID had been pouring funds into contraceptive research and distribution programs in developing countries in a highly publicized "inundation strategy" (Donaldson 1990). Its total assistance to population programs had grown from $2.1 million in 1965 to $125.6 million in 1973 (USAID 1974:2).

The U.S. emphasis on the need for strenuous population policies and programs as an integral component of development drew vocal opposition from many quarters and the American proposal for national goal-setting was rejected. As in earlier years, the United States was accused by many developing country representatives and their supporters of "neo-Malthusian rhetoric" intended to conceal the true causes of underdevelopment: the exploitation of poor countries by the rich (Mauldin et al. 1974:103–104; Finkle and Crane 1975:103). Opposition to direct intervention in Third World population growth came from nationalist, religious, and Marxist pro-growth positions, from revolutionary, anti-colonial and anti-imperialistic perspectives, and from the belief that social justice could best be served through radical transformations of social structures and political institutions. The Chinese delegation was especially vociferous in its attacks on the draft Plan of Action and on its "superpower" supporters, declaring that "of all things in the world, people are the most precious" (quoted in Johnson 1987:97). Calls for a New International Economic Order gained the headlines. Thus, although the U.S. policy statement included a reference to broadening opportunities for women's education and employment as one of a number of indirect measures to motivate couples toward smaller families, and although a consensus was reached at the conference on the importance of improving the position of women, no specific measures were proposed. "The woman question" was lost in the shadows of ideological debate.

By the mid 1970s, USAID began to change its approach to population programming by shifting from the theories of the so-called "supply-siders" to those of the "developmentalists" or "demand-siders" (Warwick 1982:45–51; Herz 1984:40–45; Jaquette and Staudt 1985:235, 252–253). The contraceptive supply-siders (not to be confused with economic supply-siders, who are a very different breed) believed that the major thrust of USAID's population program should be to expand the flow of family planning services and supplies to developing countries. The developmentalists, in contrast, insisted that broader policy reforms were needed to reduce the demand for children. Increasing the supply of contraceptive services was simply not enough.

The developmentalist approach was certainly not new. Some mainstream demographers had been contending for years that family planning programs by themselves would have little impact on birth rates in developing countries where couples continued to want large families (e.g., Davis 1967; Berelson 1969). The critical task was not only to identify those elements of the social structure that could be manipulated through development assistance to lower the demand for children, but also to determine how to achieve the greatest demographic effect (e.g., Rich 1973; King 1974; Ridker 1976; Cochrane 1979). The U.S. policy statement at Bucharest, for example, supported "developmentalist" recommendations for reductions in infant and child mortality, basic education, improved status of women, promotion of social justice, better living conditions in rural areas, provision of old age security, and the establishment of a minimum age for marriage (United States 1974:5). USAID began to emphasize projects that would bring about social and economic conditions conducive to having fewer children. A provision was added to the International Development and Food Assistance Act requiring USAID to incorporate population impact analyses throughout the full range of its development activities.

The shift to "demand-side" thinking brought the social and economic position of women more directly into focus by forcing researchers and policymakers to consider the complex range of pronatalist forces at work in most settings. In many countries, patriarchal institutions such as the arranged marriage of young girls, female seclusion, male appropriation of valued property, and discrimination against girls and women in schooling and employment, were forcing women into economic dependency and frequent childbearing. Yet, even here the demographic imperative appeared to predominate in policy-making. Although policy statements paid lip service to the idea that improving the status of girls and women in and of itself was a desirable goal (e.g., the U.S. statement at Bucharest), the motivating force behind population policy—not surprisingly—still appeared to be the search for a cost-effective method of reducing family size. The developmentalist approach did not target women's bodies, as had the inundation strategy. Rather, it targeted women's socio-economic condition where evidence suggested that certain changes might achieve the desired demographic result. If biomedical engineering had not produced the "perfect contraceptive," perhaps social engineering could identify the "perfect social variable" that might alter women's reproductive aspirations and behavior.

Following Bucharest, U.S. advocacy in the international population field lost some momentum (Jaquette and Staudt 1985:251–252; Warwick 1982:51). Although the United States remained the largest single contributor of international population aid throughout the 1970s and early 1980s, reaching almost $200 million in 1981, funding in real terms stopped growing after 1972 (Piotrow 1980:71–72). Neither President Gerald Ford nor President Jimmy Carter spoke out strongly on population issues. Responsibility for population programs within USAID was decentralized to the regional bureaus, the controversial director of the Office of Population was demoted, and professional staff was cut (Donaldson 1990:75–96).

Despite the insistence from some scientific and governmental quarters within the United States that international population growth was still an urgent issue, the political initiative with respect to population policies and programs was shifting to international agencies and to the developing countries themselves. The 1974 World Population Conference in Bucharest had triggered a surge of requests from developing countries to UNFPA for planning and program assistance (Sadik 1984:8). By 1980, 52 developing countries had official policies supporting family planning for demographic reasons (predominantly in Asia and Latin America and the Caribbean) and 65 additional countries supported family planning on health or human rights grounds (predominantly Latin America and the Caribbean, the Middle East, and Sub-Saharan Africa). Thirty-five governments gave no official support or were explicitly opposed (predominantly in the Middle East and Francophone Sub-Saharan Africa), but these countries included only 4 percent of the total population of the developing world (ibid.:151–152). The decade ended with strong international expressions of concern in the 1980 Brandt Report, "North-South: A Programme for Survival," and the 1980 International Conference on Population and the Urban Future organized by UNFPA.

THE 1980s: NEW DOUBTS, NEW QUESTIONS

By the early 1980s a mood of conservatism had swept the United States. The Equal Rights Amendment had failed ratification by the requisite number of states, and proponents of a constitutional amendment banning abortion were hopeful of achieving their goal under the administration of

President Ronald Reagan. Contraceptive services for teenagers were increasingly under attack by conservatives on the grounds that they contributed to the decline of sexual morality and the loss of parental control (Donovan 1984).

In 1982, the Reagan Administration articulated its position on the international population issue in a USAID Policy Paper on Population Assistance (USAID 1982). The population of the developing world had reached 3.3 billion in 1980, twice that of 1950, and was continuing to grow at about 2.0 percent annually, the same rate as in the 1950s. There were now 4.4 billion people in the world. Since 1965 USAID had spent over $2 billion on population assistance, about half of the total amount provided to the developing world. Intended to demonstrate the continuity of U.S. policy, the paper reaffirmed a commitment to voluntary population and family planning programs as a basic component of U.S. development assistance with two interrelated goals: (1) to enhance the freedom of individuals in developing countries to choose voluntarily the number and spacing of their children, and (2) to encourage population growth consistent with the growth of economic resources and productivity. For maximum effectiveness, family planning programs and services were to be coordinated with other development programs designed to expand access to education and employment, "especially for women" (USAID 1982: 186). Despite these assurances, however, President Reagan repeatedly attempted to cut funds for population programs overseas (Fox 1986:627–628).

According to the new USAID statement, support for family planning programs would be based on two fundamental principles: *voluntarism* and *informed choice*. All USAID-supported programs were to include "a description of the effectiveness and risks of all major methods of family planning and an agreement either to provide other family planning methods requested or to refer couples to programs offering other methods as appropriate" (USAID 1982:186).

Research and service delivery on methods of "natural family planning" (NFP)—otherwise known as the rhythm method, or periodic abstinence— were, since 1980, explicitly included in the Agency's population programming. By 1985, USAID was spending $7.8 million of its population budget on NFP training and research, a significant increase from the $800,000 spent in 1981 (Johnson and Reich 1986:277). The emphasis on NFP, although justified on the principle of expanding the range of contraceptive choices, was primarily a response to right-to-life pressure groups who were opposed to all artificial methods of contraception as well as to abortion and sterilization on any grounds. Muddying the waters that separated church and state, proponents of NFP lobbied for (and in 1985, were granted by USAID) an exemption from the informed choice provision so that NFP providers in USAID-supported church-related programs were *not* required to advise clients on methods of artificial contraception (Ben-shoof 1987). Although abortion counseling, referrals, and services pro-vided with non-USAID funds were not yet prohibited, certain restrictions on abortion-related activities were introduced such as the training of prac-titioners in abortion techniques, the procurement or distribution of equip-ment intended for induced abortion or menstrual regulation, and the funding of biomedical research on abortion as a method of family planning (USAID 1982:188).

SURPRISES AND REACTIONS: THE 1984 MEXICO CITY
CONFERENCE AND THE ANTI-ABORTION AGENDA

By 1984, when the second U.N. International Conference on Population was held in Mexico City in August 1984, most southern countries had incorporated family planning programs and sometimes even stringent pop-ulation growth reduction targets into their development plans (UNFPA 1985; 1986). The U.S. delegation to the Mexico City conference, headed by conservative and "pro-life" former Senator James L. Buckley, an-nounced a fundamental policy change that sent shock waves through the meeting. Rapid population growth per se was no longer to be considered an obstacle to economic growth in developing countries, he announced; rather, under some conditions it might even be beneficial. Claiming that there had been a "demographic overreaction" in the 1960s and 1970s, the U.S. delegation now declared that the new goal of the United States was "to encourage developing countries to adopt *sound economic policies*" based on free markets and individual initiative (United States 1984:4, emphasis added).

Whereas the developmentalists had generally favored direct govern-ment intervention in areas such as land reform, employment creation, and health and education, the Reagan policy emphasized free markets, individual initiative, and non-intervention. Once again the United States was somewhat isolated at the conference. Observers noted that "the U.S. position on the relationship between development and population was extensively discussed and broadly rejected" (Wulf and Willson 1984:228). Critics of the U.S. stance in Mexico City were not generally opposed to the idea of the primacy of economic over demographic concerns. This had been, after all, the basis of their opposition to the U.S. position at Bucharest. Rather, they were opposed to the *ideological content* of the economic agenda which defined too much government control and plan-ning rather than excessive debt burdens and protectionist international trade policies as the major cause of economic crisis in the south (ibid.; see also Demeny 1985:99–106).

Despite this startling reversal on the demographic rationale, the United States emphasized its commitment to continued funding of family planning programs on health and humanitarian grounds as a "small part" of its total development assistance. Such funding, however, would no longer be available "to any nation [engaging] in forcible coercion to achieve population growth objectives," nor could funds be used for direct or indirect support of non-governmental family planning organizations providing abortion services, counseling, or referrals, even in countries where abortion was legal. "The United States does not consider abortion an acceptable element of family planning programs," the position paper declared, "and will no longer contribute to those of which it is a part" (United States 1984:4). The U.S. position at Mexico City represented a triumph of the Reagan administration's economic and moral ideologies. It was immediately denounced by a group of congressional representatives, one of whom remarked that the delegation's "support of free market economics and opposition to abortion had such little relevance to the immediate hardships facing LDCs [less developed countries] that both AID and the State Department felt compelled to issue rebuttals to the policy" (Fox 1986:660–661).

While the U.S. policy statement recognized the negative impact that rapid population growth could have on the health of mothers and children, it contained no reference to the pervasive patterns of discrimination against girls and women that blocked their access to basic social and economic resources. Gender inequality was simply not an issue; nor were social policies that would promote more equitable access to needed services. Rather, the policy statement was devoted almost entirely to asserting the need for "sound" economic policies in developing countries and to the condemnation of abortion, which was termed "unnecessary and repugnant." The justification for family planning programs was limited to their contribution to economic and social development, to the health of mothers and children, and to the stability of the family and of society. In contrast to the U.S. policy statement at Bucharest a decade earlier, references to women's rights *within* the family and in society as a whole were conspicuously absent.

Although ignored in the U.S. policy statement, the "woman question" received considerable attention at the Mexico City conference. Throughout the discussion of the World Population Plan of Action, female delegates from many countries—especially Australia and Zimbabwe—strengthened the language that emphasized the linkages between high fertility rates and the lack of education, health care, and employment opportunities for women and their low status in general (Wulf and Willson 1984:221). Recommendations to overcome economic, cultural, and social discrimination against women were moved from a later section of the plan on "Reproduction, the family and status of women" to the front, following the section on socioeconomic development and population.

Following the Mexico City conference, population professionals within

USAID, caught in the crossfire between proponents of conflicting economic and demographic viewpoints and between pro-choice and right-to-life advocacy groups, struggled to redefine their mission. As a result of recent scientific reports and the Reagan administration's Mexico City policy statement, the economic rationale for international family planning assistance—that high rates of population growth necessarily impede economic development—was losing its political credibility. Most population professionals both inside and outside USAID continued to believe that rapid population growth was a critical problem in the majority of southern countries, however, and that well-designed family planning programs combined with other development assistance could have a considerable economic and demographic impact. Acting independently of official government rhetoric, these professionals continued their efforts in population programming, research, and technical assistance and advice.

USAID's official emphasis shifted to "meeting the interests of families," which were defined in a somewhat limited way as "(1) the desire of couples to determine the size and spacing of their family; (2) mother and child survival; [and] (3) reduction of abortion" (McPherson 1985:1). Under the new agenda, respect for "family values" and universal condemnation of abortion were the overriding principles of the government's family planning assistance. Important USAID policy statements in 1985 and 1986 still failed to raise the issue of gender inequality (ibid.; Rosenberg 1986). Freedom of reproductive choice for couples was justified as "consistent with a free enterprise system" (Rosenberg 1986:2)—that is, consistent with a conservative economic ideology—rather than as an affirmation of women's rights in a socially liberal, human rights context. Because abortion was not considered a method of voluntary family planning, it was resolutely and illogically excluded from the frequently affirmed principle of "freedom of choice."

The Reagan administration's prohibition on foreign assistance to NGOs using funds for abortion-related advocacy, counseling, or referrals was reflected in similar efforts on the domestic front. In April 1984, Senator Jesse Helms proposed legislation that would prohibit the use of Title X funds from the Public Health Service Act "by any organization which in any way engages in abortion, abortion referral, abortion counselling, abortion lobbying, [or] abortion advertising" even though Title X already prohibited direct federal funding of abortion (Rossoff and Kenney 1984). In September 1987, the Secretary of the Department of Health and Human Services announced new rules that would prohibit service providers in any Title X project (over 4,000 public and private clinics, including many in Planned Parenthood) from informing their clients either of the availability of abortion as a legal medical procedure or of places where abortion information or services could be obtained (Rosoff 1988:317). The regulations also proposed a startling redefinition of the family planning services to be included under Title X, which were rank ordered as "natural family planning methods, adoption, infertility services and general reproductive health care, abstinence and [lastly] contraception" (ibid.)

Following public comment and slight revision, the proposed Title X restrictions were announced in February 1988. A flurry of court challenges ensued, however, and the new rules were held in abeyance until the Supreme Court upheld them in the Rust v. Sullivan decision of May 1991. Domestic clinics serving low-income women and teenagers were now faced with the same dilemma as their overseas counterparts, forced to choose between offering or referring women for safe and legal abortion but losing all U.S. government funding for their health and contraception services, or maintaining their general programs but refusing a woman's request for information on terminating an unwanted pregnancy (Camp 1987). The connections between domestic and international policy were clear. Ten days after the Rust decision, the Supreme Court refused to hear a challenge to the Mexico City policy in the case of Planned Parenthood v. Agency for International Development (*New York Times,* 4 June 1991:A12). The restrictions inherent in these policies were strongly defended by Reagan's successor. President George Bush favored a constitutional amendment to reverse the Supreme Court's 1973 decision in Roe v. Wade and vetoed legislation that would add rape and incest as permissible grounds for federally funded abortions for poor women (NARAL Foundation 1991:171).

As the dust from Mexico City was settling in the late 1980s, analysts were assessing what damage had been done to international population and family planning programs by the U.S. policy (Camp 1987). In combination with legislation such as the Kemp-Inouye-Helms amendment to the Supplemental Appropriations Act of 1985 which stated that no U.S. funds shall be given to an organization that "supports or participates in the management of a program of coercive abortion or involuntary sterilization," the policy forced USAID in 1985 to stop funding the two largest international family planning organizations. The first was the International Planned Parenthood Federation (IPPF), headquartered in London with more than 120 affiliates throughout the world. IPPF was targeted because it uses a small portion of its private funds for abortion services in some countries. The second was the now renamed United Nations Population Fund (UNFPA), headquartered in New York with programs in 140 nations. UNFPA was targeted because of its assistance to China. Following acrimonious debate in Congress about whether or not the Chinese population policy was coercive or resulted in forced abortions, UNFPA was declared ineligible for U.S. support (Crane and Finkle 1989). For both IPPF and UNFPA, the jolt of the U.S. decision triggered significant increases in donor funding from other governments and from nongovernmental sources (Camp and Lasher 1989:70–71).

In Washington D.C., the Mexico City restrictions fed a political environment of uncertainty and hostility regarding the U.S. role in international family planning. Although public opinion polls continued to find core support for population funding among Americans generally, the situation in Washington deteriorated to the point that policymakers were considering international programs politically controversial even if they were personally supportive (Camp and Lasher 1989:5). Right-to-life organizations in conjunction with representatives of conservative Roman Catholic and fundamentalist Protestant churches continued to lobby members of Congress and key leaders in the executive branch on both domestic and international family planning issues. They demanded the withdrawal of funds from several U.S. population research organizations, favored (or exclusive) treatment of natural family planning over all other methods of birth control, and the elimination of family planning assistance from the foreign aid budget. Supporters urged Congress to restore support for IPPF and UNFPA in order to maintain U.S. international credibility and commitment to family planning services (Menken 1986:240–241; Crane and Finkle 1989).

FROM POPULATION CONTROL TO "RESPECT FOR FAMILY VALUES" . . . TO POPULATION CONTROL?

In the mid 1980s, developing countries were spending approximately $1.5 billion annually in support of their own population programs. This figure compared with about $500 million annually contributed by the United States and other members of the Organization for Economic Cooperation and Development (Menken 1986:235). Sixty-four developing countries had adopted explicit demographic policies favoring lower population growth rates by 1988, up from 31 in 1975 and only 15 in 1965 (Cross 1988:18). The decade ended with a world population of almost 5.5 billion people, over 4 billion of whom lived in developing countries. The world's population was growing at 1.6 percent per year in 1990 and almost 2.0 percent in the developing world despite falling birth rates. One billion more people would be added to the world's population before the century ended. In the United States, however, the political will to act intelligently on the population question seemed to be dissipating as the issues became increasingly obscured by moralistic rhetoric and political threats.

Amidst the confusion, U.S. support for the provision of birth control information and services continued to be justified on health, humanitarian, and human rights grounds. USAID's sponsorship of a review conducted by the National Academy of Sciences on the health consequences for women and children of contraceptive use and controlled fertility (National Research Council 1989) helped to substantiate its health rationale after the economic growth argument had been officially (but perhaps mistakenly) discredited. In addition, USAID's funding of the World Fertility Surveys (WFS) and the Demographic and Health Surveys (DHS) during the late 1970s and 1980s identified a significant "unmet need" among women for family planning information and services in many developing countries (Boulier 1985; Westoff 1988). Providing services to women who say they want no more children but are not using a contraceptive method offered a relatively uncontroversial basis for supporting international programs on humanitarian and human rights (the right to family planning) grounds.

There were inconsistencies, however. Prohibitions on U.S. funding of any overseas or domestic program engaged in abortion research or offering abortion counseling, information, or referrals even where abortion is legal directly contradicted the government's professed concern for protecting women's and children's health and welfare. Moroever, the continued references to supporting "family values" were disturbing to feminists in their implication that women's rights as individuals would play no role in official policy pronouncements. As long as the focus remained on strengthening the *family,* there would be little room for challenging the subordination of girls and women and the denial of their basic rights in patriarchal family systems. As long as the focus remained on *family planning,* there would be little room for a policy that would promote those economic, social, political, and civil rights that infuse reproductive choice with real meaning. And as long as the right to terminate an unwanted pregnancy safely was denied, there would be little room for a population policy that would place a woman's right to control her own body and her own life at the center, where it belongs.

A surge of public interest in the late 1980s and early 1990s in saving the global environment raised new demands for strong policies of international population control as *a* major, if not *the* major, means of stopping environmental degradation (e.g., Ehrlich and Ehrlich 1990; Brown et al. 1991). New coalitions of population, environment, and development organizations such as the Global Tomorrow Coalition, Interaction, and the Year 2000 Committee pushed the U.S. Congress for higher levels of population funding. A position paper widely endorsed by environmental organizations declared that population growth threatens to overwhelm any possible gains made in improving human conditions because of its "pervasive and detrimental impact on global ecological systems" (Priority Statement on Population 1991). USAID announced its intention to concentrate funding on the 17 southern countries (excluding China) with the largest populations in order to maximize its impact on global population growth.

This new wave of "controlista" pressure was also alarming for feminists and other critics who had long found the conventional approach wanting. The argument that population growth was the primary cause of environmental deterioriation—and thus that population control was the primary solution—was misleading and potentially harmful. It oversimplified the complexities of the relationships among population size and growth, reproductive patterns, modes of production, levels of consumption, and types of environmental damage in northern and southern countries. It was misleading in blaming overpopulation in southern countries rather than wasteful production and overconsumption in northern countries for problems such as clearcutting tropical forests and depleting ocean fisheries. (Critics of the U.S. position at Bucharest in 1974 had raised exactly this point.) It was potentially harmful in reverting to old-fashioned calls for "population control" without, in most cases, defining what was meant or how it might differ from prevailing policies and programs. The new demands ignored the progress that had been made in conceptualizing policies and programs designed to improve the quality of care and enhance women's reproductive health and rights. Indeed, they suggested that researchers and policymakers in the population field remained uniquely untouched by the social and political transformations arising from the growth of an international feminist movement.

Both the renewed calls for population control and the revisionist calls to respect family values appeared potentially damaging to women's interests. The population control mentality threatened to escalate the use of family planning programs as a tool of antinatalist propaganda rather than as a means of protecting women's sexual and reproductive rights and personal well-being. And, as suggested above, the "family values" argument was a smokescreen for the perpetuation of conservative ideologies that would deny women access to safe abortion and preserve the "harmony and stability" of the family at the expense of women's rights to self-determination. Both approaches contradicted the repeated assertions in policy documents that USAID's support for family planning would be based on the fundamental principles of voluntarism and informed choice. And, as two (contradictory) sides of the coin of U.S. international policy and programming, both sets of arguments provided fuel for their respective supporters in developing countries to justify particular political agendas. The following chapter highlights the dynamics of these forces as they are played out in the policies and protests of three developing countries. In Brazil, Nigeria, and the Philippines, women's organizations and feminist groups have found themselves struggling to define their own agendas within the contradictions of pronatalist and antinatalist ideologies expressed by increasingly powerful networks of international organizations on both sides.

4

POPULATION POLICY AND WOMEN'S POLITICAL ACTION IN THREE DEVELOPING COUNTRIES

The design and implementation of population policies in southern countries have been heavily influenced by the domestic and international policies of the United States. The influence is direct, through bilateral assistance to southern governments and non-governmental organizations (NGOs), and indirect, through USAID-funded research centers, consulting firms, family planning NGOs, and United Nations agencies such as UNFPA (until 1986) and the World Bank. The United States government has consistently been, and remains, the single largest donor for population programs (Gillespie and Seltzer 1990) even following its controversial defunding of UNFPA and IPPF in the mid 1980s (see chapter 3). Its policies have been actively promoted in forums such as the international population conferences in Bucharest in 1974 and Mexico City in 1984, with mixed results and considerable negative reaction from many Third World governments and their supporters.

Third World women's groups have also increasingly made their views known on policy issues raised in these and other settings. Resisting the ideology of population control manifested so explicitly in earlier U.S. policies and at Bucharest, they have also challenged the capitalist economic ideologies and conservative moral ideologies promoted at Mexico City and beyond. Feminists and women's health advocates in many southern countries have taken the initiative in critiquing the excesses or inadequacies of family planning programs in their own countries and in confronting internationally- and domestically-imposed threats to their reproductive health and rights.

This chapter examines initiatives in three southern countries: the Philippines, Nigeria, and Brazil. The three case studies represent different world regions, population policies, economic conditions, demographic processes, and levels of women's political mobilization. The stories are unique but not unrelated. Their uniqueness derives from the particular historical circumstances of each country. Their relatedness derives from the impact of the global economic crisis on governments' perceptions of their population problems and on their ability to provide family planning and health services; the continued interest among multilateral and bilateral donors in funding population, health, and women's programs in developing countries; and the increasingly global character of the women's movement in its various manifestations.

WOMEN'S POLITICAL ACTION IN INTERNATIONAL PERSPECTIVE

Although much has been written about the rise of feminism as a social movement in North America and Europe in the nineteenth and early twentieth centuries, parallel movements in Third World countries have been essentially ignored. Yet, there is a history of reform movements for female emancipation in most Asian and Middle Eastern countries, for example (Jayawardena 1986), and women throughout the world have played key roles in nationalist, independence, revolutionary, and democratization movements (e.g., see Jaquette 1989 on Latin America). There is no doubt that movements for women's rights in southern countries were frequently influenced by ideas and speakers from northern countries espousing ideas of female education, women's suffrage, and the reform of family laws and harmful traditional customs. But it is wrong to say that feminism in the Third World was—or is—merely imitative of western models, as so many critics of the movement have charged (Jayawardena 1986:1–24). Rather, feminists in southern countries have created their own theories and their own social movements based on their own experiences not only of sexual oppression but of oppression based on race, class, ethnicity, nationality, and decades or even centuries of economic and political domination by foreign powers.

The years since 1975 have witnessed the rise of a genuinely international women's movement (Morgan 1984; Tinker and Jaquette 1987; Shreir 1988; Wieringa 1988). Stimulated in part by the resurgence of feminist movements in Europe and North America in the mid 1960s and by the efforts of the Commission on the Status of Women at the United Nations, the designation of 1975 as International Women's Year not only raised the consciousness of women around the world but also served as a dynamic organizing tool. The decade between the 1975 women's conference in Mexico City and the 1985 conference in Nairobi witnessed a remarkable growth in the awareness, the militancy, and the organizational networks among Third World women (Mies 1986; Fraser 1987). Critical *of* prevailing social and economic policies and practices, individual women and organized women's groups in southern countries—as in the north—are increasingly demanding to be heard in many of the public debates and political decisions from which they have previously been excluded. Women's groups are also emerging as critically important *to* the success and the legitimacy of public policies that affect them because of women's growing power as a political voice.

In some countries, especially in Muslim South Asia and parts of the Middle East, the overall level of political awareness and organizational participation among the majority of women is as yet very low, even at the community level, although a few elite women may be active as professionals or volunteers in the health and family planning fields. In other countries, especially in sub-Saharan Africa, many women are active in a variety of women's organizations and some wield considerable political power, but there is as yet no recognizable women's *movement* to articulate a set of common goals and objectives or to coordinate a strategy for achieving them. In still other countries, such as India, a collective movement has clearly emerged to advance women's interests on a number of compelling political, economic, and sociocultural problems, but questions of population policy, reproductive rights, and family planning service delivery have not, by and large, been central to their concerns. Finally, there are countries, including some in Latin America, in which an active women's movement has placed sexual and reproductive rights and health at the core of its agenda for political action (Petchesky and Weiner 1990). Within all of these settings are explicitly feminist groups opposed to gender oppression in all of its private and public manifestations.

Feminists in southern countries have relied on three complementary strategies in their efforts to influence state policies on population and reproductive health and rights, each of which poses some dilemmas.

The first strategy involves building a *collective movement* that claims to represent the interests of a significant constituency of women across the major social divides of class, caste, ethnicity, religion, and region. The example of Nigeria in this chapter reveals how difficult this can be in a heterogeneous society where competing identifications obscure common interests and in which independent political action has been restricted in the past under authoritarian rule. Nevertheless, some Nigerians do consider themselves part of an international—if not yet a national—women's movement.

Although uneven in its development, the international women's movement has since 1975 engendered a number of associations linking women within and among southern countries. Among elite groups, at least, are women who meet often at regional or international conferences under the sponsorship of professional associations, governments or NGOs, and U.N. agencies. Some south-to-south networks with broad policy agendas, such as DAWN (Development Alternatives with Women for a New Era, now based in Rio de Janeiro), have developed a critical analysis of reproductive rights and population programs in the context of concurrent global issues (Sen and Grown, 1987). Others, such as ISIS-Latin America, give more explicit emphasis to reproduction and women's health. Global and regional networks such as these emphasize feminists' roles as researchers, communicators, facilitators, and catalysts for change, as well as their close working relationships with grass-roots women's organizations struggling against sexual and class exploitation in each country. Many Third World women's groups concerned with reproductive rights are affiliated with international organizations such as the International Women's Tribune Center in New York, ISIS-International, or the Women's Global Network on Reproductive Rights, based in Amsterdam, which links Third World groups with individuals and groups in industrialized countries (Tinker and Jaquette 1987).

Each of these vertical and horizontal alliances within and across countries acts as a resource for exchanging information, articulating policy positions, and planning effective political action within the broad boundaries of the international movement. Exchange and collaboration has not always been easy, however. Most groups are hampered by their lack of experience, contacts, and paid professional staff, and by their limited knowledge of political strategies, organizational behavior, and resource-seeking methods (Staudt 1981:378; Germain and Antrobus 1989). The need for financial and technical assistance from outsiders, no matter how sympathetic the latter might be, provokes fears of dependency and outside control.

A second strategy for influencing policy involves the acquisition of political skills by women who are often unfamiliar with—or suspicious of—the workings of the formal political process, government bureaucracies, and international NGOs. Assessing the first year of operation of the São Paulo state women's commission in Brazil, for example, its first president noted that "the main problems have been caused by the total lack of political experience of most of its women members. Their lack of knowledge of the way the state apparatus works, of political alliances and all the various forms of action available, leads them to take months to reach objectives that could be reached in days" (Blay 1985:303). The underrepresentation of women (particularly feminists) in key political positions in each country reduces the potential for women's interests to be forcefully articulated at the policy level. At the same time, activists in the movement are often torn between their desire to keep the movement "pure" (and thus, to engage primarily in *oppositional* politics) and the desire to institutionalize their programs (and thus, to engage in *partici-patory* politics, which inevitably involves compromise and threats of co-optation). Feminists have also found that political achievements can be fragile when the political winds shift, as the Brazilian case demonstrates.

The third strategy, building alliances with other institutional actors or constituencies around women's rights and family planning, is also simul-taneously promising and problematic. Most commonly such allies are individual physicians or organizations of obstetricians and gynecologists, other associations of health and family planning providers (e.g., nurses and midwives, family planning NGOs), civil rights advocates, social sci-ence researchers, key personnel in government ministries, and political leaders (often in opposition parties) with socially conscious platforms. Divergent views and mutual misunderstanding can make collaboration difficult, however, or reduce it to some narrowly defined content and transitory joint action such as blocking the introduction of a fetal protec-tion clause in a constitutional amendment.

Women's health advocates in developing countries have built important alliances with key personnel in some international donor organizations, however, which in some cases provides them with considerable visibility, legitimacy, and political leverage. Virtually all of the major multilateral and bilateral donor organizations and international NGOs in the fields of population, health, family planning, and development now include a few highly committed women and men who consistently advance—although not always successfully—the cause of gender-sensitive policies and pro-gramming. Some southern women's groups have been wary of collabo-rating with international agencies that they define as representing imperialistic interests or ideologies of population control, however, even on issues of mutual concern such as reducing maternal mortality. This issue appears in the Philippines case study included here. Feminists charge that some international aid agencies (as well as national governments) continue to treat Third World women in an instrumental manner under the guise of approaching population problems "scientifically" (e.g., see Sen and Grown 1985:39–42; Hartmann 1987; Germain and Ordway 1989).

The technocratic approach to policy-making, which relies on "experts" rather than on consultation with groups who will be most affected by decisions, gives the appearance of "proposing dispassionate solutions which are devoid of political bias" (Bachrach and Bergman 1973:7–8). Women activists in many countries are responding, not dispassionately, with charges of political bias aimed at the technocrats as well as the politicians. Most governmental and nongovernmental policies and pro-grams in health and family planning have not yet institutionalized the values and priorities of women themselves, critics contend. Focusing on the conditions of women's lives and on the quality of reproductive health services rather than on the achievement of demographic targets, advocates of a woman-centered perspective are attempting to transform conventional thinking about fertility policies in developing countries.

This chapter tells a story of how governments in three countries have sought to legitimize their population, family planning, or health policies in the eyes of key political constituencies, and how women's groups and other institutional actors seek to define, influence, or challenge them. Each of the three countries has undergone a process of democratization since the mid 1980s which permits us to examine women's political action under evolving conditions of popular participation. Brazil and the Philippines have emerged from long periods of repressive authoritarian rule; Nigeria's military government has lifted its ban on partisan politics as part of a planned transition to civilian rule. All three countries have created a new constitution which includes symbolically important provisions guaranteeing the equal rights of women and men in accordance with the Convention on the Elimination of All Forms of Discrimination Against Women, to which each country is signatory. The more open political environments have brought population policies along with other critical issues to the forefront of national legislative concern. Various interest groups, including women's groups, are now free to speak out on the issues that concern them.

Although Brazil's per capita income of about $2,300 in the late 1980s is almost four times higher than the Philippines' and eight times higher than Nigeria's, all three countries are experiencing international debt crises resulting in the imposition of economic austerity measures that have caused considerable popular unrest. Economic difficulties and the political tensions surrounding them impede each government's ability to improve the quality and quantity of family planning and health services in the public sector—along with most other programs—even where they are committed to doing so. Implementation thus remains a severe problem. As for their policy environments, Brazil, whose annual rate of population growth has dropped to 2 percent, does not have an official policy to reduce birth rates. Nigeria, with a growth rate of almost 3 percent, announced its first official policy to lower the birth rate in 1989 following years of pronatalist sentiment. The Philippines, with a growth rate that has stabilized at about 2.5 percent after substantial earlier fertility declines, has maintained a policy of population control, which is now being challenged, since 1971.

BRAZIL: FEMINIST CRITIQUE OF REPRODUCTIVE HEALTH AND RIGHTS

The women's movement in Brazil is dynamic, politically active, generally leftist, and explicitly feminist in its focus on gender as well as class and race relations. Women's sexual and reproductive rights are integral to its policy agenda. The movement has evolved from a unique configuration of social, economic, and political conditions that sets it apart from much of the feminist movement in the north. It draws on a critical awareness among intellectuals of the dynamics of unequal distribution of wealth and other resources in Brazilian society, a prolonged struggle against two decades of authoritarian rule which ended in 1985, and an anti-imperialist stance. The Brazilian feminist movement was inspired in part by the intense involvement of some elite women, who were in political exile during the 1970s, with feminist movements in Europe, especially in France (Schmink 1981; Corrêa 1989; Sarti 1989).

Although women's rights advocates in Brazil had campaigned for female suffrage in the 1920s and 30s, the current women's movement took shape in the mid 1970s. As in most countries, the celebration of International Women's Year in 1975 both stimulated and legitimated research and action on a wide range of women's issues such as working conditions, legal rights, child care, and sexual violence. Academic researchers had already published critical analyses of women's conditions (e.g., Saffiotti 1969) and issues such as wage discrimination and the "double shift" of women's work on the job and at home were addressed in the popular press. Many individuals and groups concerned with the rights of women of all social classes were also aligned with grass-roots movements protesting the economic policies and political repression of the military dictatorship and demanding social justice, amnesty for political prisoners, and basic infrastructural services for people living in the urban peripheries. In addition, women activists returning to Brazil during the amnesty of 1979 from over a decade of exile abroad helped to create a uniquely Latin American feminist movement by linking—both analytically and politically—the European feminists' concerns with issues such as sexuality and reproductive rights with the Brazilian leftists' struggles for economic and political rights.

With the "democratic reopening" under the military regime in 1978 of some aspects of the political process and the reorganization of political parties, women's groups flourished in many forms: feminist collectives, neighborhood residents' associations, mothers' clubs affiliated with the progressive wing of the Roman Catholic church, political groups, and women's associations within the professions and trade unions. Journals such as *Brasil Mulher* and *Nos Mulheres* appeared in the second half of the 1970s; *Mulherio* in 1980. Despite their diversity, women's groups were mobilizing as a collective movement to influence state policies (Instituto de Ação Cultural n.d.; Sarti 1989).

As opportunities for direct political participation opened, women who were shying away from the political process in order to protect the autonomy of their movement were challenged by those urging active involvement in electoral party politics (Blay 1985:300; Alvarez 1989). Feminists worked enthusiastically with opposition candidates in several state elections in 1982 to incorporate women's rights in their party platforms. The government of Tancredo Neves elected in 1985 owed a considerable amount of its popular support to organized women's constituencies who played a significant role in the movement for direct presidential elections in 1984 and in support of opposition candidates in the Democratic Alliance (Alvarez 1989). Neves died before assuming office, however, and his vice-presidential running mate, José Sarney, became president.

Brazilian feminists have developed what they call a "critical understanding of the conditions of human reproduction in Brazilian society" (Barroso 1990; Corrêa 1989; Sarti 1989). Translating theory into practice, feminist groups such as SOS-Corpo in Reçife, Pro-Mulher in São Paulo, and the Coletivo Feminista Sexualidade e Saude in São Paulo have founded centers or collectives offering self-help health care, sexuality and rape counseling, and psychological support for women as an alternative to what they see as an unresponsive and authoritarian medical establishment. Joined by some like-minded physicians (e.g., see Pinotti and Faúndes 1989), the feminists' critique of prevailing reproductive health policies and practices in Brazilian society includes the following points.

First, feminists point out that the quality of primary health care for women in Brazil is generally poor, especially for rural women and those in the urban *favelas* who cannot afford private care. Maternal and infant mortality and morbidity rates (as well as rates of illiteracy) remain among the highest in Latin America despite Brazil's relatively high per capita income, industrialization, urbanization, and abundant natural resources. Reflecting extreme inequalities in the distribution of incomes and health services, mortality conditions may worsen as national expenditures on public health and other basic social services shrink under the impact of the debt crisis and economic structural adjustment policies (Cornia, Jolly and Stewart 1987:107–109).

Second, following Brazil's participation in the World Population Conference in Bucharest in 1974, a number of state and municipal governments entered into official relations with private family planning organizations to provide services to low-income clients, especially in the economically depressed northeast (Barnett 1985:5–7; UNFPA 1989b:66–76). Disturbed by some aspects of these collaborations, feminists asserted that the largest private family planning organizations such as BEMFAM, the IPPF affiliate, appeared more interested in recruiting new contraceptive acceptors than in protecting women's physical and emotional health and rights to informed choice. The women's movement has moderated some of its criticisms of the private agencies in the late 1980s, however, in recognition of the limited capacity of the public sector to provide training and services and of the important role that the private agencies have played.

Third, feminists insist that the state has the responsibility to provide safe, accessible methods of fertility regulation in a non-coercive manner to all who want them as an essential element of reproductive health care (a social entitlement) and as a precondition for women's full citizenship (an individual freedom). The demand for services is high, yet contraceptives are still unavailable in most government health services despite the Brazilian delegation's statement at Bucharest that "birth control measures should not be a privilege reserved for families that are well off" and that "the State [should] provide the information and the means that may be required by families of limited income" (Merrick and Graham 1979:281). Most Brazilian women have a limited choice of birth control methods and service providers as attested by their heavy reliance on private physicians and pharmacies, and on only three methods: the pill, sterilization (which is legally restricted), and clandestine abortion. Barrier methods such as diaphragms and even the condom are almost impossible to obtain. According to the 1986 Demographic and Health Survey (DHS), 66 percent of women aged 15 to 49 who were currently in unions were using contraception or had been sterilized ("Brazil 1986" 1988:63). Because of inadequate screening and choice, however, many are using inappropriate methods and experiencing side effects or unwanted pregnancies. Almost half of the women interviewed in the DHS reported their current pregnancy or most recent birth was mistimed or unwanted (ibid.:62).

Fourth, abortion is illegal in Brazil except to save a woman's life or in cases of rape. Feminists have documented that even women who are eligible for legal abortions are usually denied hospital services by physicians and the courts. (Health professionals interviewed by a reporter could recall only two legal abortions performed in Rio de Janeiro, a city of six million, in three years; *New York Times*, 21 July 1991:Y5). Public health service physicians are not trained to perform abortions. Services provided in expensive private clinics by qualified medical practitioners are safe, but low-income women must often resort to dangerous self-induced or back-street procedures. In 1980, more than 200,000 women were hospitalized for treatment of incomplete or septic abortions in health clinics run by the medical branch of the national social security system, which serves about 80 percent of Brazil's population (Pinotti and Faúndes 1989:98). By 1990, the estimates had reached 400,000 hospital admissions annually for abortion complications, resulting from an estimated 1.4 million to 2.4 million clandestine abortions in all (*New York Times*, 21 July 1991:Y5).

Fifth, feminists believe that levels of female sterilization—over 27 percent of currently married women nationally—are excessive, especially in

some low-income groups, reaching over 40 percent in the North and
Central-West regions (United Nations 1988a:25). Although these national
rates are not unusual when compared with many other Latin American
countries or with the United States and Canada, feminists charge that
women are often sterilized without adequate understanding or choice of
other methods. Moreover, legal restrictions on sterilization have encouraged the excessive practice of caesarian sections at childbirth because
sterilization can be performed inconspicuously at this time and because
women with a history of caesarians can claim medical grounds for sterilization (Rutenberg and Ferraz 1988:62). Almost one-third of all deliveries
in Brazil are performed by caesarian section, ranging from under 20 percent among low-income women to almost 60 percent among women with
high incomes (Patai 1988:369). These figures compare with about 25 percent in the United States in 1988 (up from 6 percent in 1970), where
physicians have been accused of performing many unnecessary procedures (*New York Times*, 29 Aug. 1990:A12).

Sixth, feminists have questioned the ethics of contraceptive testing
programs in Brazil, such as the clinical trials for the subdermal hormonal
implant, Norplant, fearing that not enough was known about the safety
of the method and that some research subjects had not given their genuinely informed consent. More broadly, feminist health advocates have
been concerned about the limited role women have played in the design,
testing, and evaluation of new reproductive technologies and in determining ethical values and priorities (Barroso 1990).

The feminist movement in Brazil has acted as an important pressure
group in the 1970s and 1980s in advocating individual freedom of choice,
urging the government to take direct responsibility for providing birth
control information and services rather than relying on the private sector,
and demanding a more liberal abortion law. Opposed both to the pronatalist stance of Brazilian nationalists and the Catholic church hierarchy,
on the one side, and to the population control policies of the family
planning organizations and their allies in government circles on the other,
feminists insist on the primacy of a woman's right to control her own
sexuality and reproduction according to her personal needs and experiences (Alvarez 1989:216).

BRAZILIAN STATE POLICY AND THE FEMINIST AGENDA

At the time of the 1974 World Population Conference, when the U.S.
delegation was pushing to set global population control targets, the Brazilian government was encouraging population growth as a means of settling the vast frontier regions and fueling the country's economic growth
and international prestige. The Brazilian delegation to Bucharest recog-

nized family planning as a human right but denounced population control as a solution to Third World problems. A key supporter of the initiative for a New International Economic Order, Brazil criticized foreign interference in the population matters of southern countries (Nortman 1975:28).

As the widely heralded "economic miracle" of the late 1960s and early 1970s metamorphosed into unemployment, inflation, and debt crisis in the 1980s, official and private concerns about the impact of population growth loomed larger on the political agenda. At the federal level, sectors of the military drafted a plan to curb population growth in consultation with internationally funded family planning organizations such as BEMFAM who were pressing for adoption of population control measures (Alvarez 1989:223). In June of 1983, during the waning months of the military regime, the Chief of the Armed Forces spoke out publicly on the "utmost importance" of a national family planning program. Many religious, intellectual, and political leaders representing a range of ideological positions were strongly opposed, however, and the plan was not approved (United Nations 1988a:28).

When 21 years of authoritarian rule ended with the election of a civilian federal government in January 1985, the time seemed ripe for women activists to capitalize on their political support for the winning democratic candidates by playing a more direct role in policy formation at the state and federal levels. As Carmen Barroso notes (1990:10–11), "For a great part of the feminist movement it was an exciting challenge to try to affect public policies they had been criticizing from a safe distance." To be successful, however, feminists had to learn how to translate their radical critiques into feasible programs, how to gain political leverage, and how to manage the complex federal, state, and municipal bureaucracies with which they would work (e.g., see Blay 1985). This theme represents one of the most significant challenges that women's rights advocates have faced throughout the world in carrying out a policy agenda.

Appointed by the post-military Sarney government to several high-level national councils, politically favored feminists were mandated to make broad-ranging recommendations on reproductive health policies and programs and to promote their implementation. Their first major success had occurred earlier under the military regime, however. In 1983, the Ministry of Health adopted a national Integrated Women's Health Program as a specific policy alternative to the military's population control plan. Designed by feminists and physicians, the program was intended to correct inadequacies in the provision of contraception and other basic health services for women, to emphasize high quality care, and to raise the consciousness of health providers to respect women's rights and autonomy. Women's groups, most of whom initially rejected the proposal because they opposed collaboration with the military government, eventually came to its support (Barroso 1990). The women's health program was supposed to be launched in the Northeast in 1984 and extend throughout the country by 1988 (United Nations 1988a:28–29).

When responsibility for implementing the women's health program shifted in 1986 to the Ministry of Social Security (the major agency responsible for public health services throughout the country), feminists in that agency drafted a comprehensive Policy on Women's Health and Family Planning which mandated for the first time that the state should provide a full range of birth control methods through its public health services under conditions of fully informed consent. The reference to contraceptive choice was just one of many specific items in a radical policy demanding that women be protected from abuses of biomedical research, from physical and sexual violence, and from inadequate reproductive health care. The Integrated Women's Health Program was launched in 1986, but on a very small scale. Although a few committed professionals were attempting to implement its guidelines in scattered centers elsewhere, by 1989 only the state of São Paulo was offering contraception in its social security health facilities, for reasons discussed below, and even there, problems of limited contraceptive delivery and high rates of caesarian sections remained.

The presidential appointment in August 1985 of a National Council for Women's Rights marked another early achievement for feminists. The idea of a national council had arisen during the electoral campaign of the opposition candidate, Tancredo Neves, who was supported by a multiparty Democratic Alliance and was responsive to women's concerns. State councils on women's rights had been established earlier in São Paulo and Minas Gerais when opposition candidates won the 1982 state elections (Blay 1985; Alvarez 1989; Sarti 1989); by 1990 they existed in at least six states and twelve cities in addition to the federal level. The National Council for Women's Rights has supported the women's movement in its promotion of a broad range of reproductive rights. In September 1985, the new government also appointed an advisory Committee on Reproductive Rights attached to the Ministry of Health, which included representatives from the women's movement along with participants from other ministries and the academic community. Affirming the state's obligation to enable women to exercise their individual right to choose appropriate methods of fertility control (or no method at all) and to obtain safe abortions, the Committee on Reproductive Rights includes a working group that reviews the testing, use, and abuse of modern contraceptive methods such as IUDs, injectables, and implants in clinical field trials in Brazil (Barroso 1990:17, 23–24).

The National Council for Women's Rights actively promoted women's representation in the Constituent Assembly which was elected in November 1986 to write a new Brazilian constitution. Several of the 26 women elected to this 559-member body used the opportunity to put forth an explicitly feminist agenda on reproductive rights. (The 5 percent female membership of the assembly reflected the 4 to 6 percent of posts held by women in the state legislatures and at the ministerial level; see Patai 1988:373.) A significant number of members of the assembly, however, mobilized by evangelical churches and the North American right-to-life movement and supported by the conservative wing of the Roman Catholic church hierarchy, lobbied and petitioned to introduce a fetal protection clause in the new constitution (Barroso 1990). Feminists, supported by the Committee on Reproductive Rights and the National Council for Women's Rights, responded with demonstrations and a popular petition for legalized abortion on demand. Ultimately, feminists and their supporters successfully blocked the adoption of a constitutional ban on abortion by arguing that issues should not be included in the constitution that had not been publicly debated. The new constitution included neither a liberalized abortion law nor a fetal protection clause. With the active support of BEMFAM, however, family planning was declared a constitutional right.

The abortion fight symbolized the collapse of what had once been a strategic alliance of the women's movement, the Catholic church, and the political left around grass-roots struggles for social justice and an end to political imprisonment and torture under the military regime. Feminist groups and the church were both opposed to policies of population control, while "conflictual issues such as abortion, sexuality or family planning continued to be discussed privately but were not brought into public debate" (Sarti 1989). Once the democratic opposition had gained power, however, the alliance between feminists and the church collapsed. Despite the sympathetic attitudes of many nuns and parish priests toward contraceptive use, the church hierarchy—including its progressive political wing—remained firmly and actively opposed to state provision of contraception and safe abortion. Feminists resented the church's interference in matters of women's sexuality and pregnancy prevention ("Summary Report . . . 1987").

The dialogue between feminists and the state and political parties has resulted in the *partial institutionalization of a feminist perspective* on women's health and rights at the federal level. In this and other respects, the Brazilian women's movement has served as an example for feminists engaged in similar campaigns in countries such as Colombia, Venezuela, Mexico, Nicaragua, and Peru (e.g., see Portugal and Claro 1988; Portugal 1989). Implementation of the women's health program has proved difficult, however, because of the deepening economic crisis and spending cuts, the decentralization of health planning to the state level, and a lack of political support in all but a few states. According to some observers, the energies of democratization and its support by feminists have been dissipated in bureaucratic inertia and general disillusion. The continued involvement of private family planning agencies, including BEMFAM and about 135 other organizations, combined with sustained opposition on the part of the Roman Catholic hierarchy to the provision of artificial methods of birth control in public health facilities, has reduced the pressure on the state to provide costly services. In addition, political leadership at the federal level has become more conservative and feminist influence is fading. In response, activists are concentrating on influencing policies and programs in key states and municipalities such as São Paulo.

Despite their inability to guarantee the implementation of women's reproductive health and rights policies, Brazilian feminists remain deeply committed to establishing the principle of "full and democratic citizenship" across the broad spectrum of Brazilian society that is free of gender bias in all of its forms. The achievement of reproductive and sexual rights—including freedom from violence against women—is seen as central to this goal. Three "principal directions" of future feminist influence have been identified (Barroso 1989): (1) a radical redefinition of the structure and quality of women's health services; (2) a continued struggle to institutionalize women's power and voice in policy-making; and (3) the decriminalization of abortion in recognition of women's capacity to decide consciously and responsibly about their bodies, their sexuality, and their lives.

NIGERIA: EVOLUTION OF A NATIONAL POPULATION POLICY AND THE REACTION OF WOMEN'S GROUPS

Nigerian women throughout history have engaged in a variety of actions such as mass protests and strikes to protect their interests—particularly their economic interests—against encroachments by the state and other ruling elites (Mba 1982). They are used to having their voices heard. Famous for their community leadership and their dynamic market women's associations, Nigerian women of all social sectors (especially in the south) are mobilized in multiple and overlapping networks around specific cultural, social, economic, philanthropic, occupational, religious, ethnic, and class interests (Mba 1982; Enabulele 1985; Kisekka 1989b). Autonomous women's groups represent a broad range of socioeconomic statuses and educational levels ranging from the non-literate (e.g., farm women's cooperatives, village-based mutual aid societies) to the educated and affluent (e.g., internationally affiliated urban groups such as the Nigerian Association of University Women, Soroptomists, Zonta). Although most groups are independent of men's influence, exceptions include clubs of wives of professional men, especially those in the armed forces, and the women's wings of political parties (Mba 1982:302).

The decade of transition from British to local rule culminating in national independence in 1960 witnessed a surge of political activity. With the introduction of party politics in 1950, women's groups organized women's wings of political parties and mobilized women to vote in elections, especially in the Yoruba- and Ibo-dominated regions. With few exceptions, however, women were not elected or appointed to major positions and remained marginalized from the formal political process (Okonjo 1983; Yusuf 1985). In addition, most forms of independent political activity have been forbidden under the military regimes that have governed during 20 of the first 30 years of the country's independence.

As in Brazil, the celebration of International Women's Year in 1975 stimulated research and activated new constituencies of Nigerian women in universities, professions, and businesses around issues of legal rights and women's roles in social and economic development (Ogunsheye et al. 1988). Some new groups forming in the 1980s included members who defined themselves as feminists, such as Women in Nigeria, a university-based "radical feminist" and leftist organization started in 1982, and the Women's Health Research Network of Nigeria begun in 1988 (Kisekka 1989a, 1989b, 1989c). In general, however, the feminist voice has been muted. Unlike the situation in Brazil, reproductive rights and health have not become rallying points for women's protest. Despite the ubiquity of women's organizations throughout all segments of society and their activism on a variety of local issues, there is no clearly identifiable, autonomous women's *movement* in Nigeria with a collective national strategy for change. Activities are decentralized and diffuse.

The largest organization of Nigerian women, the National Council of Women's Societies (NCWS), was launched in 1959 with the merging of two national societies in order to promote women's participation and welfare in social and community affairs. Its leadership draws significantly from wives of important bureaucrats, businessmen, and politicians. From its earliest days, NCWS proclaimed itself (and was regarded by the government) as the organization representing all Nigerian women (Mba 1982:187–192). During the years from 1966 to 1979, when the previous military regime banned all political party activity, only the NCWS continued to function as a national women's interest group (ibid.:302). Concerned with strengthening public morality and family life and generally respectful of male power and privilege, the leadership of the national council has until recently spoken with a conservative voice. Indeed, in 1982 the NCWS persuaded the federal government to re-designate the annual observance of March 8 from International *Women's* Day to *Family* Day, a symbolic "highjacking" that was protested by concerned feminists and ultimately reversed (Kisekka 1989a:9). NCWS has generally played a centrist role vis-à-vis the state in complementing and supporting government initiatives, urging the government to name women to various governing councils and bodies. Its opposition to some aspects of the new national population policy in 1989, as described below, thus doubtless came as a surprise.

Nigeria did not have an official policy on slowing population growth prior to the government's formal adoption of a National Policy on Population for Development, Unity, Progress and Self-Reliance in 1989 (United Nations 1988b). The Nigerian delegation at Bucharest in 1974, like its Brazilian counterpart, expressed confidence that the country could absorb its population increase—which may have reached 3 percent annually—without difficulty (Orubuloye 1983:175). By the mid 1980s, however, the Nigerian economy was worsening following the oil-induced boom years of the 1970s and per capita incomes and agricultural output were falling (Federal Republic of Nigeria, 1988:8). Facing a full-fledged economic crisis, the Military Government of Nigeria, which in 1983 had ousted the civilian government elected in 1979, was forced to impose economic austerity measures.

In 1985 the government introduced a draft population plan devised by the Federal Ministry of Health with the participation of other ministries and several international donor agencies (including USAID) and family planning organizations. For three years drafts were reviewed and revised by various professionals, religious leaders, politicians, and other groups as part of a national "consensus-building" process. (As noted in chapter 1, the promotion of antinatalist policies in a large, socially heterogeneous and pronatalist society is politically risky, especially for a regime of fragile legitimacy.) Containing remarkably explicit goals, objectives, and targets (Federal Republic of Nigeria 1988:12–14), the National Policy was officially launched by President Ibrahim Babangida in early 1989.

Claiming they had not been consulted in the "consensus-building" process, the major national women's organizations were quick to respond. "It is no longer acceptable for planners and policy makers to develop policies and plans targetting specific communities of interest without including those communities through representative community organizations," charged the President of NCWS (*New Nigerian,* 18 March 1989:1). Coming from this long-established organization representing several hundred women's associations throughout Nigeria, the charge of neglect of women's interests was serious. Representatives of both NCWS and the Federation of Muslim Women's Associations (which was established in the north in 1985 to challenge the hegemony of the Christian- and southern-dominated NCWS) as well as of other women's organizations reacted strongly—but by no means unanimously—to several provisions of the new policy.

The first concern was the policy's target of reducing fertility from about seven children per woman in the mid 1980s to four by the year 2000. Representatives of women's groups protested widely in the press that attaching the four-child limit only to women was discriminatory because, in the policy statement, men are merely "encouraged to have limited number of wives and optimum number of children they can foster within their resources" (Federal Republic of Nigeria 1988:19). Binding only women to family limitation, some women charged, "gives license to men to either marry another wife or beget children from outside of the marriage, since according to African tradition all such children claimed by a father are recognised as legitimate" (Kisekka 1989a:5). The four-child limit also sparked the emotionally charged atmosphere of demographic rivalries among religious, ethnic, and regional groups. NCWS representatives, for example, called the new policy unfair to Christian and non-polygynous families because Muslim men are permitted to take up to four wives, each of whom could have four children.

Second, the policy explicitly states that "In our society, men are considered the head of the family and they make far-reaching decisions including the family size, subsistence and social relations. . . . *The patriarchal family system in the country shall be recognised for stability of the home*" (Federal Republic of Nigeria 1988:19, emphasis added). Nigerian feminists were particularly upset by this statement. By implication, the policy formalizes men's rights to control women's sexuality and childbearing under the guise of maintaining the stability of the family. It implies that contraceptives may be provided only with the husband's consent (the current practice in some programs) and that unmarried women may not get the services they need. In the 1986–87 Demographic and Health Survey of Ondo State, for example, about three in four Ondo women said they approved of family planning but only two in five thought their husbands would approve.

Third, as noted earlier, the president of the NCWS protested that women's associations are expected to support and promulgate the policy at the state and local levels but they were not included in its formulation. This charge of female exclusion from policy-making is a familiar one. (However, at least one writer claims that NCWS as well as the Nigerian Planned Parenthood Federation, an IPPF affiliate, was included in an inter-ministerial consultative group of high-ranking officials; see Roberts 1990:137.) Other critics questioned whether the policy was going to be "a real blueprint for action or whether it will simply gather dust" because it does not include specific recommendations for implementation (Kisekka 1989a:6). Integrating family planning into government health care services at the state level which are inadequate and starved for funds could reach only a small segment of the population, primarily in urban centers.

Fourth, conservative representatives of Moslem women's groups, many of whom observe traditional Islamic behaviors such as purdah, opposed the recommendations for educating young people in the schools and the community on population and family life because they considered such education a parental responsibility within the context of religious and moral training. Some also opposed as inconsistent with Islamic family values the goals of eliminating arranged marriages of young girls, postponing average marriage age to at least 18 years for females and 25 years for males, and avoiding pregnancies before age 18.

Despite the criticisms, however, women who have spoken out on the population policy, including NCWS representatives and feminists, have supported certain of its provisions. These include providing universal voluntary access to family planning services, reducing maternal and child mortality, and creating intensive action programs aimed at improving the situation of women and girls according to the provisions of the Convention on the Elimination of All Forms of Discrimination Against Women, to which Nigeria is a signatory (Federal Republic of Nigeria 1988:20).

ACTIVISTS IN SEARCH OF A REPRODUCTIVE HEALTH AGENDA

In an analysis of indicators of women's status in 99 countries, Nigeria ranked sixth lowest in women's overall status and third lowest on gender equality (Population Crisis Committee 1988). The government's ratification of the women's convention is consistent with its expressed commitment to improving women's status within a program of national social development. (For an alternative view, see Dennis 1987.) Some prominent women have been appointed to state and federal offices and an institutional base for women's programs has been initiated through several state policies and programs in population, health, and social development.

The Primary Health Care Program in the Ministry of Health, for example, is intended to bring health and family planning services to local populations through 40,000 primary care centers, the first phase covering 52 local government areas in 19 states (World Bank 1987:10). User charges recently levied at all government hospitals under austerity measures, a drop in governmental expenditures in health care, and inflation make these goals elusive, however. A National Social Development Policy with a special section on women's welfare sets forth a broad range of goals including the elimination of customary practices that "dehumanize women" and of religious practices that "militate against their full development" (Kisekka 1989c:7). A Commission on Women and Development has been approved (but not yet implemented) to coordinate women's affairs at the national level; similar commissions may develop at the state level. And, in September 1987, the wife of the country's president launched a Better Life for Rural Women Program to promote and support women's participation in education, training, agriculture, rural industry, credit, marketing, and health and social services.

The stage has thus been set—in principle, at least—for specific input on reproductive health programs from women's organizations at the national, state, and local levels. Most women's groups are preoccupied with other issues, however. Moreoever, reflecting the complexities and factionalism of Nigerian society, they are differentiated if not divided in their world views by ethnic, religious, regional, and occupational interests, many of which bear on issues of population policy and reproductive health.

The concept of *reproductive health* symbolizes the social value placed on women's reproductive capacity and child survival in Nigeria. Yet, in the past, women's reproductive health problems—with the partial exception of prenatal care—have not been given priority in public health services. By default or design, most women have sought care primarily from indigenous healers, pharmacists, traditional birth attendants, and spiritualists, or else have suffered in silence.

According to estimates of the Nigerian Fertility Survey (part of the WFS), only *1 percent* of married women of reproductive age in Nigeria in 1981–82 were using modern methods of contraception. The 1986–87 DHS of Ondo State (predominantly Yoruba and Christian) found only 4 percent using modern methods, a figure typical of DHS findings in Liberia, Ghana, Mali, Senegal, Togo, Burundi, and Uganda, but lower than some other sub-Saharan countries such as Botswana and Zimbabwe. Yet, traditional means of child spacing, such as prolonged breastfeeding, postpartum abstinence, and residential separation of married couples, have been eroding. Despite recent mortality declines, maternal and infant death rates remain very high: Nigeria's infant mortality rate is twice that of Brazil, for example, and its estimated maternal mortality rate is ten times as high (World Health Organization 1986:9). Female sterility or subfecundity, often resulting from sexually transmitted diseases or from infection caused by unhygienic delivery or abortion, stigmatize women because female adult identity and social status depend heavily on bearing children to enrich and empower the male lineage (Women in Nigeria 1985; Ogunsheye et al. 1988).

Some Nigerian women's associations have worked on specific aspects of reproductive health such as distributing contraceptives within market women's associations, raising money for maternal and child health clinics, or educating women in local communities about nutrition, hygiene, environmental sanitation, and infant and child care. Primarily *welfare*-oriented rather than *rights*-oriented, these activities demand neither greater sexual and reproductive rights for women, as in the Brazilian case, nor expanded social entitlements. The marginalization of reproductive health issues in most women's associations may be due in part to what sociologist Mere Kisekka (1989b:16) calls an ethic of "nobility in suffering" which is inculcated early in young girls. The dictates of cultural or religious modesty—combined with a tendency to place women's own health care needs last—prevent women from speaking out about sexual and reproductive problems. Women's groups who have raised sensitive issues such as the need for contraceptive services for unmarried adolescents or for information to prevent the spread of sexually transmitted diseases may be criticized as "immoral" or "anti-family" and opposed by other women's organizations. The abortion issue is a good example.

As in most sub-Saharan countries, abortion in Nigeria is a criminal offense for both the woman and the abortionist except when required to preserve the woman's life (Okagbue 1990). Restrictive laws reflect a colonial legacy but are rarely enforced. Maternity wards in many hospitals are crowded with girls and women suffering from incomplete or septic abortions, and many are beyond saving (Ladipo 1989). Advocates of abortion law reform, such as the Society of Gynecologists and Obstetricians, the Nigerian Medical Association, some leaders and members of professional societies such as the Medical Women's Association, the Nurses and Midwives Association, and the Federation of Women Lawyers, as well as feminists, recognize that safe services could significantly reduce prevailing high rates of maternal morbidity and mortality both among married women and among growing numbers of adolescents in urban and rural areas who are experiencing unwanted pregnancies (Nichols et al. 1986). In 1981, however, the NCWS lobbied to *block* a liberal abortion bill from being presented to the House of Representatives on the grounds that parents and the government should promote moral and religious education to prevent pregnancies among unmarried women, and that the government should improve family planning education and services for married women. No further steps have been taken to liberalize the law despite a widespread perception that clandestine abortion is increasing. Some researchers and policymakers have urged the government to grant the Specialist Hospitals the right to terminate unwanted pregnancies if and when such request is made by the individual (e.g., Orubuloye 1983:177). The dominance of USAID funding of family planning services in Nigeria (UNFPA 1989b) could block most women's access to safe services if laws were liberalized, however, given USAID's funding restrictions based on the Mexico City policy discussed in chapter 3.

In an attempt to overcome the social stigma and inherent divisiveness of some reproductive health problems and to identify a unifying programmatic theme, a group of social scientists together with some health and legal professionals and community leaders formed a new organization in 1988 called the Women's Health Research Network of Nigeria. Their purpose is to engage in research and advocacy and to mobilize women's associations, service providers (including nurses and physicians), and policymakers around women's health issues (Kisekka 1989c).

Two themes are emerging from the network's deliberations that may transcend the diversity of views among women's associations. The first is the *prevention of infertility,* which afflicts significant numbers of women (and men) in Nigeria as well as in other areas of sub-Saharan Africa (Sherris and Fox 1983:116). Infertility is a tragedy for women who experience it and a source of fear among those who have not yet borne the desired number of children. From a tactical viewpoint, it is also a rubric under which to discuss publicly such difficult issues as sexually transmitted diseases, septic abortion, the sexual exploitation of girls and women, married women's vulnerability to divorce or replacement by another wife, and harmful reproductive practices. The National Association of Nurses and Midwives, for example, has campaigned against customs such as early arranged marriage and sexual intercourse with young girls, female "circumcision" and infibulation, and the *gishiri* cut in which traditional midwives cut the birth passage in order to ease a difficult delivery or "cure" other health problems such as delayed onset of menarche.

The second theme is to ensure women an *informed choice among safe, acceptable, and affordable contraceptive methods* as a component of basic health care that emphasizes child spacing, safe delivery, and child survival. Consistent with the government's health and population policies, this emphasis requires collaboration among women's associations and health and family planning providers in the public and private sectors to improve both the availability and quality of care.

The question remains, however, as to whether a relatively small group of researchers and activists can pull together the threads of a variegated, fragmented, and sometimes competitive collection of women's organizations, persuade them to agree on a course of action despite their other preoccupations, and work simultaneously to influence service providers and policymakers at the national, state, and local levels. The planned health and family planning infrastructure could serve as a base of operations and influence for women's participation at all levels, and the policy environment for decentralized programming is favorable. In the midst of economic crisis and politically volatile structural adjustment policies, however, the implementation of this ambitious infrastructure may prove as elusive as the articulation of a set of reproductive health priorities— aside from maternal and child survival—on which diverse constituencies can agree.

THE PHILIPPINES: IDEOLOGICAL CONFRONTATIONS OVER THE RIGHT TO FAMILY PLANNING

The Philippines was among the first of the developing countries to embrace family planning for demographic as well as health and welfare reasons. A national policy of population and family planning was officially launched in 1971 under the direction of the Commission on Population (POPCOM), the chief policy-making, coordinating and monitoring body of the government's population program, with strong U.S. support. Targeting specific declines in crude birth and death rates and population growth, the Philippines Population Policy was intended to "make available all acceptable methods of contraception, except abortion," which was illegal, and to expand population education, training, research and family planning services (Peralta and Ligan 1975:62; UNFPA 1989b:467–478). POPCOM was subsumed under the Ministry of Social Services, whose female minister strongly promoted the family planning program. With substantial support from international donor agencies and the government of the Philippines under the Marcos regime, POPCOM had more than twice the budget of its parent agency.

When 20 years of martial law ended with the "four-day revolution" of February 1986, supporters of democracy hoped for the elimination of severe economic inequalities and social injustices that had permeated everyday life in the Philippines for centuries. More than three hundred years of Spanish rule had ended in 1898, when the Philippines was ceded to the United States following the defeat of a nationalist movement and Spain's defeat in the Spanish-American War. Feudalistic patterns of land-holding introduced by the Spanish along with a family code vesting all authority and property rights in the husband had created a class- and gender-stratified society that was modified only slightly under the secular influence of the U.S. occupation, which ended formally with Philippine independence in 1946. Early bourgeois women's organizations had struggled for female suffrage (won finally in 1937) and legal equality, but had not directly confronted the ideologies of patriarchy that subordinated girls and women in the family and in public life (Jayawardena 1986:158–166). Women from all classes of society came together in October 1983, however, to demonstrate against Ninoy Aquino's assassination and to oppose the martial law regime. Along with other groups and institutions who had formed a broad multi-party and multi-faceted political protest movement—including, importantly, the Roman Catholic church—women who supported democratization celebrated Corazon Aquino's election to the presidency.

In the tumultuous months between Aquino's election and the installation of a new legislature, women's rights advocates became embroiled in two major struggles relating to reproductive rights. The first was a battle over the new constitution. Reflecting on their recent history, some participants believed that the women's movement in the Philippines became a specifically *feminist* movement when activists were confronted by the draft national constitution prepared by a 48-member constitutional committee that included only two women. During the Fall of 1986 a number of women's organizations, spearheaded by GABRIELA, a national coalition of over 100 women's groups and almost 40,000 individual members, prepared a statement on the draft constitution to be submitted to the constitutional committee. Concerned with a wide variety of restrictions on their status and rights in the family, employment, and political life in addition to the economic and sexual exploitation of Filipinas in low-paid export production, prostitution, and the bar trades, women's groups wanted constitutional protections that would move beyond the simple declaration in Section 14 of the draft constitution which specified "the fundamental equality before the law of women and men."

Although at least one women's group focused on reproductive health as an issue and distributed statements on this topic to each constitutional commissioner, most representatives of the movement believed that matters of contraception, abortion, and divorce should first be discussed internally and then debated publicly before they took a position on state policy (Marcelo 1989:3). The women's movement was thus unprepared for the intense campaign to insert an article into the constitution that would protect the life of the unborn. The campaign was orchestrated by the Roman Catholic church hierarchy in conjunction with the conservative society of lay Catholics, Opus Dei, fundamentalist Christians, and organizations such as Pro-Life Philippines. In response, women's groups, family planning organizations, and legal experts who favored a more liberal abortion policy held a public seminar in December 1986 and undertook other activities to build public opposition while the draft constitution was under public review. Unable to block the fetal protection clause entirely, its opponents ultimately succeeded in inserting a guarantee of equal protection of the mother (Marcelo 1989:3). Article II, Section 12 of the 1987 Philippine constitution now reads, "The State recognizes *the sanctity of family life* and shall protect and strengthen the family as a basic autonomous social institution. It shall equally protect the life of the mother and the life of the unborn from conception" (emphasis added). The constitutional commission also defeated a provision specifying the state's responsibility to maintain population levels most conducive to national welfare, as well as an amendment introduced by POPCOM declaring that the state shall provide parents full information on all legally and medically approved means of birth limitation to enable them to arrive at an informed decision according to their conscience and religious convictions.

The second major struggle occurred over a draft executive order prepared for Aquino's signature under the auspices of the Roman Catholic church that would have abolished the Population Commission, restricted the scope of family planning service agencies, banned most contraceptive methods except natural family planning, and blamed contraception for "fomenting sexually promiscuous attitudes and behaviors" with "perverse consequences" such as "marital infidelity, prostitution and proliferation of sexually transmitted diseases" (quoted in Tadiar 1989:90). The order would also have repealed all laws or practices supporting incentives for limiting family size, setting population or family size goals or targets, and promoting or dispensing "abortifacient contraceptives" such as the pill and IUD. Intense mobilization in February 1987 of women activists and population and health professionals publicized the threat to family planning through media coverage, telegrams, and a petition to the president (Marcelo 1989:4), and the executive order was never signed. The attacks on family planning were to continue, however, and concerned women's groups mobilized around the protection of their rights.

THE ONGOING STRUGGLE

The Aquino government was caught between opposing forces on many complex issues of which the population issue was only one. It wanted to dissociate itself from the alleged excesses of population control in the Marcos regime and from the implication that rapid population growth was the root cause of poverty. However, several key senior officials along with members of the scientific, medical, and internationally-funded family planning communities contended that population growth was a critical problem and that family planning must remain a basic right. The National Academy of Science in the Philippines urged that the program be strengthened, not abolished, in order to "improve the general health of the people, decrease child and maternal death rates, and enhance the status of women by opening social and economic opportunities for them" (*Manila Bulletin*, 24 March 1987).

Aquino was lobbied by all sides. Some nationalistic and leftist leaders were insisting that the country could accommodate a population twice its current size. Adopting leftist rhetoric, the church and the right-to-life movement condemned "coercive and even deceptive" population control methods and fiercely criticized "foreign meddling" from UNFPA, USAID, and the World Bank (*Far Eastern Economic Review*, 20 Oct. 1988:25). Incredibly, the new chairwoman of POPCOM was opposed to artificial methods of family planning (*Manila Chronicle*, 21 Feb. 1989:1). She was also opposed to continuing the population program, insisting publicly that it had been a failure. Supporters of the national population program countered that it was erroneous to blame it for the failure to alleviate mass poverty. Instead, POPCOM should be moved to a more supportive institutional environment (*Manila Bulletin*, 24 March 1987).

In the midst of the confusion, POPCOM nevertheless prepared a new five-year National Population Plan in accordance with its mandate and after considerable consultation with interested parties. Approved in principle in April 1987, the plan includes a Family Planning and Responsible Parenthood Program for "married couples of reproductive age" with new demographic goals and targets, and an Integrated Population and Development Program. The program has not been fully implemented, however. According to newspaper reports, "An almost three-year struggle for control within the Government over the country's population program has culminated in a near-paralysis of a nationwide network of family planning clinics" (*Manila Chronicle,* 21 Feb. 1989:1; see also 27 July:1).

Feminists and women's health advocates have organized somewhat uncomfortably around the protection of the national population program, which is widely viewed as a mechanism for ensuring access to contraceptive services. In 1987, for example, a group called WomanHealth Philippines was formed to bring together women activists and health and family planning professionals from urban and rural areas to promote women's reproductive rights and health (Marcelo 1989:4). In addition, GABRIELA set up a Commission on Health and Reproductive Rights to maintain a critical perspective on contraceptive safety and the protection of low-income women from coercive practices and lack of informed consent.

The WomanHealth coalition made a significant attempt to shape the national policy in late 1987 when Senator Leticia Shahani, with three colleagues, introduced Resolution 39 to the Philippine Senate urging the strengthening of the national population program through the implementation of POPCOM's Policy Statement of April 1987 (Shahani 1987). Shahani, chairwoman of the Senate Committee on Population, had been an influential member of the Commission on the Status of Women at the United Nations. In consultation with several other organizations, WomanHealth (1988) proposed extensive amendments to Resolution 39 that would stress the importance of serving women's individual needs and of "humanizing" as well as strengthening the national program. Speaking in support of the revised population resolution, feminists declared that "The Resolution itself calls for popular consultation. . . . We have more points to raise about the population issue and are willing to assist the Senate Subcommittee on Population . . . in order to arrive at a national consensus. We are committed to the protection of women's health and rights" (WomanHealth 1987:2–3). The Senate eventually approved a much-diluted version of the resolution in a compromise with the Catholic church (*Far Eastern Economic Review,* 20 Oct. 1988:24).

Legislative attacks on the family planning program intensified, however, with the introduction early in 1989 of resolutions that called, first, for research on the efficacy of the Billings Ovulation Method (natural family planning) as a "universally applicable and acceptable" means of achieving or avoiding pregnancy, and, second, for an investigation into the "social costs" of using foreign funds for the national population program (Tadiar 1989). Bills were also introduced to increase the penalities for persons who performed abortions or obtained them. (The number of clandestine abortions performed annually has been estimated at between 150,000 to 750,000, in Tadiar 1989:92.) Feminists found some of their earlier critiques of the population program used against them as conservative activists opposed to artificial contraception and population control mirrored feminists' language on the dangers and abuses of particular birth control methods and of the population program as a whole (Marcelo 1989:6).

The creation of the Philippine Development Plan for Women represents a second effort by the women's movement to expand and protect the right to family planning and to shape the national population policy. Drawn up by the National Commission on Women with input from women's organizations and ministries as a companion piece to the country's Medium-Term Philippine Development Plan for the years 1989 to 1992, the plan specifies a number of sectoral targets aimed at promoting gender equality. It also reiterates the fertility and population targets of the POPCOM policy but adds measures to encourage breastfeeding, reduce sexually transmitted diseases, incorporate more comprehensive women's health services into family planning clinics, and—as in Brazil's integrated women's health policy—to train health and family planning workers to be more sensitive to issues of gender and power (*MARHIA*, Jan.–Mar. 1989:11). President Aquino moved for approval and adoption of the plan on International Women's Day, March 8, 1989.

According to its spokeswomen, the long-term goals of the women's health movement in the Philippines are to (1) monitor and defeat national legislation that threatens reproductive rights; (2) empower low-income women to demand appropriate, affordable, and accessible health services; (3) build alliances with key government personnel, researchers, non-governmental organizations, service providers, and legislators to promote high quality care; and (4) sustain reproductive health as a public policy issue despite the disarray of the government's population program (*MARHIA*, Oct.–Dec. 1988:1). The political conflict is intense, however. Continued attacks by conservative forces pose stiff challenges to the feminist health agenda. In addition, the uneasy political alliance with the family planning "establishment" as a reaction to threats by religious fundamentalists has been divisive for feminists. Some groups oppose any form of collaboration with the population control forces characteristic of the old regime or with organizations funded by the U.S. government or foundations, which they consider imperialist, while others consider such alliances essential for ensuring that all women have access to a full range of family planning information and services. The Sixth International Meeting on Women and Health, which was held in the Philippines in November 1990 and organized by Filipino women's health advocates together with the Women's Global Network on Reproductive Rights, raised many of these same issues from the perspective of women in other southern countries.

The impact of women's political action on population policies and family planning programs depends in part on the openness of the decision-making process to democratic participation, and in part on the extent to which relevant state and private agencies define "women" as an important constituency. It also depends on the ability of women's groups to act collectively to exert pressure on key agencies responsible for policy-making and program implementation. Effective pressure tactics depend, in turn, on (1) the existence and *activism* of women's organizations in each country; (2) the *political autonomy* of such organizations (e.g., as distinct from parastatal women's organizations or the "women's wings" of political parties, religious groups, or protest movements); (3) the emergence of a *shared ideology,* in the form of a women's movement, with a set of common goals and objectives and a coordinated strategy to achieve them; and (4) the *centrality of reproductive rights* and health to their political agenda.

The case studies reviewed here represent different configurations of political activism on the part of women's organizations. In Brazil, an active and explicitly feminist women's movement, capitalizing on its political support for the Democratic Coalition that defeated the military regime, has moved *creatively* and *proactively* to influence governmental policies on integrated women's health and family planning. Women's sexual and reproductive rights are central to their agenda. Successful in shaping a national women's reproductive health policy, the women's movement has been unable to see its programs implemented, for political and structural reasons, and family planning services remain almost entirely confined to the private sector. Nigerian women, organized into multiple associations with diverse orientations and in the absence of a coherent women's movement, have played a predominantly *reactive* role in their organizational response to the new national population policy, with little effect. Ambitious government plans for extending family planning and health services throughout the country will face difficulties in implementation in any case, and there are few alternatives in the private sector. Activists are trying to identify a core set of reproductive health issues that will unite Nigerian women's organizations around a policy agenda. In the Philippines, the nascent women's movement arising out of the return to democracy has been *creatively reactive* in its efforts to protect women's access to family planning services (and, indirectly, the national population program) from attacks by conservative forces, with some effect. In alliance with civil rights lawyers and members of the population establishment, women's health advocates have succeeded so far in blocking legislative and constitutional restrictions to the delivery of family planning through public and private sources, but these achievements may be tenuous in the face of continued assault.

Policy decisions relating to fertility and the delivery of family planning and health services have the potential to affect the lives of women of all social classes in fundamental, although differentiated, ways. Whether policies have a positive or negative impact may well depend on the integration into the decision-making process of the values and priorities of women from diverse backgrounds *as women themselves define them.* Whether or not women are recognized—and recognize themselves—as a primary constituency in population and family planning is therefore a key public policy issue. It is also related in fundamental ways to the realities of women's rights and women's lives.

Part Three

WOMEN'S RIGHTS, WOMEN'S LIVES

5

WOMEN'S RIGHTS AND REPRODUCTIVE CHOICE: RETHINKING THE CONNECTIONS

"How is one to understand a woman's attitudes—any woman's—on such a personal issue as the planning of births in her family without first delving into the reality of her life?" asks Perdita Huston in her book, *Message from the Village* (1978:1). "What is the situation in which she lives? What is the range of her freedom to make decisions? What are the burdens she bears, in numbers of children already born to her or in the tasks she must perform?"

These questions offer a simple introduction to part three of this book, "Women's Rights, Women's Lives." Reproductive policies and programs must be tailored to the diverse realities of women's experience if they are to engage women's trust. The three chapters in this section take somewhat different perspectives on this topic. The first considers the question of how women's abilities to exercise their reproductive rights is linked with the exercise of rights in other spheres. How does a woman's education, employment, and position within the family affect her sexual and marital choices, for example, and her ability to determine the number and spacing of her children? How severely are her reproductive choices constrained? In turn, how does the ability to delay or avoid marriage or childbearing influence the exercise of women's social, economic, and political rights? In what ways does the exercise of one set of rights act as leverage for the exercise of others?

The theme of interconnections continues in chapter 6, which looks at the linkages between reproductive rights and the right to health. Although the physical health benefits of contraceptive use and controlled fertility have been investigated, less is known about their effects on women's emotional health. Under what conditions could using a contraceptive or having fewer (or no) children engender psychosocial stress, for example? How does fertility regulation affect women's perceptions of their ability to perform those social roles upon which their survival and security depend? Identifying negative as well as positive effects of contraceptive use and controlled fertility—that is, learning about women's fears and anxieties—can provide important insights into how policies and programs could be designed to meet women's needs more effectively.

Chapter 7 addresses the relationship between abortion and women's rights to family planning and to health. Reviewing the social, legal, and medical context in which abortion occurs in developing countries, it concludes that the ability to terminate an unwanted pregnancy safely is a core element of both sets of rights. A woman cannot decide either freely *or* responsibly on the number and spacing of her children if she is forced to continue an unintended pregnancy against her will, nor can she exercise her right to health if the termination of a pregnancy is life-threatening or damaging in other ways.

If we accept the premise that a woman's ability to exercise her human rights is enmeshed with other aspects of her life, then how can the linkages between reproductive rights and other social and economic rights be most usefully investigated? What are some of the conceptual and methodological issues involved in such research? Where is the locus of control over women's sexual, reproductive, and productive capacities? Who makes the decisions, and how are women's opportunities structured?

POSING THE QUESTION: CONCEPTUAL AND METHODOLOGICAL ISSUES

The literature on the status of women and fertility is rich and extensive (e.g., Piepmeier and Adkins 1973; Germain 1975; United Nations 1975; Kupinsky 1977; Ware 1981; Anker, Buvinic and Youssef 1982; Oppong 1983; Cain 1984; Ward 1984; Mason 1987). It is also ambiguous and confusing. What do we mean by the term, "status of women," for example? Sociologist Karen Mason (1986) has documented what she calls a "bewildering variety" of treatments found in demographic studies. Among the many sources of conceptual confusion are (1) the multidimensionality of status indicators (women may have high status in some respects and low status in others); (2) the confounding of gender and class/caste hierarchies as determinants of status; (3) the changeability of status over the stages of the life course and in different locations in which the sexes interact (e.g., the household, the neighborhood, the workplace); (4) confusion between measures of absolute and relative status and of individual and family status; (5) the use of different units of analysis (e.g., the individual, the household, the nation); and (6) the difference in social meanings attached to particular characteristics, or "statuses," by researchers and by women themselves.

Some of the conceptual difficulties may be circumvented by posing the research question as one involving connections among bundles of *rights,* that is, among *specific, observable behaviors* involved in exercising these rights, rather than between the more abstract idea of the "status of women" and fertility. This approach avoids the problem of multidimensionality as well as of labeling certain behaviors as low or high status that may be considered quite the opposite by the people involved. The practice of female seclusion symbolizes high status in traditional Muslim societies, for example, and a woman who observes purdah brings honor on herself and the entire kin group (Papanek and Minault 1982). To say that she has low status because she is kept secluded is confusing. But it is not so confusing to say that she does not or cannot exercise her right to freedom of movement and association. In her dependence on maintaining the support of others for her own survival or security, she lacks the ability to act *autonomously,* that is, to make decisions on her own behalf and act on them even in the face of opposition. The concept of autonomy—which may reflect high or low status in other aspects of a woman's life—is useful for understanding the conditions under which girls and women are able to exercise their rights. What empowers a woman to act autonomously in a particular context? What resources does she require in order to circumvent the control of men or elders?

The attribution of causality poses a second dilemma. Consider the relationship between, say, the number of years of a woman's schooling (A) and her age at marriage (B). Does A "cause" B or does B "cause" A, or do they influence one another? Or, are both A *and* B "caused" by antecedent conditions such as a young woman's socialization into appropriate gender and class/caste roles that jointly circumscribe both outcomes, or the maintenance of control over both decisions by men or elders?

In trying to understand how clusters of rights are causally linked, then, we need to ask three questions.

First, *who* makes decisions about women's sexuality, childbearing, schooling, labor allocation, and so on? How much control rests with the girl or woman herself and how much with male or female relatives within the household or with elders or others (e.g., a sexual partner) outside the household? One could distinguish here among the strong patriarchal regimes characteristic of much of sub-Saharan Africa, North Africa and the Middle East, and Southern and Eastern Asia in which hierarchies of age and gender both operate; weak patriarchal regimes characteristic of Latin

America and the Caribbean marked by male dominance; and more egalitarian regimes typical of parts of Southeast Asia. Of course, strong class/
caste and regional contrasts prevail.

Second, *how* are women's sexual, reproductive, and productive behaviors controlled in specific settings? Which aspects are regulated most
tightly and which are left to chance? Patriarchal strategies may follow a
policy of *containment* or *deployment* of different dimensions of women's
sexual, reproductive, productive, and political capacities, depending on
the benefits accruing to powerful kin. A woman may be prevented from
working for pay outside the home by her husband or elders for reasons
of family honor, for example, or she may be expected or required to do
so for economic reasons.

Third, *what* is the structure of opportunities available for a particular
individual or group? Opportunity structures are created by the interaction
of individual and family strategies with the distribution of resources in
the community. If secondary or post-secondary schooling is available for
only a small minority, for example, then it is not a viable option for any
but elite families. It is not part of a woman's "opportunity structure,"
which is conditioned by the *supply* of opportunities, or options, in the
family and the community, and by the effective or latent *demand* for them
that she or her powerful kin engenders. Opportunity structures include
all of the rights discussed here: access to contraceptive information and
services, schooling, employment and incomes, property and social security, political mobilization, and equality in marriage and family life. A
function of state, community, class/caste, and family structures and ideologies, opportunity structures can be altered by public policy interventions.

Because gender relations are embedded in social, economic, and political institutions and reinforced by everyday social interactions, it follows
that reproductive behavior is more heavily influenced by systems of gender relations than by the position of individual women. Unfortunately,
the dominant mode of fertility research has been to gather information
on individual women in surveys such as the multi-country World Fertility
Survey (WFS) and the Demographic Health Survey (DHS). While providing a good source of comparative data that can be generalized to larger
populations, the survey format and the particular questions that are asked
limit the scope of analysis and interpretation (Smith 1989). Data collected
to test economic models of individual or household decision making, for
example, cannot capture the richness of theories linking social institutions
and reproductive behavior such as John Caldwell's work on kin- and wage-
based modes of production and inter-generational wealth flows (1982),
Mead Cain's work on patriarchy and environments of risk and uncertainty
(1981, 1984), and Ron Lesthaeghe's work on institutional controls over
human reproduction (1980). They cannot help us to answer the questions

we have just posed, nor do they reveal much about the reality of women's lives.

The problems of trying to fit the data to the theories will be apparent in the following review. Drawing primarily on evidence from censuses and surveys in a number of developing countries plus some speculation, the remainder of this chapter documents what is known about the linkages between specific aspects of reproductive rights and rights in schooling, employment and earnings, marriage and the family, property and security, and public life. We begin with reproductive rights. What are they, and how can they be measured?

SEXUAL AND REPRODUCTIVE RIGHTS AS A CORE CONCEPT

Reproductive rights as defined in international instruments include two components: the *freedom* to decide how many children to have and when to have them, and the *entitlement* to family planning information and services. A third component, which is not yet spelled out in international documents, is the "right to control one's own body." As noted in chapter 1, this right includes freedom from sexual assault, physical violence, unwanted or exploitative sexual relations (incest, child abuse, prostitution, coerced sex, etc.), and unwanted medical interventions or bodily mutilations. Violence against girls and women, which represents a fundamental violation of bodily integrity, is perhaps the most pervasive yet least recognized form of human rights abuse in the world (Heise 1992). The right to control one's body also includes more positive elements such as the freedom to choose one's sexual partner, to have knowledge of and enjoy one's sexuality, to initiate or refuse sexual relations, and to determine mutually with one's partner the frequency and form of sensual expression. For reasons of simplicity, however, the discussion in this chapter will be confined to the more formally defined "right to family planning."

The idea of a *right to decide* freely on the number and timing of children poses a conceptual challenge. Because surveys inquiring about a person's reproductive wishes or intentions tap into individual preferences that have been shaped by group norms, economic constraints, and the influence of partners or elders, it is almost impossible to know whether a woman is making a "free" decision. DHS data from the late 1980s can tell us that women in southern countries aged 20–24 consider an ideal family size to be approximately half to one child smaller on average than do women 20 years older, for example, and that the ideal family size of younger women ranges from fewer than 2.5 children in Bolivia and Thailand to six or more children in Mali and Senegal. But when almost all women say they want two or three children, or when almost all say they want six or eight or "as many as God sends," what economic and social pressures are governing the range of responses? How do we interpret the finding that 85 percent or more of women in Brazil and Thailand who already have three living children (or are pregnant with their third) say they want to stop childbearing at that point, compared with fewer than 15 percent in Ghana, Liberia, Senegal, and Togo? How heavily does a woman's well-being depend on achieving particular stopping/continuing outcomes as compared with others? One indicator of the "freedom to decide" would be to look for substantial variation in reproductive preferences *within* a given social class or other analytically relevant group. In statistical terms, a high ratio of within-group to between-group variance could be taken as evidence that personal preferences outweigh the strength of group norms and constraints.

A second measure of the freedom to decide is to take a woman's socially constructed fertility preferences at face value and compare them with her actual reproductive behavior. Deficit fertility, surplus fertility, and self reports of unwanted or mistimed pregnancies are all evidence of "unfreedom" in some respects. Deficit fertility may be due to fecundity impairments (a critical social and health concern for women throughout much of sub-Saharan Africa, in particular), infant mortality, absence of a responsible sexual partner, or deliberate fertility control due to economic hardship, crowded living conditions, or problems of child care, among other reasons. Fertility surveys also reveal whether a woman has more children than she says she wants or is pregnant sooner than she wants to be because of contraceptive failure or nonuse. In 21 DHS countries, 41 percent of women in marital or consensual unions who had a child in the past year or were currently pregnant said that the pregnancy was mistimed or unwanted, for example, ranging from 14 percent in Mali to 67 percent in Bolivia (DHS reports, passim.). These figures are underestimates because mistimed and unwanted pregnancies already terminated by spontaneous or induced abortion are not included.

The freedom to decide on childbearing can be roughly approximated by two measures: (1) the amount of individual variation in fertility preferences within social groups; and (2) childbearing outcomes that are consistent with these preferences. How can the *entitlement to information and the means* of fertility regulation be measured? The proportions of women who claim in surveys to know of at least one "modern" contraceptive method and where to obtain it has grown remarkably in most parts of the world since the 1960s. Except in sub-Saharan Africa and a scattering of countries elsewhere, from 80 to 90 percent or more of married women typically say they know of at least one modern method. Knowledge is even higher when traditional methods are included such as prolonged or periodic abstinence, withdrawal, or post-coital douching. (Women are almost never asked if they know how to induce a menstrual period or where to obtain an abortion, however, even though these are among the most common methods of fertility regulation.) The proportions of women who know about at least one modern contraceptive method exceed the proportions who have *ever used* such a method, which in turn exceed the proportions who are *current users*. The interpretation of data on current use (Appendix B) is complicated by the fact that many women who are not currently using a method are infecund, pregnant, breastfeeding, or hoping to have a child.

The "unmet need" for contraception is generally calculated as the percentage of all women in marital or consensual unions who say they want to delay or stop childbearing, are exposed to the risk of pregnancy, and yet are not using any contraceptive method (Westoff 1988). All contraceptive users are assumed to have their needs "met" despite the high failure rates and/or health risks or client dissatisfaction with some methods. According to this narrow definition about 25 percent of married or cohabiting women in sub-Saharan African countries with DHS data have an unmet need for contraception (primarily for spacing), about 18 percent in Latin America and the Caribbean (primarily for limiting), and about 13 percent in Asia, the Middle East, and North Africa (slightly more for spacing than limiting) (Bongaarts 1991). Inadequate health and family planning programs, many of them suffering from the effects of funding cuts due to structural adjustment programs, leave many women without the knowledge and means to regulate their fertility safely and effectively. Some women are unable to take advantage of services that do exist because services are inaccessible, inconvenient, or costly; because women fear that contraception will damage their health (the most commonly mentioned reason for nonuse); because women have no information about methods (the second most common reason); or because male partners or religious leaders are opposed, among other reasons. As expected, rural women and those with the least education generally have the highest levels of unmet need (Westoff 1988). In addition, although it is rarely measured, unmet need can be high among unmarried women who, for social reasons, are often unable to obtain birth control services. To the extent that single, separated, widowed, and divorced women in different settings are exposed to the risk of pregnancy, do not want to become pregnant, and yet are not using birth control, they too have a critical unmet need for family planning.

HOW THE "RIGHT TO FAMILY PLANNING" AFFECTS OTHER RIGHTS

The use of safe and effective methods of fertility regulation, especially those that can be used by a woman without the knowledge of her sexual partner, breaks the link between sexuality and reproduction in powerful ways. The knowledge of how to delay a first birth, space additional births, stop childbearing, or avoid pregnancy altogether gives women the means to shape their lives in ways undreamed of by those who have never questioned the inevitability of frequent childbearing or who have resorted in desperation to cumbersome, ineffective, and often dangerous methods to stop unwanted births. Knowledge of pregnancy prevention can weaken patriarchal controls over female sexuality and reproduction by enabling women to circumvent them. Indeed, this potential underlies the oft-cited fears of men in many societies that contraception will encourage women to be sexually "promiscuous" or too independent in other ways, thus threatening the very foundations of social control. Alternatively, as feminists have pointed out, contraception, sterilization, and even abortion can be used to reinforce patriarchal controls over women's reproductive capacity on the part of the state, the community, the family, or the male partner if they are imposed against the woman's will.

The potential of effective birth control for personal liberation—or, more modestly, for facilitating the exercise of other rights—depends on the environment of risk and uncertainty in which a woman lives. Some of the ways in which contraceptive use and controlled fertility impinge on women's lives are discussed in the following chapter. From what wellsprings does a woman's survival, security, or mobility flow? How does she perceive the costs and benefits of different sexual, marital, and reproductive outcomes? Are the opportunity structures in place to provide alternatives to early marriage and motherhood, for example, or to broaden her options if she has three children instead of six? Will contraceptive use and controlled fertility improve her physical health and alleviate some of the physical and emotional stress of competing role obligations? Are various options even permitted to her, or are other facets of her life—and perhaps the use of birth control itself—determined by persons or forces beyond her control? As Huston remarked in the passage that opens this chapter, the practice of birth control becomes meaningful only when considered in the context of women's lives. Because sexuality, contraception, and childbearing have such personal and social significance in all societies, it is inevitable that they will be regulated by institutional arrangements linking them with other social relations.

At the individual level, fertility regulation has the capacity to facilitate the exercise of a woman's other rights in at least six ways. The extent to which this abstract capacity is actualized in a specific context depends in large part on whether the woman has some control over the decisions that affect her and on whether the structure of opportunities in the family and community offers some choice.

First, where premarital sexual relations are common, the ability to avoid pregnancy could delay marriage and place a woman in a better position to choose a spouse or choose not to marry at all, that is, to marry only with free and full consent. Some evidence on premarital sexual behavior is summarized in a U.N. review of adolescent fertility in developing countries (United Nations 1989a) as well as in more recent individual studies. As for premarital childbearing, at least one-tenth of recently married women had experienced a first birth before their first marital or consensual union in nearly one-third of all countries surveyed by the WFS (United Nations 1989:34). The impact of effective birth control would be greatest where a high proportion of early first marriages is triggered by an unplanned pregnancy or where out-of-wedlock births are met with social criticism or economic hardship. If a premarital pregnancy is intended to ensure marriage, however, as in societies where a woman's fecundity must be proven before she is acceptable as a bride, then there would be little advantage in preventing pregnancy with an appropriate partner at this stage.

Second, effective birth planning following marriage can make it easier for couples to exercise their right to marry without incurring the costs of having a child right away. Under these conditions, the average duration between marriage and first birth tends to lengthen. Contraceptive practice could also improve a woman's chances of marrying eventually in societies where out-of-wedlock births are common, as in the Caribbean, yet where a woman without children is in a better bargaining position for marriage than is a woman who has had children by another man (Blake 1961).

Third, fertility limitation within a marriage or consensual union could improve a woman's ability to terminate an unsatisfactory relationship with less personal cost if she has the social, economic, and legal option. Although not spelled out in international documents, the right to separation or divorce is a logical extension of the right to marry only with free and full consent. Insofar as having a large family intensifies women's economic dependence, it limits her capacity to exercise equal rights with men during marriage and at its dissolution. Of course, having many children can be a valuable security strategy for women without alternative sources of support. And in societies where the husband has unilateral power to divorce his wife and take another, or where a man simply abandons a woman to whom he is not married, the fear of repudiation can motivate a woman to have many children to try to bind her partner to her. Under these conditions of risk and uncertainty, a woman with no children or with only one or two may expose herself to a higher risk of unwanted dissolution than a woman with many children. Mead Cain's research in rural areas of India and Bangladesh identifies a sequence of tragic outcomes for couples experiencing "reproductive failure" (Cain 1986). Itself a partial consequence of poverty which produces smaller family sizes and higher infant and child mortality, the absence of a surviving son increases the vulnerability of both parents to economic crisis and premature mortality. Women are particularly vulnerable because of their economic dependence: for them, reproductive failure raises the risk of divorce and widowhood as well as destitution and early death.

Fourth, fertility control should support the right to education. The most important factor here is the delay of a first birth, whether by postponing marriage, postponing the first birth within marriage, or avoiding a non-marital pregnancy or birth. The effects on school enrollment of postponing a first birth should be strongest where two conditions are met: (1) there is a high probability that a girl will continue her education beyond the typical age of first intercourse (whether marital or otherwise)—that is, the opportunity structure for schooling is otherwise favorable—and (2) marriage or the birth of a child would effectively preclude her chances of staying in school. For girls who have never been to school or attend only through the primary level—a situation typical of countries such as Papua New Guinea, Tanzania and Uganda, Pakistan and Bangladesh (see Appendix C)—postponing a first birth would make little difference. Where continuation through secondary and perhaps into post-secondary education is the norm, however, as in Sri Lanka and Hong Kong, Kuwait and South Korea, or Argentina and Chile, then a woman's ability to avoid or terminate an untimely pregnancy can be crucial. At the individual level, birth control is crucial for any woman who wants to continue: studies in several West African countries have identified a high frequency of abortions among female secondary school students who are desperate to stay in school following an unwanted pregnancy (e.g., Nichols et al. 1986). The policy of expelling pregnant adolescent girls from school (but not boys who have fathered children) intensifies the pressure.

Parental control over the decision as to which of their children will attend school, and when and whom their children will marry, may preclude a young woman from making an individual decision that attaches a higher priority to education than to early motherhood. Indeed, a girl may be withdrawn from school in order to prepare her for marriage or to keep her from becoming too independent. Yet, as literacy or higher education for women become more generally accepted and valued, parental priorities can change. Parents may keep a daughter in school longer to raise her value on the marriage market as an educated bride, which has been cited as one reason for postponing marriage in southern India (Caldwell, Reddy, and Caldwell 1983), or to raise her market wage and contribution to family earnings before she marries, which is a common pattern among the Chinese in Southeast Asia (Salaff 1981; Greenhalgh 1985).

Fifth, where opportunity structures favor female employment and where the roles of employee and mother are incompatible, women practicing effective birth planning can have significant economic advantages over those for whom early or frequent childbearing is inevitable. Delaying the first birth may enable women to complete their education and vocational training to qualify for more highly skilled jobs or to establish themselves in a profession. Controlling the timing of births permits women to combine employment and childbearing in the least disruptive way. Contraception can enable a woman in a sexual union to plan for an uninterrupted investment in an occupation (again, where such opportunities exist), perhaps even breaking out of stereotyped female jobs (Birdsall and Chester 1987). Keeping family size small makes it easier to work outside the home, especially in those countries where child care assistance is scarce or expensive. Women without children or with only one or two may face less discrimination in the labor market on the grounds that they are less likely to be absent for family reasons than women with more children. The effect of family size on labor force participation depends in large part on the children's ages, with the relationship often disappearing once the children are older or leave home. Having the last child early in the life cycle may also ease the burden on women working away from home and encourage those who have stayed at home to re-enter the labor force sooner.

Viewed in this light, a woman's ability to determine the number and spacing of her children can have a direct impact on the exercise of her economic rights. Yet, there are circumstances in which a woman may not be able to improve her chances in the labor market by delaying, spacing, or limiting her births. Employment opportunities for women are often scant in any case because of truncated or segmented labor markets. Women may face discrimination in formal sector employment on the *assumption* that they are (or will be) married and have children—regardless of their actual marital or childbearing status—and thus have less right to a job or an income than a man (Anker and Hein 1986). In informal sector employment (e.g., crafts production in the home, small-scale trading) or subsistence agricultural production, the number or spacing of children may have little effect. In some cases, higher fertility may actually facilitate her work if children assist in farming, crafts, or trading operations, as in West Africa (Ware 1977; Oppong 1983:553–554). In other cases, as suggested previously, high fertility may force her to enter the labor force or extend her work time in order to support her growing family. In Malaysia, for example, rural Indian and Chinese women who were working away from home had *more* children on average than those who worked at home or were not employed (Mason and Palan 1981). The explanation for this unexpected finding is that because children were not easily able to earn incomes on the rubber estates where most Indian families were employed or in the commercial ventures on which many rural Chinese households depended, it was wives who entered the labor force when more money was needed to support additional children.

Sixth, birth control should also enable women to exercise their political rights more fully, insofar as these involve active community work or public sector employment. Again, the usual qualifications apply with respect to opportunity structures and the locus of behavioral controls.

Several general points are also worth making here. One is that the collective impact of contraceptive use and controlled fertility can be greater than the sum of its parts. As women increasingly delay, space, and limit their births and spend shorter portions of their lives rearing children, their claims to equality in education, employment, and political life are likely to become more persistent. Reproductive rights and social, economic, and political rights are synergistic in this respect: pressure for more responsive public policies intensifies as women overcome the "biological imperative" of unavoidable motherhood. A related point is that individual actions are magnified through their intergenerational effects. A girl with few siblings, for example, is more likely to be enrolled in school (all other things being equal) than a girl with many. Fertility limitation *by her parents* improves her educational prospects, in part because resources are distributed among fewer children and in part because she is less likely to be kept home to care for younger siblings (e.g., see Knodel and Wongsith 1991 on Thailand). In turn, her own fertility limitation improves the prospects of her daughters. Intergenerational effects are relevant to all of the rights considered here: the transformations of each generation act as stepping stones for the next. A third point: spread effects are magnified and legitimized when innovations by individual "role models" are supported by public policies and programs such as family planning or nontraditional vocational training programs for girls and women.

In sum, given the right conditions, a woman's ability to regulate her fertility can have a profound impact on other aspects of her life and on the lives of others. Recognizing this, one can also turn the question around. In what ways are a woman's contraceptive knowledge and practice affected by her schooling, employment, position in the family, and the exercise of her civil and political rights? How might public policy interventions in these spheres transform the conditions of reproductive choice?

EDUCATIONAL RIGHTS: SCHOOLING AS PERSONAL, SOCIAL, AND ECONOMIC RESOURCE

The Convention on the Elimination of Discrimination Against Women declares that girls and women have equal rights with boys and men to study in educational institutions of all types, to the same choice of curricula, and to scholarships and other financial support. It also addresses other types of training such as nonformal education, adult literacy, and extension services, all of which form a cluster of rights to equal knowledge. Gender inequalities in schooling reflect and reinforce inequalities in other spheres. Yet, with the incorporation of even remote regions of the world into an overarching global economy, literacy and numeracy skills as well as specialized information are essential for workers in all sectors of economic activity, including agriculture and the rural and urban informal sectors. More advanced education is needed for entry into most formal sector jobs and for positions of political power. If women are to achieve their full productive capacity and exercise their equal rights to employment and political participation, they must first be able to exercise their equal right to an education.

Schooling prepares students to take advantage of opportunities in the public sphere. It can also transform relations within the family by challenging traditional values and weakening the authority of the old over the young and males over females (Caldwell 1982:301–330). Particularly in strongly patriarchal societies, schooling allows girls to have a wider social network, new reference groups, greater exposure to the modern world, and experience in interacting with peers and authority figures other than their parents (Kritz and Gurak 1989). Schooling may encourage a spirit of inquiry and independence; in this sense, it is not surprising that traditional parents are often ambivalent about sending their children to school. Daughters may become "unmarriable" by refusing to accept a subordinate role in an arranged marriage; sons may reject their father's occupation, move to the city, take on new responsibilities that compete with filial obligations.

A woman's schooling is among the strongest determinants of her contraceptive knowledge and use and of family size, especially in high fertility countries. The relationship is not a simple one, however, nor is it inverse in all cases (Cochrane 1979). The question is how, and under what conditions, does a woman's education make a difference to her childbearing? And what is it about schooling that has an effect?

It may be that the number of years of formal schooling is simply the most visible and quantifiable element in a cluster of interdependent forces affecting fertility. Education beyond the primary level is often associated with factors such as openness to new ideas, higher standards of living, exposure to an urban environment, higher occupational achievement, and a greater range of other options and interests outside the home. Any or all of these could be responsible for the apparent influence of education on fertility. Interestingly, most studies show that the educational level of the wife is more strongly and inversely correlated with a couple's fertility than is the educational level of the husband after controlling for other influences (Cochrane 1979; Cleland and Rodríguez 1988). Whatever way the causal mechanism works, investment in female education appears to have a greater impact in reducing family size than the same investment in schooling for males. Mother's schooling also has a greater impact than any other variable typically considered in improving child health and reducing infant deaths (United Nations 1985:286–287; Caldwell 1986).

Conclusions such as these offer persuasive arguments for affirmative action policies in countries where girls and women are currently educationally disadvantaged relative to boys and men, quite apart from the equal rights rationale per se. In many African and Asian countries young women are two to three times more likely than young men to be unable to read or write, for example, and only one-third to one-half as likely to be enrolled in secondary school (Appendix C). In most Southeast and East Asian countries and in Latin America and the Caribbean, where birth rates are generally lower, women have reached parity with men in secondary school enrollments.

Higher education for women can work indirectly to reduce fertility in at least three ways: (1) by delaying marriage and increasing the probability of non-marriage, thus reducing the time span of exposure to the possibility of conception (assuming either a low frequency of sexual contact outside of marriage or a high degree of nonmarital birth control); (2) by reducing desired family size by creating aspirations for a higher level of living for the couple and their children, and by stimulating women's interest and involvement in activities outside the home, especially employment; and (3) by exposing women to knowledge, attitudes, and practices favorable to birth control, including a higher level of communication between husband and wife that would enable them to bring their actual reproduction in line with their desired family size (e.g., see LeVine et al. 1991 on Mexico).

World Fertility Survey results reveal generally strong associations between female education and marriage age, desired family size, and contraceptive use in developing countries even when other variables influencing these behaviors are controlled (United Nations 1987:214–254). For example, women in 28 southern countries with 7 or more years of schooling married on average four years later than those with no schooling, that is, at 23 rather than 19 years. Secondary schooling had the largest impact on marriage age in sub-Saharan Africa where only a small minority of women were enrolled (a 5 year difference) and less impact in Asia and Latin America (3–4 years). Of course, decisions about marriage age and schooling tend to be jointly determined—whether by the woman herself, her parents, or family elders—and so one must be cautious about drawing causal connections. As noted earlier, parents may withdraw a girl from school as her marriageable age approaches in order to protect her reputation and improve her marriage prospects; alternatively, if literacy or higher education are valued on the marriage market, she may be required to stay.

Women with 7 or more years of schooling are also from two to four times more likely than women with no schooling to be currently using a contraceptive method. The differentials are widest in sub-Saharan Africa where overall levels of contraceptive use are low. Female education in most southern countries is closely related to family size. Among 30 countries with WFS data, women with no schooling had an average total fertility rate (TFR) of 6.9 children per woman, three children more than women with 7 or more years of schooling (ibid.:225). Contrasts between the two educational groups were least marked in sub-Saharan Africa (a two child difference, which persists in DHS surveys) and most marked in Latin America and the Caribbean (a difference of 3.6 children, which is also replicated in the DHS). Moreover, the educational differential appears to be widening as highly educated women experience more rapid fertility declines than those with little or no education.

Where higher education is confined to a small elite, its impact on overall birth rates is bound to be slight. In Burundi, for example, only 1 percent of rural women and 30 percent of urban women had some secondary education; in Guatemala, 4 and 32 percent, respectively. But even the transition from zero to three years of schooling or from three to six years has a substantial (although not necessarily linear) effect on family size in most southern countries. The exceptions are those cases where pronatalist pressures can obliterate the effects of even six or eight years of schooling. For example, Kenyan women with at least some secondary schooling interviewed in the WFS had a TFR of 7.3 children, just one child less than women with no education. In Bangladesh, the comparable figures were 5.0 and 6.1 (ibid.). In an earlier survey in rural Turkey, women with primary or higher education did not have smaller families than those with less schooling although in urban areas family size varied clearly by the level of female education (Stycos and Weller 1967). Discovering similar situations in Latin America, Joseph Stycos (1968:269) suggested that a certain amount of urbanization may be necessary "to activate the effect of education on fertility." More recent data confirm that although the general relationship between female education and family size is similar in rural and urban areas, the impact of female education is usually stronger in cities.

The urban catalyst may be due partly to a connection between female education and employment. Higher education may not motivate a woman to want fewer children if her training does not lead to salaried employment outside the home. Higher education does increase the likelihood of women's employment in most countries, although women with little or no schooling are often pushed into the labor force in even larger proportions because of economic pressures (United Nations 1987:260–262). These class-specific push-pull forces typically result in either a positive or U-shaped relationship between female education and labor force participation that has implications for fertility outcomes. Moreover, not only the number of years but also the type or quality of schooling can make a difference. Women trained in traditionally "female fields" have been shown in some studies to have more children than women in less "fem-

inine'' fields with equal or fewer years of schooling (Safilios-Rothschild
1969:595–598).

RIGHTS RELATING TO EMPLOYMENT AND EARNINGS

Everyone has the right to work (a freedom and an entitlement), to free
choice of employment, to just and favorable conditions of work, to protection against unemployment, to fair remuneration, and to equal pay for
equal work (United Nations 1973a:2). Women, married or unmarried, are
to have equal rights with men. In addition, the women's convention declares that governments are to take measures to prevent the dismissal of
women who get married or have a child, to provide paid maternity leave
with guaranteed return to the same job, and to provide childcare facilities
and other necessary social services (see Appendix A). Women are far
from achieving equal rights with men in employment, of course. Even in
countries where women constitute up to one half of the working population
they are almost invariably channeled into lower paid occupations and earn
lower wages even for the same or equivalent work (Sivard 1985; United
Nations 1991:81–100). Most employers do not provide paid maternity
leave or guarantee return to former jobs after delivery, and childcare
facilities in most countries, both industrialized and developing, are inadequate to meet the needs of working parents.

To what extent might the exercise of women's equal rights in employment contribute to greater sexual and reproductive choice? If a consistent
causal effect were to be found, the implications for development strategies
would be clear: ensuring women's rights to equal work and equal pay
would reduce birth rates while simultaneously facilitating economic development and raising household incomes. The relationship depends not
on the simple fact of gainful employment, however, but on such factors
as the sector of the economy in which the woman is employed; her occupation, income, and work commitment; whether she is a wage earner,
self-employed, or unpaid worker in a family enterprise; the duration and
continuity of employment; the location of work and whether it is full or
part time; and the availability of child care, among other influences. Different motivations for working, and the vast distinctions among women
throughout the world in the nature and conditions of their work, carry
inevitable implications for the relationship between female employment
and fertility.

Three major arguments can be found in the literature about the influence
of women's employment on fertility. The *role incompatibility* hypothesis
contends that female employment would reduce fertility where contraception is widely available and where the roles of worker and mother are
most incompatible, that is, where the job is away from home, which may
pose practical problems relating to child care, and where people believe

that mothers should care for their own children rather than relying on substitute caregivers of "lower quality" (Stycos and Weller 1967; Piepmeier and Adkins 1973). The *opportunity cost* hypothesis also assumes an incompatibility of maternal and occupational roles but is more narrowly economic. A woman should be most motivated to restrict her childbearing where the income she foregoes (if any) by having a child and staying home to rear it is highest (McCabe and Rosenzweig 1976). Expected wage rates are generally imputed from her years of schooling modified by the probability of finding employment. The *female autonomy* hypothesis contends that by providing alternative sources of social identity and economic support, employment outside the home could reduce women's dependence on men and children (especially sons); broaden girls' and women's social horizons, thus helping to counter family-based pronatalist pressures; increase women's desire to delay marriage (or to avoid or terminate an unsatisfactory union) and to space and limit births; and contribute to greater sexual and reproductive autonomy (Dixon 1978; Safilios-Rothschild 1982).

Note that although at least some of these conditions are expected to apply to women's work in industrialized countries and in urban sectors of developing countries, they do not apply to the work that most girls and women do in agrarian settings (Oppong 1983; Standing 1983). Regarding the autonomy hypothesis, for example, demographer Helen Ware points out that the idea of work as liberating "would probably seem very strange to an Indian woman working sixteen hours a day breaking stones in a quarry . . . or an Indonesian wife harvesting rice stem by stem" (Ware 1981:101). Yet, with the right conditions, even the work of illiterate rural women may produce such effects. The most substantial social, economic, and demographic benefits are likely to accrue when the employment provides income over which women have direct control, offers basic economic security, and is considered status-enhancing or status-neutral rather than status-degrading (Dixon 1978). Jobs located outside the home in a central workplace, labor-intensive light industries, cooperative work organizations with decision-making roles for women, direct access to production credit and marketing, and additional job-related services and incentives such as health education, child care, and family planning all offer possibilities for transforming women's options and enhancing their autonomy.

Research on women's employment and childbearing in developing countries has confirmed at least one finding: the relationship is "elusive" and "ambiguous" (United Nations 1987:277; see also Standing 1983). Evidence from the WFS, for example, is mixed, at best. In general, and in the aggregate, women with work experience in "modern" occupations (e.g., professional or clerical) marry from one to two years later and have fewer children than those in "transitional" or "mixed" occupations (domestic and other service work, sales, and skilled and unskilled labor), who in turn marry later and have fewer children than do women in "traditional" occupations (mostly agriculture) and those reporting no history of employment (United Nations 1987:265–266; Lloyd 1991). But there are many exceptions, especially in the least developed countries, and especially in sub-Saharan Africa. Within some countries the expected occupation-fertility relationships at the individual level do not appear at all. In others, they are diluted or even reversed when antecedent characteristics such as educational attainment or household incomes and assets, which can jointly determine *both* female employment and childbearing, are statistically controlled.

Similar results appear at higher levels of aggregation. At least five employment-marriage-fertility regimes can be distinguished at the national level: (1) a sub-Saharan African pattern combining high rates of female economic activity in agriculture and trade with early marriage and high fertility; (2) a North African-Middle Eastern pattern, including Muslim South Asia, of restricted female employment combined with early or moderate age at marriage and high fertility; (3) an Asian pattern (excluding Muslim South Asia) of high female employment in agriculture, industry, and/or services combined with generally late marriage and low to moderate fertility; (4) a Latin American pattern of moderate female employment in manufacturing and services, including the professions, combined with late marriage and low to moderate fertility; and (5) a Caribbean pattern of mixed low to high employment-fertility combinations and generally late union formation (see Appendixes B and C). These contrasting regional patterns conceal important differences across and within countries deriving in part from differences in the type of work that women do. Nevertheless, they reveal important contextual effects.

What kinds of employment are likely to have the greatest impact? Again, one must consider the question of who controls female sexuality, reproduction, and labor power and what the opportunity structures for employment are. In general, the least likely candidates for transforming gender relations and fertility decision making are those that do not confront patriarchal family relations of production and reproduction. These include unpaid work in the family fields or livestock herds (no matter how productive or valuable to the household's consumption), unpaid work in other family enterprises such as cottage industries, and self-employment in enterprises that have low returns to labor or where women depend on men for their capital, materials, or marketing (e.g., Mies 1982). In countries such as Burundi, Rwanda, Mali, Iraq, the Philippines, Thailand, and Turkey, for example, the majority of all economically active women are unpaid family workers, typically in agriculture. (If unpaid and informal-sector activities such as these were more adequately enumerated, such findings would apply to many other countries as well.) In these situations, wealth and decision-making power continue to flow from the young to the old and from women to men. "Familial modes of production are characterized by relations of production between kin that give the more powerful decision-makers material advantage," writes Caldwell (1982:159). "The struggle of the decision-makers to maintain their advantage is normally seen as the assertion of natural rights and as proper behavior; nevertheless, family economic relations are exploitative and there is potential for conflict and change."

In contrast, work for wages (what Caldwell calls the labor market mode of production) is far more likely to provide girls and women (as well as young men) with moral leverage to challenge patriarchal controls over their sexual and reproductive lives *if* the earnings contribute a substantial share of the household income or could provide an independent livelihood. (Patriarchal ideologies may demand the appropriation of the earnings of daughters or wives by elders or husbands as part of a "family wage," however, at least in transitional stages from familial to labor-market modes of production; see Greenhalgh 1985; Dwyer and Bruce 1988). This is where women's access to modern-sector jobs at equal wages is critical. Yet, in North Africa and the Middle East, women hold fewer than 15 percent of all waged and salaried jobs, on average, and in sub-Saharan Africa, from 15 to 25 percent (United Nations 1991:108–111). Corresponding figures for Latin America are 20 to 40 percent, for Asia (excluding Muslim South Asia) 30 to 40 percent, and for the Caribbean, 40 to 50 percent. These differentials are clearly related to fertility rates at the aggregate level, although both rising wage employment and declining birth rates are functions of overall development and per capita incomes (Schultz 1990).

Like schooling, participation in the labor market is likely to broaden a woman's horizons, introduce new forms of authority and social organization that compete with familial hierarchies, and offer a taste of independence. It is exactly these fears that underly the resistance of men in some cases to having their wives or daughters work away from home. In Mexico, for example, one survey found that 57 percent of the women interviewed but only 37 percent of the men thought it was acceptable for a wife to work outside the home (Folch-Lyon et al. 1981:415). In a separate study, 40 percent of husbands opposed their wife's decision to look for a job. Among other reasons, husbands feared that "once women were allowed to work—especially outside the home—'they lose respect for their husbands' and the husbands themselves lose face or are criticized by (male) relatives and friends . . . '' (Benería and Roldán 1987:146). These concerns lead directly to the question of what rights women have at the time of marriage, during marriage, and at its dissolution.

RIGHTS ON ENTERING MARRIAGE

The principle of equality in marriage has elicited considerable controversy in international debates over women's rights. As noted in chapter

1, the Declaration on the Elimination of Discrimination Against Women which preceded the Convention cautioned that women's rights within marriage were to be exercised "without prejudice to . . . the unity and harmony of the family . . . " The idea that daughters and sons should have the right to choose whom and when to marry, and that wives and husbands should have the same rights and responsibilities in marriage, collides head-on with the customary rights and privileges of men and elders. In many countries equality within the family has not yet been recognized in civil law and upon marriage a woman may be deprived of many rights such as the independent ownership of property or the right to work or travel without her husband's consent. Even in countries where legislation favors equal rights, traditional cultural patterns of male dominance in marriage and the family are slow to change.

Consider, first, the rights of women and men on entering marriage. The U.N. Convention on Consent to Marriage (1962) prohibits the customs of child marriage, the betrothal of young girls, and the inheritance of widows (the levirate) by a male relative of the deceased husband. Minimum standards for age at marriage are to be set in every country at not less than 15 years and all marriages are to be officially registered (United Nations 1973a:92–93). The emphasis on marrying at full age and with free and full consent conveys the idea that both women and men have rights over their own bodies and their own futures. A woman cannot be married against her will or to a person she does not accept, a practice the United Nations terms "similar to slavery." Because marriage sanctions and indeed obliges sexual intercourse, the choice of whether, when, and whom to marry is an important element of a woman's rights over her sexual body.

Although most countries have established or changed their legislation to meet international standards, more than 30 countries worldwide continue to permit girls to marry legally below the age of 15. In some countries the marriage age is tied to ethnic custom or religious law and differs for each group. (There are nine separate codes in Lebanon, for example.) In the 1980s, civil and religious codes allowed the marriage of girls under 15 among some groups or in some states in at least four nations in sub-Saharan Africa (Ethiopia, Kenya, Madagascar, Nigeria); 15 in Latin America and the Caribbean (including Chile, Argentina, and Peru); two in the Middle East (Lebanon and Iran); two in Asia (Malaysia and Sri Lanka), and the United States and Canada (United Nations 1989a:42–43). Approximately 75 countries have legislated inequality by setting a lower minimum marriage age for brides than for grooms.

The decades since 1960 have seen a dramatic rise in female age at first marriage and a slight rise in proportions never marrying in many southern countries under the influence of urbanization, education, and economic change (Henry and Piotrow 1979; United Nations 1989a, 1990a, 1991). Although many young girls continue to marry as children and bear children as children, especially in sub-Saharan Africa and in South Asia, contrasts are marked in every region. In the 1980s from half to two-thirds of women ages 15 to 19 in Afghanistan, Bangladesh, and Nepal were already married, for example, but only one in ten in Sri Lanka married this young (Appendix C).

How does the timing of marriage affect the ability of girls and women to exercise their sexual and reproductive rights, apart from its association with higher education and premarital employment? First, early entry into a marriage or consensual union often contributes to (or results from) limited contraceptive knowledge and practice, at least in the early years. It is also associated with higher completed fertility: a gross difference of two to four children, on average, between those who marry before age 18 and at 25 or older (United Nations 1987:96). In this sense, delayed marriage appears to facilitate control over the timing and number of children.

Second, early marriage, especially before age 16, escalates the health risks of pregnancy and contributes disproportionately to maternal death and disability where medical resources are scarce (Zimicki 1989). In Bangladesh at least one woman in five gives birth before she is 16, for example, and reproductive complications can be severe. In Ethiopia, half of a sample of women interviewed at health and family planning clinics said they first had intercourse with their husbands before having menstruated, and one in five had done so before age 13 (Duncan et al. 1990:339). Early intercourse was associated in the sample with a higher prevalence of sexually transmitted diseases and of cervical cancer. Thus, delayed marriage can facilitate the exercise of a woman's right to reproductive health.

Third, in most southern countries the earlier a woman marries, the more likely it is that her husband is considerably older. This is especially true of arranged marriage systems where a daughter may be married off to a widower or to a polygynous husband who already has another wife, where patrilocal residence is the rule, and where contractual transfers of wealth between families in the form of dowry or brideprice serve to legitimize the claims of the male lineage to the couple's offspring.

Surveys in several sub-Saharan African countries found that recently married women were 6 to 8 years younger than their husbands, on average, compared with about 2.5 to 5 years in Latin American and Asian countries but up to 9 years in Bangladesh (Cain 1984:41). Early marriage for girls combined with a wide age gap can perpetuate a situation of powerlessness between the daughter whose marriage is arranged and the parents or elders who arrange it, and between the young bride and her husband and his kin. Indeed, this is precisely the intention. As Mead Cain notes, "[a] large age difference . . . connotes a potentially powerful means of male control over women, and is further indicative of the kind of control that derives from the interaction of age and sex hierarchies . . . '' (1984:40).

Cain's analysis of the consequences of the age gap between spouses in a number of southern countries demonstrates that it acts as a ''filter'' through which social and economic changes in society affect the couple's fertility. Regions of strong patriarchal family structures where husbands are at least five years older than their wives on average (sub-Saharan Africa, South Asia, and the Middle East) have higher fertility than do weak patriarchal regimes with smaller age differences (Southeast and East Asia, Latin America) even when other factors affecting fertility such as infant mortality, per capita income, female secondary school enrollments, and female age at first marriage are statistically controlled. Fertility rates in weak patriarchal regimes respond in the expected way to variations in the other factors whereas in strong patriarchal regimes they are resistant. In this sense, then, both the timing of marriage *and* the age difference between spouses appear to be important determinants of fertility behavior as well as of other rights.

The loss of parental control over the arrangement of their children's nuptials, insofar as such control is associated with early and universal marriage in an extended family system, should serve to delay marriage on the average and to increase the probability of nonmarriage for some women, either voluntarily or involuntarily. Courtship, after all, takes time, and an independently contracted marriage requires a degree of maturity not needed or even desired of a young girl whose primary obligation is to obey the wishes of her husband and her elders. The free choice of a spouse—even with a considerable amount of parental guidance—also implies a degree of equality between husband and wife at the time of their marriage that may be important for effective communication about family size desires and the practice of family planning.

GENDER EQUALITY WITHIN MARRIAGE

According to the women's convention, husbands and wives have equal rights and responsibilities *during* marriage, including equal rights and duties in matters relating to their children, the same right to choose a family name and occupation, and the same rights of ownership and disposition of property. They have the same right to decide on the number and spacing of their children and to the information and means to do so. Under what conditions are women likely to decide equally with their husbands on contraceptive use and the timing and number of children? What impact does (or might) such equality have on reproductive outcomes? This area is a rich and fascinating one to explore, for it is in the everyday interactions between women and men that extraneous factors such as education and employment are translated into actual reproductive patterns through birth planning behavior (Beckman 1983; Hollerbach 1983; Hull 1983). Unfortunately, we can touch on it only briefly here.

Resource theory argues that the greater are the material and social resources that a woman brings into her marriage relative to those of her husband (e.g., education, paid employment, personal assets, a strong network of social support from her relatives), the greater is her power or influence over family decisions (Weller 1968; Safilios-Rothschild 1982). Legal rights are also resources. Gender inequalities in the public sphere are thus mirrored in the private sphere, with implications for the nature of family decision making. Yet, there are at least two possibilities of overriding their effects. First, gender role ideologies may support or negate the importance of relative resources. A "modern" educated couple may believe strongly in the ideal of equality in decision making despite a large difference in their incomes, for example, whereas a more traditional couple may believe that the husband should make the major decisions even though his wife earns as much or more than he does. Second, the possibility of using contraception, sterilization, or abortion surreptitiously permits a woman with fewer resources to prevent an unwanted pregnancy or birth unilaterally without having to confront her partner or other decision makers directly. (The fear of discovery may inhibit this option, however; in addition, evidence suggests that contraceptive acceptance and continuation are related to the husband's approval; see Beckman 1983:417–418; Pariani et al. 1991.)

A related approach looks to the degree of gender *role segregation* as a key to understanding the decision-making process. Some studies suggest that married couples who share a more equitable division of labor within the home—that is, who have joint rather than segregated role relationships—are more likely to communicate with one another about sex, family size desires, and birth planning, which in turn leads to more empathy with the partner's feelings, greater sexual satisfaction, a desire for fewer children, and more effective contraceptive use (e.g., Rainwater 1965; Hollerbach 1980). Empirical support for these findings in developing countries is sketchy, however, and the causal paths are unclear (Beckman 1983). And, as for resource theory, the disadvantages of role segregation may turn to advantages for women if contraception and childbearing decisions fall under their "natural" sphere of responsibility. As Mason points out, "some cultures may give wives a relatively strong voice in fertility decisions, even though wives are given little power in other areas, because childbearing is regarded as a female domain" (1987:736).

A third approach looks at the *situational advantage* of key family members in fertility decision making. Drawing on Caldwell's work on intergenerational wealth flows (1982, 1983) as well as on earlier cross-cultural studies of the perceived costs and value of children (e.g., Arnold et al.

1975), this approach emphasizes that the costs and benefits of childbearing as well as the power to decide depend on a person's location within the household or kin group. Patriarchal control over the reproductive and labor capacity of adult children enhances parents' abilities to enjoy positive economic benefits and/or to substantially defray the costs of children, while the control of men over women enhances men's ability to shift a significant portion of the cost of children to women (Folbre 1983). In situations such as these, "husbands benefit from children's labor but bear few of the costs of their rearing, and so have little incentive to reduce fertility; women bear most of the costs of children, but do not see family size decisions as one of their basic rights" (Kritz and Gurak 1989:10).

The key question is whether husbands and wives have different reproductive goals. If the goals are similar, then the wife's relative power to postpone or limit births should make little difference. (Alternatively, a woman's lower fertility goals would make little difference if she lacked the capacity to influence contraceptive use.) A review of women's and men's reproductive goals derived from surveys in a number of southern countries concluded that, more often than not, men's and women's fertility goals are similar *in the aggregate* (although often based on different reasons) even though there is considerable variation across countries and studies (Mason and Taj 1987; see also Fawcett 1983). In a few settings women wanted more children than did men; in others, men showed a stronger son preference and thus a slight tendency to want additional children more often than women did. These aggregated findings do not permit an analysis of how differences between husbands and wives within individual couples are related to their relative resources, role segregation, or situational advantage, however. In addition, it is important to note that women's reported fertility goals reflect current patterns of sex discrimination.

Couples may concur on their fertility goals for a number of reasons, only some of them related to communication and joint decision making (Beckman 1983). Concurrence may be strictly coincidental, for example, or reflect the joint influence of narrowly defined social norms or the expectations of elders. If only one partner is interviewed, she (or he) may impute her own goals to her partner or guess at her partner's goals and report them as her own. Or, concurrence may result from consensus, a joint agreement based on discussion. Even here, however, the influence of one partner over the other may predominate.

There are strong a priori reasons for arguing that relative resources, role segregation, and situational advantage are important determinants of reproductive outcomes, and some find substantial empirical support. However, a fuller understanding requires knowledge of the cultural and structural conditions of each society. The relationship between women's rights and fertility may differ according to the type of union, for example, such as legal marriages compared with consensual or more casual unions, monogamous compared with polygynous unions, and independent nuclear households compared with extended households. Evidence regarding the effect of these differences is also somewhat inconclusive and the direction of causality uncertain (Burch 1983). Couples in nuclear households do not necessarily bear fewer children on average than couples in extended families in the same social setting even though one would expect a higher level of communication and joint decision making. Women in monogamous unions may bear more children than women in polygynous unions, where long taboos on sexual intercourse are more easily observed during lactation; yet polygyny can increase the overall birth rate by ensuring that all women marry, marry young, and remarry quickly. Women in visiting or consensual unions may have their first sexual experiences earlier and begin childbearing earlier, but because such unions are more unstable their pregnancies tend to be spaced at wider intervals and lead to fewer children than those of women in formal marriages. The woman's legal and de facto rights in each type of union as well as the relative instability of unions also need to be specified in order to understand how gender inequalities affect reproductive behavior. In this context, a woman's right to property and social security offers some insurance against risk and uncertainty.

RIGHTS TO PROPERTY AND SOCIAL SECURITY

Whereas a great deal of attention has been paid to the effects on women's sexual and reproductive choices of education and employment, the effects of rights to property and other forms of support have not been systematically addressed. How does the denial of the right to own, inherit, or bequeath property affect a woman's perceptions of the need to stay married, for example, or her desired family size? Is a woman who bears no children, or only one or two, or only daughters, disadvantaged under some legal systems more than others? The U.N. convention states that women and men, married or unmarried, have the same rights to acquire, own, enjoy, manage, and dispose of property; to obtain bank loans, mortgages, and credit; to receive benefits such as unemployment, welfare, and social security; to have title to land (and presumably to houses, livestock, and other assets); and to benefit from agrarian reform. Women have the same legal status as men to conclude contracts and testify in court. Like the other bundles of rights mentioned above, these rights confront patriarchal practices that deny females control over the means of production and subsistence. The question of use rights raised earlier is relevant here. Full equality requires that women have equal *control* over resources, either jointly with men or in their own names as independent "contractors." This notion is very different from that of use rights contingent upon maintaining a filial or marital relationship or some other patron-client obligation. The loss of land rights at the time of divorce or widowhood, for example, can plunge a woman into destitution if her livelihood is based on subsistence agriculture and she has nowhere else to go.

The question of property rights and public support is crucial for both married and unmarried women. According to DHS findings from 21 countries, fewer than two-thirds of all women of reproductive age (15 to 49) in the late 1980s were currently married or cohabiting. Over one-fourth had never (or had not yet) married or entered a consensual union, and an average of one-tenth were widowed, separated, or divorced. At ages 60 and over, the proportions of women not in unions typically rise to 50 to 70 percent (United Nations 1991:26–29). Because women's life expectancy exceeds men's in almost every country and because women typically marry at younger ages than men, women whose marriages are terminated by the death of a spouse can generally expect to spend from 5 to 15 years or more as a widow.

It is often assumed that widows in most societies are protected by strong extended family systems: by their sons, perhaps, or by their husband's kin. This may be true among the affluent, but research suggests that households facing economic crisis are increasingly unable or unwilling to support additional dependent members (Cain 1978). In short, rather than veneration a widow may face ill treatment, exploitation, or neglect at the hands of her relatives. Alternatively, she may be forced into exploitative labor markets, often with limited skills and experience. With highly imbalanced sex ratios at older ages, most older women's chances for remarriage are slim. Considering the probability of divorce as well as widowhood, and the higher propensity for divorced and widowed men in most cultures to remarry, the number of divorced, separated, or widowed women can greatly exceed the number of men. In Bangladesh, for example, formerly married women of all ages outnumber formerly married men by nine to one (Population Crisis Committee 1988:5).

Many of these women—as well as those who have never married or cohabited—are heads of households living alone or with their children. Sometimes termed the "ignored factor in development planning" (Buvinic and Youssef 1978), the growing number of households headed by women in both northern and southern countries derives from a mixture of rising rates of delayed marriage, non-marriage, divorce, desertion, and out-of-wedlock births in many countries; the breakdown of kinship obligations that formerly absorbed single or previously married women into ongoing households; male outmigration from rural areas that leaves many wives as de facto heads of households; and the inability or unwillingness of husbands to support their families in times of economic crisis. The proportions of all households headed by women run typically from 10 to 20 percent in Asia, 15 to 30 percent in sub-Saharan Africa (but 45 percent in Botswana), and 20 to 40 percent in Latin America and the Caribbean (United Nations 1991:226–229). In view of these trends, the elimination of discrimination against women in all aspects of property rights and social security as well as in education and employment becomes especially compelling.

Nondiscrimination in property rights is also compelling from another point of view: its impact on women's marital and reproductive goals. The limited research that has been done on this subject—primarily in rural Bangladesh and India—suggests that the production of children, especially sons, is a form of insurance for women who are denied independent access to income and land (Cain 1978, 1980, 1984; Ahmad 1991). Facing a high probability of divorce, desertion, or widowhood, and with no public assistance for the destitute and no pensions in old age, rural women in resource-poor households have little option but to turn to their sons for support. Discrimination against women in labor markets and property rights exacerbates their vulnerability. Although these examples are drawn from a particularly discriminatory setting, the general questions they raise are important from a policy viewpoint. How do particular environments of risk and uncertainty shape women's sexual and reproductive goals, and what role do property and old-age security rights play in this calculus? Are women who control property independently more likely to delay or forego marriage, to terminate an unsatisfactory union, or to regulate their fertility? Unfortunately, these questions cannot be answered here. Comparative research is needed to explore these relationships in diverse settings.

SUMMING UP: THE NEED FOR AN INTEGRATED REPRODUCTIVE POLICY

The relationship between the status of women and fertility has attracted considerable interest at international population conferences and among some multilateral and bilateral donors and non-governmental organizations involved in population assistance. As described in chapter 3, most attention has been paid to the possibility that improving women's positions in the family and society—especially through the expansion of female educational and employment opportunities—could significantly reduce birth rates in developing countries with rapid population growth. The World Population Plan of Action adopted at the World Population Conference in Bucharest in 1974, for example, urged "the full integration of women into the development process, particularly by means of their greater participation in educational, social, economic and political opportunities . . . " as a development goal that would also create conditions favorable to smaller family size (Mauldin et al. 1974:386). Similar recommendations were made at the 1984 International Population Conference at Mexico City (Isaacs and Cook 1984:139). In this context, raising the status of women represents one means among many of achieving the demographic goal of lower birth rates.

Less attention has been paid to the impact of fertility regulation on women's rights, that is, on family planning as one means among many for reducing gender inequalities as a social goal. The 1974 Bucharest population conference touched on this briefly with its statement that " . . . the opportunity for women to plan births also improves their individual status" (Mauldin et al. 1974:387), while the 1984 Mexico City conference noted more strongly that "The ability of women to control their own fertility forms an important basis for the enjoyment of other rights . . . " (Isaacs and Cook 1984:139). The heavier emphasis placed on the demographic rather than the human rights side of the equation is understandable in view of the concern with population dynamics expressed at international meetings and in population program assistance. Yet, as we have noted in this chapter, a woman's ability to determine the number and spacing of her children can influence in fundamental ways her ability to complete her schooling, to take full advantage of employment opportunities, and to acquire greater control over the terms of marital or nonmarital sexual relationships.

The crucial factor shaping the relationship between reproductive choice and other rights is the structure of opportunities that girls and women face. A rural woman who has never been to school gains no educational advantage from delaying her first birth, for example, nor does an illiterate woman forced by economic hardship to labor in the fields or factories for minimal wages improve her chances for advancement by having fewer children. By the same token, a woman kept secluded in her husband's household is denied the right to work regardless of her reproductive behavior. Thus, it makes little sense to promote policies encouraging contraceptive use and smaller families without simultaneously addressing other legal, social, and economic constraints on women's rights. Similarly, it makes little sense to promote policies advancing women's integration in development without addressing their fundamental need for sexual and reproductive choice.

According to the women's convention and other international documents, women have the same rights as men to vote, to hold public office, to participate in policy-making and implementation, to engage in community activities, to organize self-help groups and cooperatives, to join non-governmental organizations, and to associate freely with men and with one another. The importance of female solidarity groups as a determinant of women's status has been documented cross-culturally (Sanday 1974) and emphasized as a source of individual autonomy and collective power (Safilios-Rothschild 1982). Indeed, as we have seen in the preceding chapter, the ability to mobilize politically around a variety of mutual interests and activities acts as a catalyst for changes in other spheres.

The role of public policy in this context is twofold. In the first instance, women's rights to participate equally with men in policy-making and implementation need to be fully recognized. In the second instance, substantive policies need to be designed to eliminate gender discrimination in health care, schooling, employment and income generation, property rights, family law, and public life. Government ministries can set specific targets in all sectors and invest selectively in promoting women's participation until equal access has been achieved. Within this framework, a reproductive health program offering women the means to choose how many children to have and when to have them takes on real meaning.

6

OBJECTIVE AND SUBJECTIVE DIMENSIONS OF THE RIGHT TO HEALTH

The idea of human rights as expressed in the Universal Declaration includes the enjoyment of "the highest attainable standard of physical and mental health" (United Nations 1973a:5). According to the World Health Organization (WHO), health is "a state of complete physical, mental and social well being and not merely the absence of disease or infirmity" (United Nations 1990b:62). This broad-brushed definition is useful for understanding the relationship between fertility regulation and women's health. How does a woman's ability to use contraception and to space, limit, or avoid childbearing affect her physical and emotional health and well-being? Put another way, can we consider family planning as an "enabling" ingredient in the exercise of a woman's right to health? It was, after all, the physical and emotional suffering of women unable to cope with frequent pregnancies that drew Margaret Sanger into the fight for birth control: a woman's death from clandestine abortion symbolized for her the excruciating cost of ignorance and inaccessability.

Most research on the health consequences of contraceptive use and controlled fertility has focused on physical effects as measured by rates of maternal (and infant) morbidity and mortality (Maine 1981; Rinehart and Kols 1984; Trussell and Pebley 1984; National Research Council 1989). The narrowness of this focus is due in part to the relative ease with which mortality can be measured, even though the collection of data on maternal deaths is fraught with difficulties in many countries (WHO 1986). The universal recognition of the positive effects of family planning on maternal and child health has led to the redefinition of family planning as a vital preventive and positive health measure. Several international conferences have highlighted these connections, such as the International Conference on Better Health for Women and Children through Family Planning, and the International Safe Motherhood Conference, both held in Nairobi in 1987 (Black 1987; Starrs 1987). In addition, some governments support family planning programs primarily on health grounds, particularly in sub-Saharan Africa where economic or demographic rationales are less politically persuasive.

In exploring the relationship between reproductive choice and women's health, it is helpful to cast a wide net in order to capture the full array of costs and benefits of alternative reproductive behaviors as women themselves experience them. Considering the effects of fertility regulation on women's mental health and social well-being can provide insights that the physical health equation—and particularly the mortality equation—cannot capture. Women alone bear the physical risks of pregnancy and childbirth. Women also bear the physical risks of using female methods of contraception—the oral pill, the IUD, injectables, implants, and tubal ligation, for example—and of abortion. But women also experience emotional hardships associated with their sexual and reproductive lives resulting from their low status in many societies and from feelings of shame that cause them to suffer in silence. Few investigators have looked systematically at how gender inequalities within the household affect girls' and women's sense of self-worth, that is, how girls and women feel about themselves and how they relate to others within a given "moral framework" governing the intra-household distribution of entitlements (Papanek 1990). Similarly, few investigators have considered systematically how different patterns of reproductive behavior affect women's sense of self-worth and the fabric of their social relationships. Yet, these "psychosocial" consequences may be equally as important to women—if not more so—than the morbidity and mortality outcomes that are so commonly addressed.

Reproductive events and conditions impinge in major ways, both positive and negative, on a woman's ability to perform key social roles on which her survival, security, and emotional well-being depend. Reproductive behaviors that are innocuous or beneficial from a physical health perspective, such as using a contraceptive, delaying the first birth, or limiting the number of children to two or three, could cause some women considerable psychosocial stress in settings where such behaviors are considered deviant within a particular ideological or moral framework. That is why, ideally, one would study women *in situ* in order to understand how using contraception or postponing or preventing a birth impinges on their right to health in concrete situations.

This chapter has two objectives. The first is to review evidence of the effects on women's survival of delaying, spacing, and limiting childbearing and of practicing contraception. Demographic and epidemiological studies address the "objective" aspects of reproductive benefits and risks. The second objective is to present a conceptual framework for analyzing the psychosocial consequences of contraceptive use and controlled fertility as they affect women's role performance. The empirical literature on this second topic is scant. Instead, the analysis draws on speculative logic and on ethnographic and anecdotal reports of how women talk about their lives. The inclusion of these "subjective" psychosocial effects as well as the physical effects of fertility regulation, and of the costs and benefits of using contraception as well as of having or not having a child, should present a more nuanced view of what appears at first to be a set of simple relationships. It may also help to explain why many women are reluctant to practice contraception despite its "obvious" health benefits.

DEATH FROM PREGNANCY-RELATED CAUSES

The World Health Organization estimates that at least half a million women die each year from maternal causes, that is, from complications associated with pregnancy, abortion, and childbirth (WHO 1986:2–3). Over 98 percent of these deaths occur to women in developing countries. The most frequent causes are hemorrhage, pregnancy-induced hypertension (toxemia or eclampsia), infection (sepsis), obstructed labor, and unsafe induced abortion (Zimicki 1989). Frequent childbirth can also aggravate the incidence of other debilitating conditions such as malnutrition, high blood pressure, epilepsy, severe anemia, and diabetes (Rinehart and Kols 1984:673).

African women face the highest risks of maternal death, particularly in Western and Middle Africa. Asian women face somewhat lower risks overall, higher in Southern Asia but lower in East Asia. The risks to Latin American and Caribbean women are lower still, and lowest of all in North America and Europe. Whereas a woman in northern Europe has a lifetime chance of dying from maternal causes of only one in 10,000, a woman in some areas of sub-Saharan Africa faces over *one chance in 20* (Herz and Measham 1987:7). In general, women in southern countries risk death from *each* pregnancy at a rate that is 15 times higher than for women in northern countries. Put another way, complications of pregnancy and childbirth account for between 10 and 30 percent of all deaths among women of reproductive age in parts of Asia, Africa, and Latin America, but less than 2 percent in North America and Europe (Rinehart and Kols 1984:657).

The vastly different pregnancy-related risks across nations—and among social classes and other subgroups within nations—derive from at least four factors. First, the quantity and quality of reproductive health care available to pregnant women, as well as women's knowledge of and ability to take advantage of the services that *are* available—are unequally distributed in favor of wealthier nations, urban locations, and social groups with higher education and incomes. At the national level, for example, fewer than one woman in ten was attended by a trained birth attendant at the time of her most recent delivery in countries such as Cameroon, Somalia, Ethiopia, Afghanistan, Bangladesh, and Nepal. Yet, virtually all women were assisted by a trained practitioner during childbirth in most (but not all) northern countries, in several Caribbean nations and Gulf states, and in Cuba, Chile, Dominican Republic, Uruguay, Mongolia, and Singapore (United Nations 1991:67–70). The typical range across countries of assisted births is about 95–100 percent in Europe, 50–95 percent in Latin America and the Caribbean, 10–100 percent in Asia, and 10–80 percent in Africa. For *any given pregnancy*, then, the risk of complications and death is dramatically higher for women in countries with inadequate health services, and, within these countries, for low-income and rural women.

Second, the more pregnancies a woman has, the more frequently she is exposed to the risk of reproductive complications and death. This is a simple, additive effect: women with more pregnancies are more likely to suffer or die from pregnancy-related causes, and maternal mortality is higher in high-fertility populations. Third, certain *types* of pregnancies are riskier than others, such as pregnancies at a very young age (under 16) or older age (over 35), pregnancies of high parity (e.g., beyond the fifth or sixth child); and pregnancies among women with major health problems such as hypertension, diabetes, heart disease, and malaria (National Research Council 1989:32–33). The extent to which these high-risk pregnancies are unequally distributed by social class, urban or rural residence, and other socially differentiating factors alters the likelihood of death or disability in systematic ways. Early motherhood carries especially high risks: girls under age 15 are five to seven times more likely to die in pregnancy and childbirth than are women in the lowest-risk age group of 20–24 (Starrs 1987:15), and two to four times more likely to die than those aged 16–19 (Rinehart and Kols 1984:673). Dangers to maternal health are compounded when two or three high-risk conditions occur simultaneously and when they are associated with poverty, poor nutrition, poor hygiene, illiteracy, and lack of access to medical advice and services. Good socioeconomic and medical conditions can override the negative effects of age and parity (Winikoff and Sullivan 1987:139). Fourth, complications from unsafe abortion currently account for one-quarter to one-half of all maternal deaths in some countries (Starrs 1987:16). Women with unwanted pregnancies face significant risks to their survival and health in countries where legal restrictions or inadequate services force them to resort to unsafe abortion.

What effects would altering the number and timing of pregnancies have on women's survival? Demographers have estimated that about one-quarter of all maternal deaths worldwide could "theoretically" be avoided if women's existing need for family planning could be fully met, that is, if all women wanting to postpone or stop childbearing used contraception (Winikoff and Sullivan 1987:141). Perhaps one-fifth to one-quarter of deaths could be avoided if women in the high-risk age and parity categories did not get pregnant, especially young girls. An additional one-quarter of deaths could be avoided if women with unwanted pregnancies had access to safe abortion services. The remaining deaths occur to women within the so-called *low-risk* pregnancy categories, however, among whom complications cannot usually be predicted. Reducing the number of these deaths requires improvements in the quantity and quality of prenatal and delivery care at the community level together with improved systems for referring complications to more advanced facilities. In addition, of course, safer pregnancy and childbirth depend on basic improvements in women's nutrition, knowledge, socioeconomic conditions, and access to prenatal and delivery care.

Alterations in the timing and number of births have unambiguous benefits for women's health and survival, especially for women who otherwise face the highest maternal risks. Health policies need to address those pervasive inequalities in service delivery that place certain groups of women at severe risk of maternal death or disability. Access to health care is a social *entitlement,* and access to safe and effective family planning is an essential ingredient of this entitlement.

Given this simple conclusion, let us add some complexities. First, the positive health consequences of postponing, spacing, and limiting births must be weighed against the health risks of trying to *prevent* a birth. Second, they must also be weighed against the *social and emotional* costs and benefits to women of using contraception and altering their fertility. Analyzed in the context of women's restricted social and economic opportunities in many societies and of the centrality of childbearing to their personal security, we can see that the pressures for reproductive conformity are often great and the penalties for reproductive failure severe.

PHYSICAL HEALTH RISKS OF SEXUALITY AND BIRTH PREVENTION

Pregnancy, abortion, and childbirth under adverse conditions (and, to a lesser extent, under all conditions) carry risks of death that can be alleviated by having better timed or fewer pregnancies. But having sex and preventing pregnancy can also be physically risky. The concept of *reproductive* rather than *maternal* mortality and morbidity recognizes this broader range of risks.

The major health risk of sexual intercourse is infection from sexually transmitted diseases (STDs). If left untreated, some STDs can result in pelvic inflammatory disease, sterility, ectopic pregnancy, cervical cancer, and even death (Wasserheit 1989). Some STDs also cause miscarriage, stillbirth, low birthweight, premature birth, and congenital infection of the infant, the latter including AIDS. Not only are the health consequences of most STDs more serious for women than for men, but a woman is typically more likely to be infected from a single sexual encounter with an infected male partner than is a man from a woman (Hatcher et al. 1989:96). The prevalence of STDs is surprisingly high among some female populations in southern countries as well as in the north. For example, studies of women in family planning or general health clinics in Africa have found gonorrhea rates as high as 40 percent; in Asia, 12 percent; in Latin America, 18 percent (Dixon-Mueller and Wasserheit 1991:6). Many infected women remain untreated through lack of information, understanding, or capacity to seek medical help.

Practices such as the early initiation of forced or consensual sexual intercourse in young girls, the use of vaginal medications and inserts to treat diseases or heighten the man's sexual pleasure, and female circumcision also contribute to reproductive morbidity. It has been variously estimated that from 10 to 30 million girls and women—mostly in Africa— have undergone genital operations at or before puberty, for example. Procedures range from minor clipping of the external genitals to severe infibulation that can cause painful intercourse and difficulties in childbirth or even death (Koso-Thomas 1987). In addition, girls and women in virtually all societies are subjected to various forms of sexual violence. Physical and sexual assaults of husbands on wives and the incestuous sexual exploitation of young girls within the family are especially difficult to discover and treat because family honor is at stake and outsiders are often reluctant to interfere. In the community at large, the act of rape may be viewed as a manifestation of male power and "entitlement" to the female body. Physical damage resulting from these behaviors is part of the calculus of reproductive morbidity. Psychosocial damage should be considered in the broader definition of reproductive health.

Women attempting to *prevent* pregnancy also confront health risks from some contraceptive methods and from tubal ligation. The decision about which method to use confounds the decision about whether to use a method at all. Which contraceptive is the safest from a health viewpoint, in general and for a particular woman? How is safety weighed against efficacy, that is, against the possibility of an accidental pregnancy? How do the perspectives of medical experts differ from those of women in diverse circumstances who are trying to make rational decisions about their own lives?

The medical and demographic literature contains two types of risk assessment that are relevant here. The first compares the relative risks of mortality and morbidity of different methods of pregnancy prevention (National Research Council 1989:36–52). Whereas all of the hormonal methods (e.g., pills, injectables, implants) plus IUDs and tubal ligation carry some health risks and are contra-indicated for some women, most also have some noncontraceptive health benefits such as preventing the spread of STDs (condoms) or reducing the risk of endometrial and ovarian cancer (the pill; see Lee, Peterson and Chu 1989). Because health effects are difficult to quantify, most comparisons use contraception-related *mortality* to measure relative risk. In the United States, for example, one in 16,000 women on the pill who are smokers dies each year, one in 20,000 women obtaining laparoscopic tubal ligation, one in 63,000 pill users who are nonsmokers, and one in 100,000 IUD users (Hatcher et al. 1989:201). These rates compare with one death in 50,000 resulting from sexual intercourse alone (deaths from sexually transmitted pelvic inflammatory disease), one in 100,000 for a legal abortion between 9–12 weeks gestation, and one in 400,000 (the lowest risk of all) for women terminating pregnancies of less than nine weeks.

Contraceptive methods such as condoms, diaphragms, and vaginal foams carry no mortality risks but their lower efficacy raises the likelihood of accidental pregnancy and maternal death if the pregnancy is continued (e.g., one maternal death in 10,000 live births in the United States). If couples were to use a safe method correctly and consistently, such as a diaphragm with spermicide, condoms, spermicide alone, contraceptive sponge, or even withdrawal, fewer than 5 percent would become accidentally pregnant during the first year of use (Lee, Peterson and Chu 1989:51). But about 20 percent of American couples experience accidental pregnancies using these methods due to imperfect use or method failure. Method failure rates for the pill, IUD, injectables, implants, and female and male sterilization—which allow little room for incorrect use, except for the pill—are 1 to 2 percent or less.

Most of the reliable data on contraception-related morbidity and mortality and on contraceptive failure are drawn from samples in North America and Europe. It is likely that both the adverse health effects of most contraceptives *and* the failure rates are higher for women in southern countries (examples from the Philippines are given in chapter 7) and among low-income women in some northern countries, many of whom face a limited choice of family planning methods, inadequate medical screening, and poor or non-existent follow-up care. The risks of pregnancy-related death or disability are also higher for these women, of course, which leads us to the next comparison.

The second type of relative risk assessment compares contraceptive-related mortality (or morbidity) with the risk of dying from pregnancy, abortion, or childbirth. "Compared with other drugs and surgical procedures and compared with childbearing," runs a typical statement, "family planning methods are safe and free from substantial risk of major complications" (Rinehart and Kols 1984:666). An Egyptian woman is 13 times more likely to die from pregnancy or childbirth than from using the pill, for example; a Thai woman 27 times more likely to die from maternal causes than from using the IUD (IMPACT 1988:20). Not surprisingly, contraception and sterilization almost always look good under these circumstances: the higher are the prevailing rates of maternal mortality, including death from unsafe abortion, the "safer" the contraceptive method appears. Comparisons such as these are often used to justify the health risks of hormonal or surgical procedures for women in developing countries, particularly the use of long-acting, provider controlled methods such as the IUD, hormonal implants, or tubal ligation.

While the argument that contraception is almost always safer than pregnancy and childbirth is technically true, the comparison raises important questions about how the perspectives of medical experts differ from those of women who are trying to decide what to do in their personal circumstances (WHO 1991). When experts minimize the dangers of certain contraceptives on the grounds that they are lower than chidbirth or unsafe abortion, for example, the comparison fails to ask why the risks of childbearing or abortion are so high in the first place and how contraceptive safety and service delivery could be improved. Moreoever, women have very different views from medical experts and from one another on the relative risks of pregnancy, abortion, and contraception in their own life circumstances. For example, how much risk of contraceptive side effects or failure a woman is willing to take depends on the intensity with which she wants to avoid having a child or an induced abortion. For many women, risks that affect her everyday life may be far more pressing than the remote chance of death. Anxiety about going to a family planning clinic, humiliation during a physical examination, a partner's anger, the threat of social criticism, and other concerns make contraception difficult for some women, and perhaps for all women at some point in their lives (Scrimshaw 1976; Bruce 1987). Fears of contraceptive side effects and of possible infertility, whether founded or not, contribute to contraceptive discontinuation or non-use even among women who want to avoid pregnancy. Evidence from 10 southern countries in the late 1970s suggests that from 10 to 30 percent or more of married women of reproductive age who were not using contraception even though they wanted no more children said that fear of contraceptive side effects was the main reason (Schearer 1983:122).

Calculations of relative risks of contraception compared with childbearing point almost invariably to contraception as the "safer" choice. Yet, dying taps only the extreme of physical health and measures of physical health tap only one dimension of the experience of contraception and childbearing. In assessing the overall impact of contraception and fertility on women's lives in diverse circumstances, the whole range of personal experience must be brought to bear.

PSYCHOSOCIAL STRESS AS A HEALTH ISSUE

The physical health benefits of controlled fertility and the health benefits and risks of contraception are fundamentally important to the quality of women's lives. Most research has paid little attention to the broader implications of reproductive behavior for women's health and well-being, however—that is, to their *psychosocial* consequences—as reflected in the way women in differing socioeconomic circumstances feel and talk about themselves and their family and work situations. The discussion becomes more speculative here in the absence of hard data. How might different patterns of childbearing and contraceptive use affect a woman's sense of her own value, for example, which derives in part from her capacity to perform important social roles? Are there circumstances in which contraceptive use and controlled fertility might cause greater psychosocial stress?

Given the evidence on the connections between psychosocial stress and physical health (albeit mostly from industrialized countries; e.g., Monat and Lazarus 1977; Cohen and Syme 1985; Barnett, Biener and Baruch 1987), it is remarkable that the literature on health consequences of contraceptive use and controlled fertility essentially ignores this question (for an exception, see Bogue 1983). Concepts of health and illness are highly culture-bound, of course (Newman 1985; Whelehan 1988). Developing a set of indicators of how women perceive their physical health, let alone their mental health and social well-being, would not be easy. Nevertheless, conceptual and methodological difficulties should not prevent this aspect of women's reproductive lives from being incorporated into theoretical frameworks and research.

Psychosocial stress can manifest itself in at least three types of mental disorder: depression, anxiety, and hostility. Each of these disorders may be related to—or perceived and expressed as—physical disorders, as when a woman anxious about whether she can provide adequate food for her children complains of "dizziness," "headaches," or "nervous exhaustion." Of the three dimensions of psychosocial stress, anxiety is probably the most common disorder that women experience in relation to their sexual and reproductive capacities (Ford 1964). As one review of the cross-cultural literature on pregnancy and childbirth concludes (Harrison 1983:69), "The major, single, unifying theme that runs through both cultural accord and divergence on the subject of childbearing is that the entire experience is not only a time of discomfort but a time of danger, the source of which may be physical or supernatural. In consequence, *it is a time of vulnerability and anxiety,* and the penalties for failure are high'' (emphasis added).

Why does reproduction create such anxiety? One could argue that events or conditions such as the failure to bear a child, the fear of an unwanted pregnancy, or the expectation of ill health from contraceptive use threaten women's perceptions of their ability to perform those essential social roles upon which their survival, security, and well-being depend. The penalities for failure can indeed be high, and they are firmly embedded in the social system.

The relationship between social structures, social roles, gender, and psychological distress has been studied in northern countries (e.g., Barnett, Biener and Baruch 1987). But how does one attempt a comparative analysis? Studying a sample of educated Ghanaian women, Christine Oppong and Katharine Abu (1987) have constructed a framework that is useful for analyzing the impact of contraceptive use and controlled fertility on women's lives (see also Oppong 1983). The framework distinguishes seven social roles which can be examined for their effects *on* reproductive behavior and the ways they are affected *by* reproductive behavior. These are the maternal, occupational, conjugal, domestic, kin, community, and individual roles. Elaborated further below, each of the seven roles involves (1) particular sets of activities, expectations (rights and obligations), and social relationships; (2) different patterns of decision making; (3) the investment of time and other resources; and (4) the possibility of psychosocial and perhaps economic rewards. These various attributes can best be described as *role content*.

In addition, the seven roles in combination represent a *role profile*. Like role contents, role profiles include elements that are common to the social group (however the group is defined) and elements that are unique to each woman. Ascertained through individual interviews or focus group discussions, a role profile reflects a woman's perception of the varied demands made upon her and what aspects of her life she finds most difficult and most satisfying. The profile allows a researcher to identify which roles have the highest priority at any given time in a woman's life cycle, which roles offer the least and the greatest rewards, and which roles constitute sources of strain and conflict.

The concepts of role strain and role conflict are particularly important as potential sources of psychosocial stress. *Role strain* refers to the extent to which a woman feels unable to cope with the demands of a particular social role with the resources at her disposal (for example, time, energy, money, or social networks). *Role conflict* refers to the extent to which a woman perceives the demands of two or more roles as incompatible (for example, working outside the home and caring for young children). In a slightly different formulation, role conflict can also refer to the extent to which people disagree among themselves about the normative content of a particular role, for instance when a mother-in-law and husband (or a husband and wife) hold contradictory views of what it means to be a "good wife." The former definition is more salient to the present discussion.

The seven-roles framework presents a useful analytic approach for investigating the psychosocial consequences to women of contraceptive use and controlled fertility. In every society, reproductive events or conditions such as puberty, menstruation, sexual intercourse, the use or non-use of a contraceptive method, pregnancy, infertility, or the birth or death of a child are charged with personal and social meaning. Indeed, such events often form the object of elaborate social rituals reflecting the depth of a family's or community's investment in reproductive conformity (Paige and Paige 1981). Whether the impact of such events or conditions on women is positive, negative, or neutral should depend on how they transform the content of particular roles in a given structural and ideological context. It follows that reproductive behaviors that *intensify role strain or role conflict*—particularly among those roles that a woman defines as crucial to her security and survival—would be likely to cause the most stress.

Psychosocial stress may be mediated by adaptive or coping behavior, particularly in settings where women can draw on social support networks or on other material and social resources to counter or dilute the negative effects of threatening events or conditions (Cohen and Syme 1985). Intervening mechanisms include relying on interpersonal networks (seeking social support for a decision to terminate a pregnancy, for example), having access to economic resources (being able to give adequate food and shelter to a newborn child, for example), receiving accurate information (such as learning about contraceptive side effects), and controlling outcomes by making structural changes (such as finding a good child care provider). Malay women in rural Brunei were found to rely on three major mechanisms for coping with common stress disorders, for instance: the use of traditional healers, assistance from extended female kin; and religious practices (Kimball and Craig 1988:170).

Despite the ameliorating effects of adaptive strategies, it is probably safe to say that most women in most socioeconomic circumstances are likely to experience extreme stress at some time in their lives that is triggered by sexual or reproductive events or conditions. The resulting psychosocial distress may or may not translate directly into physical disorders. One study of Saraguro Indians of southern Ecuador found that *all* adult women claimed to have suffered from a condition of "nervios," with symptoms that included depression, loss of appetite, sleeplessness, fatigue, and headaches (Fineman 1988). The condition was often triggered by pregnancy, child death or illness, or marital conflict. Poor women in rural El Salvador revealed high levels of psychosocial stress related to (in decreasing order of frequency) excess births, contraception, and miscarriage (Harrison 1983). When we consider that poverty, powerlessness, and physical illness also cause psychosocial stress, we can better understand how certain reproductive events, interwoven as they are with other risks and uncertainties, can engender high levels of emotional disturbance. This is particularly true of low-income women with limited resources.

THE EFFECTS OF FERTILITY REGULATION ON CONJUGAL STRESS

Defining a woman's relationship with her husband, the conjugal role is considered here to include relationships with sexual partner(s), whether in a casual or "visiting" union, a consensual union (cohabitation), or a formal marriage (monogamous or polygamous). Oppong and Abu (1987:58–59) found that educated married women in their Ghanaian sample ranked their satisfaction with their conjugal roles on average *below* their parental, occupational, kin, and individual roles. They also ranked the amount of "role deprivation"—that is, the gap between what they expected of their conjugal roles and what they experienced—as significantly higher than for any other role. Yet women defined the conjugal role as high priority (second only to the parental role) for their social status and personal happiness. The combination of importance and dissatisfaction is a potent one for psychosocial stress.

Patterns of contraceptive use and controlled fertility should have an immediate impact on the conjugal relationship. Some research has attempted to identify qualities of conjugal roles that influence sexual and contraceptive practices and fertility outcomes, such as the effects on contraceptive use of joint or segregated role relationships, male-dominant or more egalitarian patterns of decision making, and female autonomy (Beckman 1983). Few investigators have turned the causality in the other direction. How, for example, do different patterns of *contraceptive use* (including indigenous methods or no method at all) affect a woman's conjugal role performance and the levels of stress associated with her sexual relationship?

Ethnographic literature from both industrialized and developing countries suggests that the conjugal relationship itself is frequently a source of psychosocial stress. Perdita Huston's informal interviews with rural and urban women, both literate and illiterate, in Egypt, Kenya, Sudan, Tunisia, Sri Lanka, and Mexico sometimes elicited ambivalent if not hostile statements from the women about men in general and their own marriages in particular (Huston 1979). These themes also surface in studies of El Salvador (Harrison 1983:59–61), Mexico (Benería and Roldán 1987:127–163), and Jamaica (Brody 1981), among many others. Women's complaints often focus on their husband's or lover's violations of the implicit "terms of trade" of the marital or sexual agreement, such as his excessive physical abuse or authoritarianism, flaunted infidelity, failure to provide financial support, threats of abandonment, or extreme lack of consideration for the woman's feelings.

Contraceptive behavior can also elicit conflict, for a number of reasons. Some conflicts relate to the question of who has the right or the responsibility to use birth control; others relate to manifest or latent disagreements about sexuality, childbearing intentions, or other aspects of the relationship such as women's resentment of men's power and privilege.

For a woman who wants to delay or terminate childbearing, the unwillingness of her partner to use birth control consistently or at all can cause strong feelings of anxiety, depression, or hostility. Wives who received little if any sexual pleasure from their husbands were particularly likely to be resentful about birth control in a study of low-income families in the United States (Rainwater 1960:122–141). Women participating in a study of attitudes toward natural family planning (NFP) in the Philippines complained that it was difficult to get their husbands to cooperate when the men got drunk and became sexually aggressive or lost control (Verzosa, Llamas and Mahoney 1984:76). Fear of unwanted pregnancy may extend to fear of intercourse: from half to three-quarters of women in a Lebanese survey said they had refused their husbands at least once in the past five years for this reason (Chamie 1977:306). Refusing sex poses its own anxieties, however, and some women would never consider it. "What is the good of refusing, they will never let us alone" says a woman in Sri Lanka. "He will go to some other woman and then what will become of me and my children?" (Ryan 1951:376). The anger of some Latin American women who complain of their menfolk, "He uses me," often centers on a man's refusal to practice birth control despite his persistent sexual demands (Shedlin and Hollerbach 1981). A Mexico City study found that a major cause of women's resentment about their marital situation was "a sense of deep depersonalization, humiliation, and physical dissatisfaction caused by their husbands' treatment during sexual relations" (Folch-Lyon, de la Macorra and Schearer 1981:415).

In some circumstances women's negative attitudes toward sexuality and toward their partners could be moderated if the fear of an unwanted pregnancy is removed. Indeed, this should be one of the major psychosocial benefits of contraceptive practice. There is little evidence on the effects of different methods on women's sexual enjoyment and orgasmic capacity, but there is some suggestion that the use of coitus-dependent methods such as withdrawal or the condom may reduce the frequency of intercourse and/or the sexual pleasure of one or both partners as compared with coitus-independent methods (Verzosa, Llamas and Mahoney 1984; Coleman 1981). Women whose husbands can be trusted to practice periodic abstinence or withdrawal consistently tend to express more positive attitudes about the conjugal relationship. The expression "he takes care of me" as compared with "he uses me" suggests far more than relief of anxiety about bearing an unwanted child.

A woman who decides on her own to use birth control—either in accordance with or defiance of her partner's wishes—incurs a different type of stress from the woman who depends on her partner's cooperation. On the positive side, she may feel in control of her body and confident in her ability to determine her own sexual and reproductive behavior. But, depending on the method used and on what she has heard or experienced, her anxieties about real or rumored side effects and about accidental pregnancy can adversely affect her own sense of well-being and the conjugal relationship. Moreover, she may be resentful at having to carry the burden of health risks in order to be sexually available to her partner (especially if she experiences little sexual pleasure herself), or anxious about other effects of contraceptive use on the relationship such as her partner's perceptions of her as "like a prostitute" or "no longer a woman" (Warwick 1982:113). If she uses a method against her partner's will, she may be accused of sexual promiscuity or threatened with violence, desertion, or divorce. The extent to which such threats or experiences become personally devastating depends in part on her access to adaptive mechanisms such as independent economic resources and social support.

The effects of *controlled fertility* on conjugal roles are also pervasive. Postponing the first birth can eliminate the psychosocial stress associated with a premarital pregnancy resulting in an out-of-wedlock birth or a forced marriage in which one or both partners feel trapped, or the stress incurred within marriage by an early birth for which a couple is emotionally or financially unprepared. Similarly, child spacing and limitation may place less stress on the relationship between sexual partners, other things being equal, leaving more time for couple-oriented activities. This should result in less role strain or conflict for women and in higher reported levels of conjugal satisfaction.

In settings where elders in the kin group place a high value on having a child soon after marriage and on having many children, however, a couple's (or woman's) decision to postpone or limit births may produce some anxiety if being a "good" wife conflicts with being a "good" daughter, daughter-in-law, or family member. Moreover, in circumstances where a woman is afraid that her husband or sexual partner might leave her (for example, where she may be unilaterally repudiated through divorce, as in Islamic custom, or when a lover in a visiting union can simply move on to someone else), she may have additional children to bind him more securely to her. In this sense, voluntarily controlled fertility or childlessness could leave women feeling more vulnerable to desertion. Such fears relate not only to the number of children born but also to child survival. As an Egyptian village woman told an interviewer, "Of course it's important to have more than one child. Do you know what my husband did after our first two children died, one after the other? He went to his mother and asked her to find him another wife" (Warwick 1982:109). Less drastically, some respondents in the multi-country Value of Children surveys stressed the importance of children for strengthening the marital bond (Fawcett 1983:437). It is not clear how this effect might be linked to the timing or number of children, however.

In considering how childbearing patterns influence the conjugal relationship and woman's sense of her value as sexual partner or wife, it is often those situations over which the woman has no control that cause the greatest stress. The failure to bear a child at all, or to bear a son, is considered a transgression of the marriage contract in some cultures and a personal misfortune in others. Almost always it is the woman who is blamed. Among the Yoruba of Nigeria, researchers found that many men want to ensure that a woman can become pregnant *before* they marry her (Feyistan and Pebley 1989:353). If a young bride in Iran does not get pregnant right way, her father may be discredited because he has passed on "inferior goods." "Sterility is a broken contract," a researcher explains (Vieille 1978:457). "The young wife who is, habitually and without proof, taken to be responsible for the sterility of the couple, will do everything to change her state: pilgrimages, magic practices, potions. . . ." Sterility—or the failure to bear a son—is first attributed to the woman because people believe that a sexually potent man cannot be sterile (again, a common theme in the literature) or fail to produce sons. Yet, studies in Bangladesh, Singapore, Indonesia, Nigeria, and Brazil have found that male factors are a major cause of infertility in about 25–30 percent of infertile couples and contribute to infertility in another 15–20 percent of cases (Sherris and Fox 1983:127–131). As for the sex of the offspring, the male factor is of course entirely responsible.

Reproductive events can have a dramatic impact on the conjugal relationship, strengthening or undermining it. But in many cases their effects cannot be anticipated. Sexuality, contraceptive behavior, and pregnancy can become fraught with anxiety for a woman who fears that a relationship on which she depends for economic, social, and personal support may be threatened. The sexual imbalance in the attribution of blame for reproductive failure, combined with the centrality of childbearing to the achievement of full adulthood in virtually all societies, creates an especially volatile situation for the stability of the conjugal role.

CHILDBEARING AND OCCUPATIONAL STRESS

As noted in chapter 5, women constitute well over one-third of the world's labor force as formally measured. With increasing proletarianization of the rural workforce, women in rural areas of many southern countries engage in heavy outdoor work for wages in cash or kind, such as laboring in the fields and plantations or carrying earth or bricks. Women in industrial or service jobs tend to be concentrated in small-scale, labor-intensive enterprises not covered by labor laws regulating wages or working conditions. Those who are working in larger industrial and agro-industrial enterprises most often endure hazards such as cotton dust in textile mills, toxic chemicals and fumes, shattering noise on assembly lines, or pesticides in the fields. Although men are also exposed to hazardous working conditions, girls and women experience gender discrimination, sexual harassment, repetitive tasks, job insecurity, low pay, and the difficulties of combining work with pregnancy, childbearing, and caring for young children.

Women's occupational roles offer perhaps the clearest examples of how contraceptive use and controlled fertility can reduce psychosocial stress. Postponing a first birth or spacing and limiting subsequent births (or avoiding childbearing altogether) frees women to pursue job opportunities and advancement—if they are available in the first place—less encumbered by the stress of conflicting child care demands. Anxiety about having to interrupt or terminate employment because of pregnancy can be alleviated by the practice of safe and effective contraception and the availability of safe abortion. Effective contraception introduces an element of choice, or *control*, which is generally associated with lower levels of stress. In an example from the United States, low-income mothers of young children in Boston who participated in a study of family stress reported that the most common reasons for stopping work were events such as pregnancy, birth of a child, or problems with child care arrangements'' (Belle and Tebbets 1982:184). Most of the women associated work with ''confidence, self-esteem, accomplishment, dignity, and independence,'' even if it was not highly skilled. Women who wanted to be working but were *unable* to do so because of child care problems experienced more symptoms of depression than did employed women or those who did not want to be employed.

Whether fertility limitation is actually translated into better occupational performance, lower psychosocial stress, and improved emotional and social well-being depends on the priority a woman places on the occupational role relative to other roles, on the structure of the labor market which determines the demand for her labor and the returns she is likely to earn, and on her class position (economic need), among other factors. The women interviewed by Huston in developing countries perceived themselves, in general, as ''having primary responsibility for the economic well-being of their families . . . *provided that society gives them the opportunity* to participate in income-generating economic activities'' (Huston 1979:147; emphasis added). Indeed, they defined the opportunity to work for pay as of top priority in solving their economic problems, followed by education that would lead to employment, and access to family planning. Whether fertility limitation actually reduces the stress of combining employment with child rearing depends on mediating factors such as the hours and time of day spent at work, locational flexibility of the job, and the availability and cost of acceptable child care.

In certain circumstances, not having enough children or having children of the "wrong" sex may create occupational role strain. Examples include secluded Hausa women in northern Nigeria who prepare foodstuffs in their homes that their children sell door-to-door, or West African women traders or cultivators for whom young sons and daughters may provide essential labor. Occupational stress induced by a shortage of child labor is sometimes resolved by structural changes, however, such as recruiting other family members, hiring wage workers, or adopting (fostering) the children of kinswomen. Moreover, as noted in chapter 5, in some circumstances childrearing may *not* constrain women's labor force participation, as evidenced by the lack of a statistical relationship between fertility and some forms of female employment. Occupations such as home-based manufacturing (crafts) or agricultural work on the family holding, for example, are said to be "compatible" with child care. What is missing from these conclusions, however, is insight into the psychosocial and physical stress women experience when they try to breastfeed an infant or keep track of toddlers while engaging in activities that must constantly be interrupted.

MOTHERHOOD

Perhaps no role presents women with such rewards and anxieties as motherhood. The sample of educated Ghanaian women ranked the maternal role as *highest priority* for their well-being and as most satisfying. At the same time, motherhood was associated with high levels of strain (inadequate resources of time, energy, other resources) and a gap between expectations and reality (Oppong and Abu 1987:58–59). Any parent will identify with the stress as well as the pleasures of rearing children. As a woman interviewed in Mexico remarked, "My children are my greatest source of happiness, but also my greatest worry" (Warwick 1982:113). The theme of women's ambivalence about the maternal role weaves throughout much of the ethnographic literature (Harrison 1983:62–75). Cross-cultural survey research on the value of children suggests that wives often place more importance than husbands do on the social and economic benefits from children, but wives are also more sensitive to the personal costs of raising them (Fawcett 1983:437). The question of interest here is whether contraceptive use and voluntarily controlled fertility might contribute to lower levels of anxiety, depression, or hostility associated with the maternal role.

The psychosocial benefits of contraceptive use and controlled fertility to women who are at high risk of pregnancy-related disabilities or even death are obviously great. These risks may be associated with a woman's personal characteristics, her class position, or the availability of health care services. Women often express fear of disability during pregnancy and of excruciating pain or death in delivery. As Harrison notes (1983:69), "... childbirth is often prolonged and painful, particularly for primiparas [first births], and all societies have developed special techniques for dealing with difficult births." "Fear of pain" she continues, "is accompanied by apprehension about the wholeness and viability of the fetus, about whether fetal presentation will be favorable to an easier birthing, and about survival itself. The ethnographic evidence simply does not substantiate the claim that the fear and pain associated with childbirth is an artifact of Western civilization." Women also express anxieties about miscarriage, stillbirth, birth defects, and infant and child illness and death, all of which have the potential of causing intense emotional distress. Other things being equal, then, controlled fertility should reduce levels of psychosocial stress associated with *becoming* a mother.

The ethnographic literature reveals that women in a variety of social groups are often extremely worried about their ability to provide adequate care for their children, or are depressed by their apparent inability to do so, or hostile about the failure of other persons or institutions to help them. Voluntary postponement of the first birth, longer spacing of subsequent births, and the termination of childbearing at an earlier age should ease the stress of the maternal role by reducing women's anxieties about providing adequate care. In Huston's interviews, for instance, most women considered smaller families (however defined) to be more desirable and identified the availability of modern contraceptives as a positive change compared with their mothers' lives. "In expressing their views about planning their families," says Huston, "the women seemed to be less concerned about themselves than about their ability to provide for their children [especially education for good jobs]. When they did speak about themselves, it was in terms of their health and the fact that child spacing would give them strength (Huston 1979:144).

On the other hand, controlled fertility may not reduce the stress associated with raising children if role expectations escalate with regard to the time or intensity of maternal investment, along with aspirations for children's success. The oft-cited anxieties of Japanese mothers who are preoccupied with their children's academic achievements even before kindergarten is just one example. The nature and severity of the stresses relating to maternal role performance are strongly related to social class and to cultural expectations. Stresses induced by maternal role strain or conflict can be mediated by adaptive mechanisms such as support networks (assistance from a husband or other family members with child care, for example) and structural changes such as fostering a child in from or out to another family (a West African pattern).

FERTILITY REGULATION IN THE DOMESTIC, KINSHIP, AND COMMUNITY ROLES

The *domestic* role refers to women's housekeeping obligations such as cooking, cleaning, washing, shopping, and so on. The Ghanaian women ranked this the second lowest of the seven roles in priority, the lowest in derived satisfaction, and the highest in role strain (Oppong and Abu 1987:58). Household time-use studies in southern countries and from urban samples in northern countries show similar results: women almost always work longer hours than men do and have less time during the day for rest and leisure (Szalai 1972; Goldschmidt-Clermont 1987).

Women throughout the world complain of the stresses of the "double day" when conjugal, maternal, and domestic role expectations are heaped on top of occupational roles with little modification. Among rural Malay women in Brunei, for example, investigators remarked that "Underlying the stress of overwork is the stress of never receiving a reward for one's efforts. After tirelessly working from dawn to dusk, there is always something left undone. The Brunei Malay woman is subject to frequent interruptions. These interruptions produce stress because the woman may then be unable to perform all the necessary tasks of the day, and thus feel *malu,* shame, at not doing all her appointed duties" (Kimball and Craig 1988:174). Women's anger at this state of affairs is often palpable: "I work in the field, opposite the men, seven hours of hard work, and then I go home, and I am required to play the role of a housewife 100 per cent—cooking, cleaning, and washing for the children" (Huston 1979:135). Says another, "I am working outside and inside. I am doing a dual job. Some people think that work is liberation of women. It is not liberation. Sometimes it is just that women are more exploited."

The extent to which controlled reproduction eases the stress of the domestic role depends on many factors, including the number, age and gender of household members, standards of upkeep, and the availability of help from family members or from other relatives, neighbors, or paid workers. Having fewer children and spacing them wider apart should ease the strains of domestic role performance. Yet, as in the case of child care, standards for domestic role performance can escalate with rising incomes and changing tastes. Moreover, the literature on sex preferences and the value of children indicates that most women hope to have at least one daughter even in countries with very strong preferences for boys, partly because girls help around the house more than boys do. Failure to bear a daughter could exacerbate domestic role strain if there are many sons and little help from others.

The *kinship* role refers to a woman's relationship with her affinal and consanguineal kin and, in some cases, with fictive kin (e.g., godparents to herself or her children) upon which much of her social and economic security and survival may depend. Good relations with kin can endow women with considerable satisfaction and self-esteem. The kinship role can also be divisive: a woman may resent her husband's filial obligations to his parents or elders if they interfere with his responsibilities to herself and their children, for example. She may be caught in a dispute between her own and her husband's kin over a dowry or brideprice, or with her husband's brothers over property when she becomes widowed, or with co-wives over the allocation of resources to children in a polygamous marriage. The expectations of kin regarding a woman's contraceptive practices and childbearing may conflict sharply with her own wishes, particularly when elders expect to maintain control over the sexual and reproductive decisions of the younger generation through mechanisms such as arranged marriages and extended household residence. As noted in chapter 1, contradictions such as these form the "stress points" of the patriarchal family system.

The impact of contraceptive use and controlled fertility on a woman's relations with her kin would depend on whether powerful family members support such behavior, ignore it, or criticize it. A woman whose behavior is viewed as deviant may experience considerable stress when she seeks contraceptive services or fails to produce a child, or the socially appropriate number of children, or a son. Such examples are common. A wife interviewed in the Nile delta region of Egypt said, "I stayed four months after marriage without getting pregnant. I was very worried. Everyone was anxious to find out whether I was pregnant or not. Every time I had my period my husband's family talked about me" (Warwick 1982:109). Fulfilling the reproductive expectations of the kin group can bring real satisfaction. The Egyptian woman continues: "My husband's family treated me differently after I had the first child. I felt settled and secure among them. *I became one of them.* They all called me 'mother of Hassan' " (emphasis added).

Women's concerns about who will support and take care of them in their old age could also be included in the consideration of kinship relations, although such concerns are perhaps more specific to maternal and conjugal roles. The absence of sons or daughters who are able and willing to care for an aged parent is likely to strain a woman's relations with her in-laws or other kin who may have to take on the responsibility of her care, willingly or not.

Beyond the kin group, women play a role in *community* relations that may be extensive or limited and of high or low priority, depending on many factors. Community activities include participation in religious and ceremonial events, political meetings, sports and recreation, entertainment, community projects, and general public socializing. Contraceptive use may be stressful or not depending in part on community norms, such as the judgment of religious leaders and the prevalence of contraceptive information and practice in the community. Fertility limitation may or may not ease women's participation in community affairs. It could act in a manner similar to the occupational role, that is, primarily facilitating, or it could diminish community involvement if children form the locus of public socializing. Generalizations are not warranted at this point; what is needed is some attention to the effects of variations in reproductive behavior on women's participation in those community activities they value most.

CONTRACEPTION, REPRODUCTION, AND THE INDIVIDUAL WOMAN

The role of woman as "individual" is considered last because it is so often submerged by other responsibilities. The content of this role includes pursuing personal interests, relationships with friends, and identities relating to women as persons, as individuals, as "themselves." Separating the individual role from other roles is difficult because a woman's self-perception often derives primarily from the performance of her other roles, especially if she has been socialized within a moral framework that ennobles the idea of female self-sacrifice and the abnegation of her individual needs (Papanek 1990:173). The educated Ghanaian women rated the individual role as lower priority on average than their parental, conjugal, occupational, and kinship roles (in that order) but among the most satisfying (Oppong and Abu 1987:58).

How does contraceptive use affect a woman's sense of herself as an individual? Certainly it can contribute to heightened self-esteem where women believe they are now in greater control over their sexuality and reproductive capacity and thus, perhaps, over other aspects of their lives as well. In this sense, effective contraception is a component of self-actualization. Yet, as noted previously, contraceptive use also has psychosocial costs. A woman may think of herself as "unnaturally" or perhaps "sinfully" trying to avoid or terminate a pregnancy, for example. Encounters with service providers often cause emotional distress and lowered self-esteem. Women attending a family planning clinic in Morocco complained bitterly of degrading and dehumanizing treatment by clinic personnel: "If you make a mistake, if you mispronounce a word, the name of a syrup or a pill, the nurse laughs at you, calls her colleagues to tell them the story and points at you. You feel the floor crumble away under your feet" (Mernissi 1975:424). Another woman adds, "When we are waiting to get into a gynecological service, they will shout at us. 'Take off your pants before going into the doctor's office.' You take off your pants in the hall and sit there waiting. There are . . . people walking by. You feel inhuman." Psychosocial stress induced by the act of obtaining birth control services needs to be considered in addition to the stress engendered by their use.

We turn finally to the question of how women's roles as individuals are affected by fertility limitation. Delaying the first birth, spacing subsequent births, and limiting the total number should leave women more time to pursue their individual interests (other things being equal) and, perhaps, to develop a stronger individual identity. This is particularly true of women who avoid childbearing altogether. Yet whether fertility limitation translates into a more individualized role or a more positive or negative self image depends on factors such as the opportunities for individual role behaviors in each society and the relative priority that a particular woman places on the individual role compared to others (particularly, marriage and motherhood) in her role profile.

Where individualized opportunities are plentiful and priorities are high, fertility limitation should reduce role strain and thus the stress engendered by having "no time for myself" or wondering, "who am I?" Yet, marriage and motherhood are highly valued in all societies. Women who remain childless by choice or who have one or two children may be viewed as selfish, irresponsible, or unnatural, while those with larger families are often seen as warm, loving persons who are willing to make sacrifices and take on adult responsibilities (see Rainwater 1960, 1965 for examples from the United States). (Of course, having "too many" children may also be viewed as selfish or irresponsible in some settings.) Women may become anxious about their worth as persons if their reproductive behavior deviates significantly from the social norms of their group. Once again, however, stress can be diluted by the adaptive mechanisms identified previously. In particular, if the environment offers some choice and she has the resources, a woman can seek out those activities and social networks that offer the strongest confirmation of her individual identity.

In sum, the relationship between fertility regulation and women's health takes on different forms and meanings depending on how the "right to health" is defined. Using the narrowest definition of physical health, risks of maternal morbidity and mortality correspond closely to the timing and number of births, to the availability of safe abortion, to variations in socioeconomic conditions, and to the quality and accessibility of maternal health services. *Contraceptive use and controlled fertility are key elements of women's rights to maternal health.*

This simple fertility-health equation is complicated by the physical risks of sexuality and of some methods of pregnancy prevention, however, and by the sociopsychological aspects of sexuality, contraceptive use, and controlled fertility. Consideration of these factors expands the definition in two ways: "maternal" health becomes "reproductive" health, and "health" becomes not only physical but also emotional. As the scope of inquiry widens, the "objective" quantitative evidence becomes scarcer and the "subjective" qualitative observations predominate. Despite the anecdotal nature of many of these observations, they do raise important questions about areas of inquiry that need more systematic analysis. The vantage point also shifts as one moves from the calculus of epidemiologists and other demographic and medical experts to the calculus of women themselves, many of whom are struggling for survival and security within environments of risk and uncertainty. Indeed, the world views could not be more different.

How does this broader definition alter the relationship between reproductive choice and women's health? And what are its implications for population policy and family planning service delivery? In response to the first question, it would seem that, at the very least, relationships become more complex and more unknown (and perhaps unknowable) to the outside observer. The clear statistical association between fertility and health becomes clouded by the many other considerations women bring to bear on their contraceptive and reproductive decisions. The seemingly irrational becomes rational when viewed in the context of the *meanings* women ascribe to sexuality, pregnancy prevention, and childbearing in their own life circumstances. Once again, the analysis suggests that human rights are interconnected: although family planning is a component of the right to health, the health benefits may be sacrificed to behaviors such as early marriage or frequent childbearing that serve women's needs for survival and security in more immediate ways.

The implications of this analysis for population policies and family planning programs are addressed more fully in chapter 8. Essentially, policies and programs need to be more responsive to the realities and diversity of women's lives. Health policies need to address the glaring inequalities in many countries in the provision of basic maternal health care so that becoming pregnant, having a child, or terminating an unwanted pregnancy are not life-threatening conditions. Family planning programs need to address a broader spectrum of reproductive health problems such as women's fears about contraceptive side effects, infertility, and sexually transmitted diseases in a manner that speaks more directly to their concerns. Contraceptive use and controlled fertility are not only health issues but also fundamental economic, social, and personal issues. Medical personnel may know a lot about the former but very little about the latter; professionals are expert in one area and program clients (actual or potential) in another. As Judith Bruce points out (1983), what the woman knows about her own body, her own preferences and fears, and her own life is very different from what the provider knows about contraceptive methods, medical contra-indications, and the mortality risks of pregnancy and birth prevention. The exercise of a woman's reproductive rights requires a fundamental transformation of the provider-client relationship so that both sources of knowledge are brought to bear in the negotiations.

Finally, the psychosocial aspects of contraceptive use and controlled fertility are embedded in the network of economic and social roles on which women's survival, security, and emotional and social well-being depend. Each of these roles involves, in theory, certain individual freedoms and social entitlements that are infringed, in practice, by structures and ideologies of class, caste, and patriarchy. An examination of the impact of family planning on women's rights to health must recognize the denial of women's rights in other spheres.

7

UNNECESSARY DANGER: ABORTION AND WOMEN'S HEALTH IN DEVELOPING COUNTRIES

Perhaps 20 to 25 percent of all recognized pregnancies worldwide are terminated by induced abortion. An estimated 40 to 50 million women obtain abortions every year of which somewhere between 25 and 45 percent are illegal, most of them in developing countries (Henshaw and Morrow 1990:76). Health officials estimate that from one to two hundred thousand women in developing countries die every year from the effects of clandestine abortion (Liskin 1980:110–114; Winikoff and Sullivan 1987:139; Starrs 1987:16). In addition, millions of women suffer physical and emotional anguish and social stigma from their clandestine attempts (whether successful or not) to terminate an unwanted or mistimed pregnancy. In Latin America, where abortion is illegal in most countries on almost all grounds, a Colombian psychologist points out that "women who undergo abortion do so against judge, priest, and generally the family and public opinion, in the face of loneliness and guilt feelings, because this is a dissident act with far-reaching political connotations ... " (Lodoño E. 1988).

Abortion is probably the principal means by which women throughout the world have limited their fertility (Davis and Blake 1956:229). It was widely practiced in Europe and North America during the fertility transition of the nineteenth century. In 1890, doctors estimated that two million abortions were performed in the United States each year, a figure thought to be an underestimate (Petchesky 1984:53). If the current global estimates of 40 to 50 million abortions for the late 1980s are correct, then abortion ranks among the most common methods of family planning along with barrier methods (about 50 million users), the pill (60 million), the IUD (80 million), and male and female sterilization (150 million; see National Research Council 1989:36–52). Viewed in this light, the efforts of abortion opponents to define abortion as *not* a method of family planning, thereby excluding it from any discussion of the right to family planning at international meetings, seem oddly misplaced.

More than two-thirds of all women in southern countries, excluding China, have no access to safe legal abortion. As a consequence, estimates of induced abortion are scarce because most are clandestine. Among countries for which some reliable data are available, proportions of known pregnancies terminated by induced abortion range from under 10 percent in Bangladesh, Tunisia, and Vietnam (and the Netherlands, for comparative purposes), to between 25 and 40 percent in China, Singapore, and Turkey (along with the United States and Sweden, among some other northern countries), to 40 percent or more in Cuba and South Korea (along with Japan, the former Soviet Union, and several Eastern European countries; see Henshaw and Morrow 1990:78).

Abortion rates and ratios differ widely across nations and among social classes depending on factors such as premarital sexual activity and contraceptive use, the frequency of unintended pregnancies among married women, how women and their partners react to these pregnancies, and whether women have access to safe abortion services. Demographic and Health Survey (DHS) evidence from 21 southern countries in the late 1980s reveals that, on average, 22 percent of all married women who were currently pregnant or had a child in the last 12 months said they had wanted the child later but not now, and an additional 17 percent said they had wanted no more children at the time they became pregnant (DHS reports, passim.). In other words, four in every ten recent births or current pregnancies was mistimed or unwanted, ranging from less than two in ten in Mali, to over half in Bolivia, Dominican Republic, Mexico, and Botswana. These figures represent pregnancies that were *not* terminated by abortion, of course, thus underrepresenting the true extent of unwanted pregnancies to an unknown degree. In the United States in 1987 a national survey found that over half of all pregnancies were reported by women as "unintended" and almost half of those were terminated voluntarily (*Wall Street Journal*, March 8, 1990:8).

The thesis of this chapter is that abortion as a method of fertility regulation falls clearly and logically under the rubric of "the right to family planning." Women use abortion like other methods of family planning to regulate the timing and number of their births, that is, to try to ensure that a child is born into circumstances where it will be welcomed and cared for. The provision of safe legal services for voluntary pregnancy termination is an essential ingredient of the personal *freedom* of individuals and couples to determine the number and spacing of their children, and of the social *entitlement* to the information and means to do so safely and effectively. Safe abortion is also an essential ingredient of the right to health. As noted in the previous chapter, safe abortion services could prevent from 20 to 25 percent of the half a million deaths to women that occur worldwide each year from pregnancy-related causes. Safe services could also prevent widespread reproductive damage resulting from botched clandestine procedures which require costly emergency hospitalization. It is difficult to understand how the refusal of many governments and medical practitioners to consider legalizing the termination of unwanted pregnancies can be justified when viewed side-by-side with their professed concern with protecting women's lives and health.

ABORTION AS A METHOD OF FAMILY PLANNING

Throughout the ages and in virtually all societies, women have used a variety of methods—effective or not—to prevent or destroy unwanted conceptions or births (Himes [1936] 1970; Devereux 1976). Indigenous and modern techniques can be arrayed on a spectrum from prevention to "cure," such as abstaining from sexual intercourse during presumably fertile periods; having sexual relations without vaginal penetration; using magical incantations or herbal potions to prevent conception or induce menstruation; suppressing ovulation with breastfeeding or hormonal treatments; blocking the passage of sperm by practicing coitus interruptus or using chemical or mechanical barriers; altering the uterine environment with mechanical devices or contragestive drugs; obtaining surgical sterilization; inducing miscarriage or having an abortion; and killing an unwanted infant or letting a child die. The act of preventing conception is clearly distinguishable in a scientific sense from the act of destroying the conceptus or developing fetus. But the sharp legal and moral distinction that some experts have made between them seems to impose an artificial duality on what has historically been—for many women—a more graduated approach to fertility regulation.

The ethnographic and demographic literature suggests that the crucial distinction for women in many societies is not between regulating fertility before or after a conception has occurred but between having or not having a surviving child. With the knowledge at her disposal, each woman may be said to look (consciously or not) for a method of family limitation that has the least negative impact on her life in a given socioeconomic context (Rogow 1990). Conception has not always been the "cut-point" in this regard. Women in pre-industrial Europe took their herbal potions before or after a missed period; it was "animation" or "quickening" rather than "conception" that had meaning for them (ibid.; Petchesky 1984:29–30). Even a live birth may not be the event that fully defines life: in some societies, a newborn child is not considered a full member of society until it has passed through a ritual presentation or naming ceremony some days or months later. The widespread practice in eighteenth- and nineteenth-century France of abandoning infants to foundling homes or sending them to the countryside for wetnursing (from which few returned) demonstrates the use of disguised infanticide—in addition to abortion—among the working and middle classes (Petchesky 1984:45–49). It is possible that the higher mortality risks of infants born "too early, too late, too many, or too close" that have been identified in studies of child survival also represent to some degree the effects of disguised infanticide resulting from the pregnancy having been unwanted (Scrimshaw 1978). A study in rural Thailand, for instance, found that children wanted by one or neither parent were twice as likely to die during their first year as children wanted by both parents, after other factors influencing child survival were statistically controlled (Frenzen and Hogan 1982:402).

The distinction between contraception and abortion becomes especially blurred when we consider that women in virtually all societies know about and use a variety of methods for "removing female irregularity" or "bringing down the period." An astonishing array of "menstrual-inducing recipes"—as distinct from abortifacients—has been identified throughout the world in studies of indigenous fertility-regulating methods (Jöchle 1974; Musallam 1983; Newman 1985). Botanical agents include (among others) preparations of pineapple, crocus, mungbean, banana, cinnamon, chamomile, thyme, celery juice, parsley, and lemon. Some women take quinine pills, extra oral contraceptives, estrogen or projesterone injections, various over-the-counter pills, and other medications in an attempt to induce menstruation. More drastic measures such as inserting leaves, roots, catheters, or sticks into the uterus, massaging the abdomen, or taking more dangerous substances (many of which are life-threatening poisons) may be resorted to if milder methods fail and the woman is determined to induce bleeding. These latter extremes are more clearly intended to cause miscarriage, however, whereas the former "recipes" are emmenagogues—that is, menstrual inducers—of ambiguous interpretation.

Whether menstrual regulation (MR) is a deliberate euphemism for abortion or is simply perceived as a means of ensuring a "healthy" or "non-pregnant" state depends in part on perceptions in different cultures regarding the possible causes of a delayed period, when a pregnancy is determined, and when life begins. As Rosalind Petchesky points out (1984:29), "The very concept of an abortion is a particular way of constructing an event whose boundaries and content have differed in different situations. Can we always identify the markers on the continuum between a 'spontaneous' abortion and one that is 'helped along,' or between the latter and a whole series of possible interventions through different means and at different points during a pregnancy?" Can we even identify the markers between methods of regulating fertility and of maintaining good health? Women in most countries tend to view menstruation as "a natural, vital, physiological occurrence indicative of good general health" (WHO Task Force 1981:13). In many cultures the monthly period is widely believed to rid the body of "bad blood" and "poisonous wastes"; thus, its absence or "stoppage" could lead to (or be a sign of) serious illness. The possible causes of a delayed period and the ways women may interpret them are revealed in a study of indigenous fertility regulation methods in Cali, Colombia. "For most Latin women," concludes anthropologist Carole Browner, "delayed menstruation is an ambiguous sign: it may indicate pregnancy, a natural change in body state, or a potentially harmful *atrazo* (menstrual delay)" (Browner 1985:105). The *atrazo,* in turn, may be caused by accumulated impurities in the menstrual blood or the womb, among other possibilities. Thus, having regular menstrual periods is a reassuring sign of reproductive health. "Since it is difficult to distinguish a late period from an early pregnancy," Browner continues, "unwanted pregnancies may be surreptitiously terminated through use of privately administered remedies. Women find this an effective and culturally acceptable method to practice fertility control" (Browner 1985:118).

The practice of menstrual induction may not be considered abortion at all. Among rural Chinese in Malaysia, for example, "When a 'pregnancy' is to be 'prevented' from occurring, a woman may 'induce her menses' to ensure her 'nonpregnancy'.... When menstrual flow resumes, she is no longer ill or pregnant.... To the woman ... an abortion can take place only after the fetus is formed, which in local beliefs may take up to two months after a missed menses" (Ngin 1985:27, 35). Similarly, some women in Afghanistan—as elsewhere—believe that terminating a pregnancy before the unborn child has a "soul" is not abortion. Indeed, the Hanafi school of Islamic jurisprudence distinguishes between menstrual induction "prior to ensoulment" of the fetus, which is permissible, and abortion, which is not (Hunte 1985).

WHEN ABORTION IS NECESSARY OR PREFERRED

The question of whether a particular pregnancy is wanted or not is also better represented by a continuum rather than a dichotomy. A pregnancy may have been wanted at the time of conception but become unwanted later because of changed circumstances. It may have been wanted by one partner but not the other, or by neither or both, or wanted later but not now (Hass 1974; Luker 1975). A woman who wanted to become pregnant may resort to abortion because she simply cannot have the child in her current circumstances. An unwanted pregnancy may become a wanted child, accepted and even welcomed despite its inauspicious beginnings. Some unwanted pregnancies result from unwanted intercourse (rape, incest, emotional or physical coercion), some from unprotected intercourse, others from contraceptive failure. Abortion may be a man's decision with little regard for the woman's wishes, or a parent's decision made for a daughter whose illegitimate pregnancy threatens the honor of the family as well as her future marriageability. A woman may seek independently to terminate her pregnancy despite her partner's (or the state's or church's) insistence that she bear the child. Abortion in this context represents her ultimate veto of patriarchal or state authority as well as a personally desperate act.

Under what conditions are women most likely to terminate a pregnancy with induced abortion? In a 1975 study of 108 women living in three working-class barrios in Cali, Colombia, who had at least one pregnancy that they described as unwanted at the time of conception, most women reported that it was the response of the lover or husband that was the major determining factor in their decision (Browner 1979). Most critical was the question of whether the man was willing to accept social and financial responsibility for the child and whether the relationship appeared stable. Abortion is illegal in Colombia except to save a woman's life. Yet of 123 unwanted pregnancies in the sample, 44 were aborted either spontaneously or with the use of folk remedies, 42 were terminated by surgical intervention, and 37 resulted in live births. Only 28 women made no attempt to interrupt the pregnancy. Women who used major or multiple minor interventions (half of the sample) were significantly more likely to be under 25 years of age, to be single or separated, to be experiencing their first pregnancy, and to have been using a contraceptive when they became pregnant.

Studies in other social settings would reveal different configurations of events than those described for the women of Cali (e.g., Kabir 1989; Mashalaba 1989). Nevertheless, some generalizations pertain. In general, recorded abortion rates are higher in urban areas of developing countries and among the better educated, where knowledge and access are likely to be greater (Liskin 1980). Most illegal abortions in southern countries are performed on married women with several children who wish to stop childbearing or postpone the next birth. This pattern is typical of India, Bangladesh, Singapore, and other Asian countries, as well as Eastern Europe (Henshaw and Morrow 1990). The pattern of young, unmarried women wanting to delay the first birth is more common in North America and Western Europe, with Latin American and African patterns typically falling somewhere in between. Although the *proportion* of all pregnancies that are unwanted and the proportion of unwanted pregnancies interupted by abortion are significantly higher among unmarried women, the absolute numbers are higher for married women.

With changing sexual norms and delayed marriage, rates of unwanted pregnancies among single women are rising rapidly in many southern countries. The phenomenon is particularly visible in sub-Saharan Africa where the typical patient admitted to an urban hospital for complications of clandestine abortion is likely to be young, usually unmarried, often a student, with no previous births (Liskin 1980:142). In Mali, for example, only 18 percent of women admitted to hospital for the treatment of complications from induced abortion in 1981–82 were married compared with 86 percent of women admitted for treatment of spontaneous abortion (Binkin et al. 1984:9). Four of every ten women admitted for induced abortion were students and 62 percent were reported as having major complications. In Thailand, a 1978 survey of rural providers estimated that at least 300,000 illegal abortions were performed that year. Almost half of the rural practitioners who were interviewed stated that they served mostly single women (Narkavonnakit 1979:227). Problems of unwanted pregnancy and illegal abortion are particularly severe for adolescents. According to two Latin American physicians, "They have less social support, greater doubts, less financial capacity to pay for an interruption and take longer to realize that they are pregnant. Consequently, they have more severe complications, a high rate of infection, and greater risk of mutilation and death" (Pinotti and Faúndes 1989:98).

Abortion is a necessity for some women and a preferred method of family planning for others. International fertility surveys have shown that many couples who are not contracepting do not want to have a child right away. Many of these women are candidates for abortion if they become pregnant. Some get pregnant while believing they are safe because they are breastfeeding or for other reasons; others are ambivalent about using contraceptives or have discontinued using them because of inaccurate or misunderstood advice, experience with side effects, or fears of future illness or infertility. In addition, high rates of contraceptive failure typical of some methods and population subgroups underscore the need for safe abortion as a backup. In the Philippines, for example, a sample of pill users experienced a pregnancy rate of 19 percent during the first year of use despite a "theoretical" method failure rate of well under 1 percent (Laing 1984). Four percent of IUD users become pregnant during the first year of use, 33 percent of those using periodic abstinence (NFP), 44 percent using withdrawal, and 60 percent using condoms. Demographers have estimated that the rate of accidental pregnancies among contraceptors can be anywhere from under 1 percent to over 50 percent in a given population depending on which contraceptives are most commonly used and how effectively. "Given the reality of contraceptive practice," concludes one review, "one is faced with the problem of contraceptive failure on a rather large scale. Thus, the requirement for [maternal] health care services (prenatal care, delivery, and abortion services) is raised directly by the needs of the women who have *accepted* family planning, as well as by the majority who have not" (Winikoff and Sullivan 1987:136; emphasis added).

Abortion is not only *necessary* as a backup for contraceptive failure or non-use, it is also a *preferred* method of family planning for some women. Depending on a woman's personal circumstances, abortion can offer several advantages over contraception (Davis and Blake 1956; Rogow 1990). First, abortion permits the greatest control over the timing of childbearing: it allows a woman to decide about a pregnancy if and when she is actually pregnant. Second, as a curative rather than preventive method its outcome is more certain than a contraceptive that may or may not be effective or even necessary. Third, a woman can in theory use abortion without the knowledge of her sexual partner, which is not true of all contraceptive methods. Fourth, some women may also prefer abortion if they are afraid to contracept or afraid to ask their partner to contracept. Fifth, in some settings "bringing down the period" or inducing a miscarriage may seem more natural to a woman than taking a pill every day, getting periodic injections, having a device inserted into her uterus or under the skin, or being surgically sterilized. Sixth, where abortion is properly performed within the first 12 weeks of pregnancy the resulting mortality rate is lower than for other family planning methods such as the IUD, tubal ligation, or hormonal methods (Hatcher et al. 1989:201). A sexually active woman might rationally choose a barrier method with early abortion by trained providers as a backup because, *in combination,* they offer the safest method of preventing an unwanted birth.

Many women also prefer abortion over contraception at certain points in their lives because of conflicting social norms and sexual relationships. Some young single women want to avoid the dilemma of being contraceptively "prepared" for sexual encounters that they or others may consider immoral. Getting pregnant with the option of safe termination enables a woman to test her own fecundity or to test her partner's commitment to maintaining the relationship and raising a child (Luker 1975). For all of these reasons, some women will continue to prefer abortion over contraception, at least at some point in their lives, and in some personal circumstances.

Will the demand for abortion among women in southern countries fade as contraceptive services become more widely available? This assumption is probably based less on hard evidence than on wishful thinking. First, the percentage of couples who are protected by "modern" methods of contraception and sterilization remains extremely low in many countries among the poor, the young, the less educated, and those living in rural areas. Many women and their partners cannot hope to have access to effective contraceptive information and services for years to come, especially given the rapid growth in populations of reproductive age who need services. Second, as family size desires change and women are increasingly motivated to space or limit their births, more pregnancies will be mistimed or unwanted. The risk of contraceptive failure also rises as women spend less of their reproductive years pregnant or breastfeeding and more time trying to prevent a pregnancy. Third, the experience of northern countries shows that the demand for abortion often remains high among some subgroups even given widespread contraceptive availability and generally effective use. In France in the early 1980s there were about 15 legal abortions each year for every 1,000 women in the age group 15 to 44; in Sweden, 18 to 20; in Denmark, 20; in Japan, about 22; in the United States, 24 to 29 (Tietze and Henshaw 1986:30–42). These figures represent about 22 to 40 abortions for every 100 live births. Fourth, the demand for abortion often *rises* along with contraceptive use, and where it falls, as in Chile, it is never eliminated (David 1983). As the 40 to 45 percent of the total population of many developing countries now under 15 years of age enters its reproductive years and desired family size continues to drop, the number of abortions attempted is likely to increase. The key policy question is whether women must continue to risk their lives in order to regulate their own fertility or whether they will be offered safe and affordable services.

LEGAL AND PROGRAMMATIC RESTRICTIONS ON SAFE ABORTION

As noted in chapter 2, widespread legal prohibitions in Western Europe and North America banning all but medically indicated abortions were largely a feature of laws and statutes adopted in the nineteenth century. By 1900 the general legal prohibition against abortion had spread throughout the colonies of European powers as well as China and Japan. Then, slowly and unevenly, a few European countries began to liberalize their laws beginning in the 1930s, with a significant groundswell in the 1950s in Eastern and Central Europe. Since the 1960s there has been a pronounced liberal trend in abortion laws (as well as in divorce legislation) in Europe and North America, primarily as a response to an intensified concern with women's health, women's rights, and social justice (Field 1983; Cook 1989a). In most cases eligibility for abortion has been extended from total prohibition or medical emergency (saving the life of a pregnant woman) to broader maternal health grounds. Some northern countries have also extended eligibility to social or socio-medical indications such as serious economic difficulties or personal distress. Others such as the United States, Canada, and Sweden have made abortion available to women on request within the first trimester subject to restrictions to licensed practitioners or facilities. By 1990, only Ireland among all northern countries limited abortion to saving a woman's life, while 15 countries (that is, over half) offered some form of abortion on request (Henshaw and Morrow 1990:77). The remainder permit abortion at least on health grounds and in cases of fetal deformity and rape or incest, if not on broader social or socio-medical grounds.

The contrast between the north and south in the availability of legal abortion is stunning. Many developing countries have maintained restrictive codes long after their former colonizers liberalized their own laws. Compared with only one northern country, over 50 southern countries prohibit abortion entirely or permit it only *in extremis,* including at least 21 in Africa, 16 in Asia, and 14 in Latin America and the Caribbean (Henshaw and Morrow 1990:77). *One-third of all women in the developing world live in countries where abortion is essentially illegal on all grounds* (see Appendix D). Ironically, these are often countries in which women face the highest risks of death or disability from childbirth. At the other end of the continuum, a number of southern countries have liberalized their laws. The most permissive states are Togo, Tunisia, China, Singapore, Turkey, Vietnam, Cuba, and Puerto Rico, where abortion is available on request with certain qualifications, and Burundi, Zambia, India, Taiwan, the Democratic Republic of Korea, and Uruguay, where it is available on broad social or socio-medical grounds (ibid.).

The legal status of abortion tells only part of the story, of course. Abortion is widely practiced in some countries with restrictive laws, while in other countries only a small minority of eligible women have access to safe services despite more permissive legal codes. In the middle range, abortions that are technically allowed for maternal health reasons or in cases of rape or incest may be rarely or frequently performed depending on how individual practitioners and other moral, legal, and medical "gatekeepers" interpret such provisions.

The category of *restrictive* regimes includes a number of "lapsed law" countries such as Mexico, Colombia, Brazil, Egypt, Nigeria, and Indonesia where abortion is nominally illegal but, according to observers, is readily available (sometimes with the acquiescence of the government) for those who can afford to pay (Camp 1987). Physicians, midwives, and other trained professionals in addition to untrained practitioners and quacks offer their services in private offices, clinics, a borrowed space, or someone's home despite the threat of criminal penalties. Prior to the liberalization of abortion in the Republic of Korea in 1971, for example, a household survey estimated that about 100,000 illegal abortions were performed in Seoul that year, a ratio of 750 per 1,000 live births (Hong and Tietze 1979:161). Estimates of the annual number of clandestine abortions in Brazil range from 1.4 to 2.4 million, as noted in chapter 4, with 400,000 women hospitalized in 1990 for incomplete or septic procedures. In Indonesia estimates range from 750,000 to one million illegal procedures annually (Jacobson 1990:31); in Colombia, perhaps 280,000 (Isaacs, Holt and Hill 1990:38).

As was the case in the United States prior to the decriminalization of abortion in 1973, governments and local law enforcement agencies often close their eyes to known violations unless they are forced to prosecute because of a formal complaint or a woman's death. As a consequence, criminal penalties are rarely if ever imposed. Clients themselves are often unaware that they are breaking the law. The 1971 Seoul survey found that approximately 30 percent of respondents did not know that abortion was illegal at that time (Hong and Tietze 1979:161). Similarly, a 1976 survey of women in five villages in the Philippines found that 57 percent believed that abortion was legal and only 4 percent were unsure, when in fact abortion was illegal on all grounds (Flavier and Chen 1980:70). Despite the rarity of prosecutions, however, it is important to emphasize that criminalization of abortion creates a climate of fear, subterfuge, profiteering, discriminatory and restricted access to safe medical procedures, and unnecessary danger, disability, and death for those who cannot afford to buy safe services.

Even in countries with more *permissive* legislation, safe services are sometimes unavailable to the majority of women. India offers the most vivid example of this shortfall. Abortion has been allowed in India on broad medical and social grounds since the Medical Termination of Pregnancy (MTP) Act was passed in 1971. But, MTPs may be performed only in approved institutions by authorized physicians. More than a decade later, in a country with over 160 million women of reproductive age, only 4,600 medical facilities and fewer than 15,000 physicians had received official approval (Tietze and Henshaw 1986:27). This bureaucratic bottleneck has made it impossible for the formal health system to handle the demand. Despite the increase in legal abortions, illegal abortions were estimated at 4 to 6 million yearly because of the shortage of approved hospitals and personnel (Liskin 1980:135).

Bangladesh presents a unique example of a restrictive abortion law combined with a permissive policy that provides menstrual regulation services on request in government clinics within 8 to 10 weeks of a woman's last menstrual period (Dixon-Mueller 1988). MR is not considered abortion because it is done early, without a pregnancy test, as a means of bringing on the period and ensuring that the woman is in a "healthy, non-pregnant state." This interpretation follows some schools of Islamic thought in which terminating a pregnancy before the fetus takes on "human form" is not forbidden. It also supports the indigenous practices of women who attempt to "wash out the uterus" or "clear the period" with various herbal remedies when an unwanted pregnancy is suspected.

The Bangladesh law permitting MR is based primarily on concerns for women's health. In 1978, a national study estimated that almost 800,000 illegal abortions were done that year resulting in the deaths of almost 8,000 women and untold misery to thousands of others (Measham et al. 1981). As is typical of many southern countries, about half of all admissions to gynecology units of major urban hospitals were for abortion complications, as were about one-quarter of pregnancy-related deaths. In 1979, the Government of Bangladesh declared that early menstrual regulation by vacuum syringe would not be subject to the penal code restricting abortion. By the mid 1980s, a nationally representative survey of MR providers in governmental and non-governmental facilities estimated that perhaps 240,000 MRs (as distinct from abortions, which remained restricted to life-threatening cases) were performed yearly in addition to approximately 200,000 illegal abortions (Begum, Kamal and Kamal 1987; Khan et al. 1986). Clinic records show that at least one-quarter of potential clients come too late for legal MR, however, which cannot be performed later than 10 weeks because of the limitations of the hand-held vacuum syringe. Many of these rejected women subsequently resort to clandestine abortion, which is especially dangerous in the second trimester. In addition, women who have *no* access to MR services in rural areas not yet served by trained providers continue to use traditional unsafe methods.

Bureaucratic regulations in many countries and programs also restrict women's access to safe services where abortion is permitted on health or social grounds (Isaacs, Holt and Hill 1990). The written permission of a husband or guardian may be required. A woman may be required to obtain authorization from two or even three doctors, or a gynecological specialist, which is virtually impossible for all but a privileged few in countries where physicians are scarce (e.g., Turkey). Often only hospitals are licensed to perform abortions. The liberal abortion law of Zambia, for instance, which permits abortion up to 12 weeks on broad health and socio-medical grounds, requires approval by three medical practitioners, including one specialist. Yet in 1975 there was only one physician in Zambia for every 10,000 inhabitants (Liskin 1980:142). It is impossible for all but a tiny minority of women to negotiate the bureaucratic maze or even to obtain an abortion once permission is granted. Consequently, illegal procedures greatly outnumber legal ones (Jacobson 1990:15).

The cost of legal abortions performed in hospitals and private clinics can also be prohibitive unless there are subsidies for low-income clients. In the Republic of Korea, a typical charge for a first-trimester legal abortion in Seoul in 1977–78 represented about 10 percent of the monthly earnings of a construction laborer, and for a second-trimester procedure up to 35 percent (Hong and Tietze 1979:161). Where abortions are illegal, however, clandestine practitioners (especially physicians) charge fees in equivalents of hundreds of dollars.

In a 1988 symposium in Rio de Janeiro on unwanted pregnancies, two medical experts concluded that because the risks of abortion result not from medical factors but from its illegality, "the logical step to prevent deaths among women who have an unwanted pregnancy is to decriminalize abortion" (Pinotti and Faúndes 1989:101). The legalization of abortion on request without bureaucratic obstacles is undoubtedly a *necessary* condition for the provision of safe services to all women who need them. It is clearly not a *sufficient* condition, however. Shortages of facilities and trained providers, programmatic restrictions, and the reluctance or refusal of some health professionals to perform abortions, combine to block women who meet the legal conditions of eligibility from obtaining safe services in many countries.

According to one legal analyst, a major problem in countries with permissive legislation is that governments "are almost invariably reluctant to place health professionals and facilities under *positive duties* to perform abortions" where the procedure is legal (Cook 1989a; emphasis added). The United States experience is a case in point: in 1982, abortions were provided in only 26 percent of all non-Catholic general hospitals and 16 percent of public hospitals (Tietze and Henshaw 1986:121). About one-third of these facilities performed fewer than two abortions per week. In more restrictive regimes, governments are also generally reluctant to clarify through their executive, legislative, or judicial branches the precise conditions under which abortions *can* legally be performed (Cook 1989a). In these cases, women who do meet eligibility requirements, such as those who are pregnant as a result of rape or incest, or for whom the pregnancy or birth poses medical problems, are often not served because medical professionals (and the courts, if they become involved) are reluctant to take the risk in what they perceive as a "chilling" political environment. In *both* permissive and restrictive regimes as well as in the intermediate ranges, then, the structure of health care delivery systems and the training and attitudes of health care providers are vitally important to the provision of safe services.

THE MEDICAL ENVIRONMENT: ACCESS, SAFETY, AND TECHNIQUE

Despite international initiatives promoting primary health care, family planning, child survival, and safe motherhood, many women in developing countries are marginalized by vertically structured medical institutions— most of them concentrated in urban areas—that pay little attention to their general reproductive health needs (Germain 1987). Problems of overall scarcity of medical facilities and personnel are often compounded by the maldistribution of resources in ways that deny access to basic care to a majority of women, especially the young, the poor and less educated, and those in rural areas. Only half of all births to women in southern countries in the mid 1980s were attended by trained personnel, for example (including midwives), and in many countries fewer than one-third of pregnant women visited a trained health worker at least once before childbirth (WHO 1985).

It is widely acknowledged that stronger community-based health care systems are needed to remedy these deficiencies (Starrs 1987; Black 1988). The community-based approach to women's reproductive health relies heavily on paramedical personnel such as family planning workers, village health workers, and nurse-midwives for birth control counseling and services, identification and treatment of common reproductive tract infections, basic prenatal and postnatal care, midwifery, and referral of women with high-risk pregnancies to advanced medical facilities. Community-based programs counteract the tendency to over-medicalize birth control and childbearing in high-technology centers serving a limited clientele and help to overcome clients' fears of seeking treatment. Paramedical personnel are essential where physicians are scarce and are important under all circumstances. When properly trained, they are usually more effective providers of basic health care because they are closer to their clients in social background and more familiar with the everyday needs and concerns of the people they serve (Beeson et al. 1987). Paramedical personnel may also specialize in tasks that physicians consider of little challenge and low prestige. These tasks often constitute the "dirty work" of a profession; considered degrading or morally questionable, they are allocated to others unless they bring profit or some other reward (Joffe 1986). The termination of unwanted pregnancies is one of these tasks.

From the medical viewpoint, the termination of a suspected pregnancy within the first few weeks of a missed period by vacuum aspiration of the uterine lining is safe and relatively simple. Prior to 1970, the medical profession relied primarily on the technique of dilation and curettage (D&C) using sharp instruments to scrape the walls of the uterus after a missed period. The development in the late 1960s of the Karman syringe and flexible cannula—a simple and cheaply produced hand-held plastic instrument—allowed the "induction" or "extraction" of the menses by vacuum aspiration of the uterine lining. The no-touch technique, which reduces the risk of infection, is relatively easy to perform and has low complication rates when done early (van der Vlugt and Piotrow 1973:15–18). Menstrual regulation by these mechanical means can be performed without anesthesia or sedation by trained paraprofessionals on an outpatient basis in about five to ten minutes. (The special case of contragestive agents such as RU 486 is discussed below.) In Bangladesh the majority of MRs are performed by female paramedics (Dixon-Mueller 1988). The technique can also be used as a diagnostic tool in cases of excessive uterine bleeding, and for treating women with potentially life-threatening incomplete abortions, either induced or spontaneous, if the pregnancy is of short gestation. The availability of MR services at the primary health care level thus contributes to the reduction of reproductive morbidity and mortality in at least three ways. In addition, it acts as an entry point into the health and family planning systems for many first-time clients.

The risks of abortion rise steeply with the duration of pregnancy. Early vacuum aspiration by hand-held syringe (up to 10 weeks since last menstrual period, or LMP) or electric aspiration pump (up to 12–13 weeks) is far safer than the sharp curettage of D&C (up to 16 weeks) and the saline injections and other medical methods used to induce miscarriage in advanced cases. Practitioners need more skills and training for more advanced pregnancies, complications occur more frequently, and general anesthesia—a potential cause of death in itself—is used more often. In the United States in the early 1980s, for example, deaths per 100,000 legal abortions rose from 0.2 at eight weeks or less LMP to 0.3 at 9 to 10 weeks, 0.6 at 11 to 12 weeks, 3.7 at 16–20 weeks, and 12.7 at 21 weeks or more (Henshaw and Morrow 1990:81). (These figures compare with 6.6 deaths per 100,000 live births from maternal causes excluding abortion and ectopic pregnancy.) About one-quarter of abortion deaths in the U.S. resulted from the use of general anesthesia rather than from the procedure itself.

The illegality of abortion greatly increases its risks. Not all illegal abortions are unsafe, of course: depending on the country and the social class of the client, many may be performed under hygienic conditions by physicians or trained midwives in private clinics. This "medicalization" of illegal abortion reduces maternal morbidity and mortality, but safe procedures are usually available only for a small minority of women who can afford them. In general, clandestine abortions are associated with high risks of female death and disability because most are self-induced or performed by unskilled practitioners using crude methods. Where abortion is subject to criminal penalties, even practicing physicans often lack the necessary training and use outmoded methods such as sharp curettage for early procedures. Death rates from illegal abortion in developing countries can reach as high as 400 per 100,000 procedures, according to some estimates, compared with 6 deaths per 100,000 procedures where abortion is legal (Sai and Nassim 1989) and only 0.6 deaths per 100,000 procedures in 12 northern countries with permissive abortion laws (Henshaw and Morrow 1990). Illegality also makes it more likely that abortion complications and deaths will be undercounted in official statistics because they are attributed to spontaneous abortion or some other cause. The dangers of illegal abortion can be up to 100 times greater than those of legal abortion. As one panel of experts concluded in recommending reform, "Nowhere else in health care can such a marked change be brought about

by a single legal/administrative decision; that is, in no other area can legal
change reduce individual health risk to 1% of its alternative level'' (Cook
and Senanayake 1978:16).

Of special relevance to women in developing countries are the short-
term and long-term complications—both physical and emotional—resulting from clandestine procedures. Common physical complications include incomplete abortion requiring evacuation of the uterus, pelvic
infection that may cause infertility from scarring, hemorrhage, shock,
poisoning, tetanus, and damage to the pelvic organs from mechanical or
chemical inserts or from heavy abdominal massage (Liskin 1980:113). The
emotional costs include social isolation, panic about what to do, fear of
the procedure itself, anxiety about health consequences, resentment of
the sexual partner, fear of discovery, and shame and humiliation. Where
safe abortion is illegal or inaccessible, the time spent experimenting with
folk remedies and then searching for a skilled provider elevates the danger
of complications as the pregnancy becomes more advanced. Followup
care is generally nil. Women who experience infection, heavy bleeding,
or severe pain after an illegal procedure are often reluctant to seek medical
help because they believe they have committed a crime. Those who wait
too long suffer or die without treatment, while those who do seek medical
help are often treated with impatience or contempt in maternity wards
crowded with other victims of botched or incomplete abortions.

Both the *risks* to women's lives and health and the unnecessarily high
costs of treating abortion complications through emergency hospitalization could be significantly reduced by providing early, safe services on
an outpatient basis. The argument that medical resources in many southern countries are too limited to provide safe abortion must be weighed
against the evidence of the costs in hospital space, physicians' time,
emergency blood supplies, and other resources of providing emergency
services. A hospital study in Thailand in 1977–78 found that women seeking treatment for complications from abortions induced outside the hospital (80 percent of which were self-induced or performed by nonmedical
personnel) were hospitalized on average 2.2 days but sometimes up to a
week or more, compared with 0.2 hospital-days on average for women
obtaining abortions within the hospital on an outpatient basis (Chaturachinda et al. 1981:260). Safe early abortion is cost-effective not only relative to the treatment of septic abortion but also relative to some other
methods of birth prevention. For instance, a study of MR services provided in clinic settings by paramedical personnel in the Bangladesh Wom-
en's Health Coalition found that the cost of an ''adjusted birth prevented''
through MR was U.S. $7.08 for the coalition clinics compared with $68.25,
$58.10, and $32.20 for other family planning programs that relied primarily
on contraception (Kay and Kabir 1988). The average cost of providing
services to an MR client who left a coalition clinic with a contraceptive

method was $3.75, although clients received free services or paid only a few cents.

The *attitudes* of physicians and other health care providers also influence the availability of safe services within any given legal policy or program. Even within the constraints of restrictive legislation, medical professionals usually have considerable flexibility to act individually or collectively to provide services. The risk of criminal prosecution or professional censure, however slight, is bound to have a chilling effect on some practitioners. Others choose to interpret permitted medical exemptions liberally. Many perform safe abortions under the guise of treating incomplete spontaneous abortions or diagnosing uterine bleeding or menstrual irregularity. Countering the reluctance of some physicians to perform abortion for personal reasons, others have declared on ethical grounds that "as medical doctors, we are obliged before any other consideration to attend to the health of our patients and to put their interest before our own" (Villarreal 1989).

Most often, medical professionals and women's health advocates in developing countries with restrictive laws who provide safe services do so because their own attitudes are more liberal than state policy. Physicians practicing in rural Bangladesh, for example, where abortion except for MR is authorized only to save a woman's life, were found overwhelmingly to approve of abortion to protect a woman's health (95 percent), in cases of premarital pregnancy (79 percent), and rape (66 percent; see Rosenberg et al. 1981:320). Reflecting the patriarchal nature of Bangladeshi society, however, physicians were extremely conservative on the question of abortion for a married woman for reasons acceptable to the physician but without her husband's consent: only 12 percent approved. Nearly half of the physicians interviewed reported performing abortions in the past year, almost all of which would have been illegal.

In contrast, in countries where abortion is legal on health or social grounds or on request, many individual and institutional health care providers refuse to provide the appropriate medical services. Some hold personal religious or ethical values that define abortion on some or all grounds as morally unacceptable or inappropriate. For others, as noted earlier, abortion represents a low-status practice lacking in technical challenge or professional, financial, or personal rewards. In these settings, a woman's legal "right" to terminate an unwanted pregnancy can be a hollow one indeed.

THE SPECIAL CASE OF RU 486

The development of the menstrual-inducing pill RU 486 highlights the hazy legal status in many countries of inducing menstruation in the weeks following a late period as well as the volatility of the abortion debate.

During the 1970s, the Office of Population of USAID had been deeply committed to the search for a "once-a-month pill" or vaginal suppository or injection that could induce menstruation, thereby ensuring a state of nonpregnancy. Many publicly and privately funded researchers in Europe and North America were engaged in this quest. After years of experimentation, in the late 1980s the French pharmaceutical company Roussel-UCLAF launched its new product, RU 486. The pills can be taken before the onset of a menstrual period, at the time a period is due, or within several weeks following a missed period. The new technology further blurs the distinction between contraception and abortion, much to the delight of its proponents and the horror of its opponents. For its supporters, the drug promises to expand women's access to safe abortion throughout the world. It might even remove abortion from medical and legal control altogether by offering a simple method that a woman could use on her own in complete privacy. For those opposed to abortion on religious or moral grounds, the new drug threatens exactly what its supporters hoped for. But the situation is more complicated than that. Caught in the middle, once again, are groups of women's health advocates, medical practitioners, and proponents of human rights (among others) who strongly support legalization of abortion and the provision of safe services but who fear that the health infrastructures of many countries are inadequate to the task of providing the high quality of service delivery and followup care necessary to protect women's health and ensure method safety.

RU 486 is an antiprogestin drug that blocks the activity of progesterone, a hormone necessary for establishing and maintaining gestation. It induces bleeding and sloughing off of the uterine lining, including the embryonic tissue. By 1990 more than 60,000 women had taken RU 486 under medical supervision, primarily in France where—in combination with a prostaglandin—it was used by about one-fourth of all women who elected to terminate their pregnancies.

What effect is RU 486 likely to have on the health and lives of women in southern countries? At first glance, it seemed that the new drug might save many of the 100,000 to 200,000 women in developing countries who die every year from unsafe abortion along with countless others who experience severe abortion complications. These hopes may be unwarranted, however, for several reasons.

First, the technology already exists for providing safe early abortion by vacuum aspiration with a manual syringe or electric pump. RU 486 offers an important alternative method that many women will prefer, but the major impediments to safe abortion, as we have seen, are *political* and *administrative,* not technological. Second, Roussel-UCLAF intends to permit marketing of RU 486 only in countries where abortion is *legal* and where public, medical, and political opinion is supportive (Cook

1989b). In southern countries where abortion is already legal and accessible, such as China, RU 486 (or an equivalent drug) is unlikely to save lives because almost no women die from abortion complications in any case. In countries such as Brazil, Indonesia, or Nigeria where abortion is legally *restricted,* the drug will not be available unless an international agency such as WHO is able to distribute it directly under different guidelines. Access to RU 486 through an illegal black market might save some women's lives if it substitutes for dangerous clandestine abortions, but many women's health advocates are concerned that the drug could also cause harm if used incorrectly. Where abortion or MR are *legal but not yet generally accessible,* as in India and Bangladesh, respectively, RU 486 may not make much difference either. For various reasons, RU 486 will likely be distributed through the same medical channels that currently provide vacuum aspiration. To the extent that these outlets are limited by registration requirements or lack of health facilities or trained providers in many areas, women's access to RU 486 may be just as restricted as is their access to current procedures.

Third, many aspects of RU 486 need to be better understood with regard to its safety, effectiveness, and acceptability in developing countries. For example, when first introduced RU 486 was to be administered only up to 49 days LMP, that is, *within three weeks of a missed period* (Baulieu 1989). This leaves women little time to recognize the signs of a possible pregnancy and to decide what to do and where to go. Many women experiment first with herbal remedies or other means of inducing menstruation before seeking clinic services. Although the upper limit for RU 486 may be raised to eight or nine weeks LMP with no loss of effectiveness, it still offers a relatively narrow window of opportunity. An RU 486 client must also visit a clinic *three times:* the first for counseling, a medical examination, and administration of the pills; the second, within 36–48 hours, to receive an injection or vaginal suppository of a synthetic prostaglandin to induce uterine contractions, and to be held for observation for several hours; the third, about 7–10 days later, to be checked for completeness and undergo vacuum aspiration if necessary. The success rate of RU 486 in clinical trials *without the prostaglandin* is about 60–85 percent, depending on the duration of the pregnancy (Baulieu 1989). The prostaglandin raises the efficacy of RU 486 to about 95 percent, with less than 1 percent chance of complete failure (the woman is still pregnant) and 3–4 percent chance of incomplete expulsion. Used alone, RU 486 initiates bleeding within 24–72 hours, with expulsion of the embryo taking 7–10 days on average but occasionally up to several weeks. The prostaglandin shortens the time to expulsion, resulting in greater predictability, but some women will expel the conceptus after they leave the clinic. Bleeding continues for 9–10 days, on average, with individual variations from 1–40 days (ibid.; Silvestre et al. 1990). What problems is the prolonged bleeding likely to cause for those women who do not use protective pads or who must observe cultural restrictions associated with menstruation, both of which make privacy difficult?

As is the case for hormonal contraceptives, women seeking to terminate a pregnancy with RU 486 (a steroid) and prostaglandin (a hormone) need to be carefully screened for a long list of contraindications to both drugs. Health problems such as hypertension and anemia, which are contraindications, are common among poor women in many developing countries. Moreoever, as is the case for other abortion methods, providers must be able to diagnose and treat emergency complications such as hemorrhage or ectopic pregnancy. Vacuum aspiration is essential for women who present too late for RU 486, as a backup for method failure, and as a method choice, which means that facilities and trained personnel for routine mechanical procedures must be available. Considering a not unreasonable hypothetical example in which 10 percent of women present too late for RU 486 but early enough for vacuum aspiration, 10 percent experience method failure (including some who do not return for the prostaglandin), and 30 percent choose vacuum aspiration voluntarily because it is quicker and requires only two clinic visits (the initial procedure and a followup visit), it may be that the introduction of RU 486 will have far less impact on the use of existing procedures and facilities than is sometimes alleged. RU 486 is not a substitute for vacuum aspiration or a way of getting around current legal and programmatic restrictions. More realistically, it is an additional method of fertility regulation that will be appropriate for some women in those countries that have the necessary laws, policies, and health infrastructures for monitoring the technique and providing followup care. Despite the volatility of the political debate, RU 486 promises less than its enthusiasts hope and threatens less than its detractors contend.

INTERNATIONAL ABORTION POLITICS AND POLICIES: IS WOMEN'S HEALTH IMPORTANT?

We turn finally to the question of whether the protection of women's lives and health in southern countries has generated international pressure for the reform of restrictive abortion laws and policies. With few notable exceptions, the answer is, quite simply, no. In 1974, official delegates to the world population conference in Bucharest avoided the issue by relegating abortion to the morbidity and mortality section of the World Population Plan of Action, which quietly urged the "reduction of involuntary sterility, subfecundity, defective births and illegal abortions" (Mauldin et al. 1974:385). The subject attracted greater attention in the 1984 Mexico City conference because of the controversial U.S. policy position; ultimately, abortion was once again mentioned only in the maternal morbidity and mortality section of the plan. The *wording* of the recommendation was nevertheless hotly debated. "Governments are urged . . . to take appropriate steps to help women avoid abortion, which in no case should be promoted as a method of family planning," it stated, "and whenever possible, provide for the humane treatment and counseling of women who have had recourse to abortion" (Wulf and Willson 1984:230). The word "promoted" was a compromise. The Vatican (which has formal status as a U.N. observer) and its conservative supporters had tried to introduce language stating that abortion should in no case be provided as a method of family planning, which was defeated on the grounds that countries have a sovereign right to make their own policies (Finkle and Crane 1985:13). Abortion opponents *were* succesful in removing the word "illegal" before the last word, however, which obliterated the distinction between legal and illegal procedures by deploring both.

The reluctance of many official government representatives to endorse safe abortion as a health and family planning measure frequently reflects the political realities and restrictive laws in their own countries. It is more difficult to understand how experts participating in international conferences on maternal and child health could avoid doing so. Nevertheless, the final recommendations of the International Safe Motherhood Conference and the International Conference on Better Health for Women and Children through Family Planning, both of which were held in Nairobi in 1987, did exactly that. While deploring the dangers of unsafe clandestine abortion and even insisting that "it is unethical for scientists and service providers to shut their eyes to this waste of human life" (Black 1988), both conferences concluded formally only that humane treatment of septic and incomplete abortion was needed in all countries and that, *where legal,* "good quality abortion services should be made easily accessible to all women (ibid.; see also Starrs 1987). The United Nations Population Fund (UNFPA) was even more cautious at the International Forum on Population in the Twenty-First Century held in Amsterdam in November 1989. Lamenting the serious threat to women's lives and health posed by dangerous clandestine abortion, UNFPA insisted nevertheless that it "does not take a position either for or against" the legality of abortion (UNFPA 1989a:99). Indeed, citing an undocumented "strong societal consensus against abortion" as limiting the programmatic responses of health and family planning professionals in developing countries, UNFPA warned that providing safe services could pose "the risk of legitimization" (ibid.:101–102). In sharp contrast, physicians and women's health advocates from 35 countries meeting in 1988 in Rio de Janeiro at an International Symposium on Women's Health in the Third World: The Impact of Unwanted Pregnancies concluded with a statement urging governments to eliminate on health and human rights grounds all legal constraints to voluntary abortion, and to generate the necessary health policies and resource allocations to guarantee safe and accessible procedures to all who need them (International Women's Health Coalition 1989:175).

The international environment for abortion law reform is a hostile one. With a lack of commitment on the part of the major international agencies, a reactionary policy on the part of the U.S. government from the Reagan-Bush administrations, and an increasingly active transnational coalition of anti-abortion organizations operating in southern countries such as the International Right to Life Federation (which also has U.N. consultative status) and Human Life International, the struggle to establish women's rights to safe services is likely to be prolonged (Jacobson 1990; Crane 1990). As noted earlier, more than 50 southern countries continue to restrict legal abortion to medical emergencies and even these are rarely performed. In most cases having inherited their restrictive laws from former colonial powers, many governments now face resistance to change on the domestic front from religious fundamentalists, organized right-to-life groups, and other political opponents. At the same time, medical and family planning associations, legal experts, women's organizations, and public health officials in some countries are calling for reform.

In many southern countries, particularly in sub-Saharan Africa (e.g., Senegal, Burkina Faso, Mali, Zaire), there have been no organized efforts at abortion law reform even though problems of clandestine procedures have entered the public discourse in some cases (Isaacs, Holt, and Hill 1989). In other countries, advocates have made substantial but as yet unsuccessful efforts at reform. Recall from chapter 4 that a reform bill in Nigeria was defeated by the legislature in 1981, while in Brazil, feminist groups and their supporters were defeated in their efforts to legalize abortion in the new constitution. The Indonesian government has considered liberalizing the law, encouraged in part by recommendations of its national medical associations, but the political environment has not been considered sufficiently supportive as yet (Holt 1989a). Indeed, fears of political backlash which could result in a more repressive environment for abortion have been cited by government officials in Indonesia as well as by medical practitioners in Thailand who are otherwise supportive of reform efforts in that country (Holt 1989b). In Mexico, the incoming president in 1982 dropped the recommendations of the National Council on Population Activities to decriminalize abortion (Holt 1989a), while representatives of the Catholic Church hierarchy blocked reform efforts in Colombia and Costa Rica (Tietze and Henshaw 1986:19).

Despite the various obstacles to reform, however, a number of southern countries *have* adopted permissive laws. China legalized abortion on request within the first 10 weeks of pregnancy by a directive from the Ministry of Health in 1957 despite opposition from the medical profession (Tietze and Henshaw 1986:25). Abortion has been available on request in Singapore since 1974 and Vietnam since 1975. Tunisia's permissive law was enacted by presidential decree in 1973; Turkey's by the passage of a Population Planning Law in 1983. The permissive policy on MR in Bangladesh was established by the government on the basis of a legal interpretation in 1979. In Cuba, elective abortions have been available in government hospitals since the mid 1960s. Elsewhere, some southern countries have successfully modified their laws to include broad medical or socio-medical grounds while stopping short of abortion on request, such as India, Hong Kong, and Taiwan; Burundi and Zambia; and Barbados, Belize, and Uruguay (Cook 1989a). In Zambia, the Termination of Pregnancy Act of 1972 was adapted almost verbatim from the English Abortion Act of 1967 (Isaacs, Holt and Hill 1990). Further efforts are likely to require substantial support from national and international coalitions of women's groups, family planning organizations, medical practitioners, and family welfare organizations in cooperation with strategically located government ministers and political leaders.

The evidence is overwhelming that clandestine abortions are a major cause of disability and death among women in most southern countries. In both the south and the north, rates of maternal mortality have been shown to decline when abortion laws are liberalized (Tietze and Henshaw 1986; Henshaw and Morrow 1990). Where eligibility is tightened or eliminated (e.g., Romania in 1966), mortality rises. As recently as the early 1960s, complications of illegal abortion were the leading cause of maternal mortality in some parts of the United States, such as the state of Louisiana (Ward 1986:22), yet by 1990 abortion-related deaths were almost unknown. The political act of decriminalizing abortion combined with a health policy of making early procedures available in the public and private sector on a routine basis virtually eliminates reproductive mortality from this cause.

The protection of women's lives and health in developing countries requires that abortion be fully decriminalized, that unnecessary bureaucratic restrictions be removed, and that all women have access to skilled providers under affordable conditions as a normal part of their reproductive health care. "If the State is to do all in its power to protect the health of its citizens," a United Nations report concludes, "then it would be appropriate to repeal all laws impeding access to medical termination of pregnancy, leaving abortion subject only to those regulations surrounding other medical procedures of a similar nature. In this way, a safe, legal abortion would become part of the general medical care to which all persons are entitled" (United Nations 1975:89).

Much can be done in improving women's access to safe services *within* the constraints of prevailing laws if the laws are liberally interpreted in order to provide the necessary medical care (Cook and Senanayake 1978; Cook 1989a). In countries with *permissive* legislation, accessibility can be improved if governments revise unrealistic regulations (e.g., requiring written permission of specialists) and enact appropriate health policies and resource allocations for training and services. The curative treatment of incomplete or septic abortion is already considered by WHO as an essential element of medical service at first-referral level facilities. Teaching the preventive techniques of menstrual regulation to paramedical workers at the community level can almost eliminate the need for emergency treatment, at great savings in hospital utilization and human suffering. Policies can also be adopted to require medical practitioners who are unwilling to perform legal abortions to refer eligible candidates immediately to other providers.

Where abortion is unlikely to be liberalized for political reasons, much can still be done to expand current services. In countries where abortion is permitted on health grounds, medical professionals can adopt—individually or in their professional associations—WHO's definition of health as a state of complete physical, mental, and social well being. Under more restrictive laws, they can adopt a more realistic concept of life-threatening pregnancies so that a woman who is desperate to terminate an unwanted pregnancy need not risk her life at the hands of an unskilled practitioner to do so. Women's organizations and other committed groups can support service providers, refer clients, and maintain informational networks.

Governments can also clarify the scope of national abortion laws by specifying the circumstances under which the termination of pregnancy can be presumed not to violate prevailing laws. For example, some statutes expressly or implicitly require proof of pregnancy as an element of criminal prosecution (e.g., Spain, Argentina, Brazil, Mexico). Under such statutes, menstrual regulation by vacuum aspiration or contragestive drug, which is performed early after a missed period and at a time when pregnancy tests are unreliable or are not performed, may represent a safe and legal alternative (Lee and Paxman 1977). In addition, judiciaries can agree to interpret prevailing laws liberally and law enforcement officials can be slow to prosecute. In many countries safe services are now provided or could quietly be offered in women's centers, family planning clinics, or maternal and child health facilities with little risk of prosecution because they are supported and utilized by respected members of the community.

More broadly, policymakers in governments with restrictive laws and in medical institutions with restrictive policies can examine critically the legal, medical, and ethical principles upon which these restrictions are based. Medical ethicist Ruth Macklin (1989) proposes three "moral principles" for governing decision making in a pluralistic world: the principle of *liberty* (an individual right to freedom of action); the principle of *utility* (achieving the greatest good or welfare for the greatest numbers); and the principle of *justice* (ensuring equitable access for all persons to goods and services that fulfill basic human needs). Each of these principles rests on what Macklin calls "an underlying moral requirement," that is, the pre-requisite of *toleration* of the beliefs and practices of others in a hetero-geneous world.

From this ethical perspective, one can raise several questions about the termination of unwanted pregnancies. First, given the safety of modern methods of pregnancy termination and the hazards of most clandestine procedures, how can restrictive policies be justified on health and human welfare grounds? Second, given that family planning has been defined as a basic human right consistent with individual liberty and responsibility, how can restrictive policies be justified on human rights grounds? Third, given the professed commitments of many governments to promoting equality of access to basic social services, how can the denial of safe abortion to those classes of women who cannot afford safe private services be justified on grounds of social justice? Finally, if the principle of tol-eration is indeed a moral prerequisite for ethical decisions, then why must so many women in southern countries continue to face anguish and death in their attempts to regulate their fertility?

Part Four

TOWARD A FEMINIST POPULATION POLICY

8

WOMEN'S RIGHTS AND REPRODUCTIVE HEALTH: A POLICY AGENDA

One of the major challenges for feminists and others concerned with population and human rights has been to formulate a set of principles on which population policies and family planning programs could be based. The women's movement in the south and the north has raised its voice in opposition both to the crisis mentality of the antinatalist forces, which can lead to program abuses and distortions in funding, and to the crusading mentality of the pronatalist forces who often draw on ethnic, religious, or nationalist ideologies in their exhortations to be fruitful and multiply. Both approaches, when taken to extremes, result in violations of basic human rights. Both, too, degrade women by treating them as objects of manipulation rather than as subjects of their own fate.

What would a responsive reproductive policy and service delivery system look like? From an ethical standpoint, critics point out that policy choices must balance the demands of personal freedom, distributive justice, and security/survival (Callahan 1981; Macklin 1989). A feminist perspective stresses these themes with specific attention to women (Tangri 1976; Overall 1987). Given the ideological differences among feminists over many issues, it is not possible to draw up an agenda on which everyone can agree. As the international feminist group Development Alternatives with Women for a New Era (DAWN) emphasizes, "feminism cannot be monolithic in its issues, goals, and strategies, since it constitutes the political expression of the concerns and interests of women from different regions, classes, nationalities, and ethnic backgrounds. There is and must be a diversity of feminisms, responsive to the different needs

and concerns of different women" (Sen and Grown 1987:13). Nevertheless, it is possible to propose some general principles. The policy goal
would be to empower women to gain control over their own sexual and
reproductive capacities in the context of a broad program of social transformation that advances the freedom and security of women of all social
classes. Fertility reduction is likely to result from these transformations,
but it is not a primary goal.

Reproductive policies that are genuinely supportive of human rights recognize that personal freedoms and social entitlements are essential to the
advancement of human welfare. They respond *not* to a crisis mentality
about the perils of overpopulation, which can trigger damaging and ultimately self-defeating efforts at massive population control. Rather, they
evolve from a thoughtful engagement of the difficulties women face around
the world in their struggle to take control over their own fertility and their
own lives. For many women in the world the most important aspect of reproductive freedom is to be able to *have* the children they want, and to be
confident that their children will survive, be provided for, and go to school.
For others the issue is to avoid unwanted childbearing. For these women,
the choice of *whether and when* to have children and how many to have is
still to be realized. There is much to be done, not only in the broader context of transforming the material and social conditions that shape reproductive decision making, but also in the more specific context of providing high
quality reproductive health services for all who need them.

This chapter proposes a framework for thinking about population policies that departs from the conventional view. It builds on the ideas presented at the outset which traced the evolution of two "streams of
thought." The first stream was the historical development of ideas about
human rights, which were subsequently elaborated as ideas about equal
rights for women and men and, more recently, as ideas about reproductive
rights and freedoms. The second stream of thought evolved from ideas
about economic growth (e.g., the "wealth of nations"), to ideas about
the role of population in development (e.g., "optimal populations"), to
ideas about the role of family planning in controlling population growth.
The evolutionary "arrows" flowed downward through time in the parallel
streams:

human rights	economic growth
↓	↓
equal rights for women	population growth
↓	↓
reproductive rights	population control through family planning

Previous chapters have explored the relationships among ideas, social
movements, policies, and practices in each of these areas. They have
identified sources of conflict between advocates of women's rights on the

one hand and of population control on the other, and between supporters of reproductive freedom and of target-driven family planning. This final chapter brings the two streams of thought together. Introductory comments on the elements of a responsive reproductive policy lead to a critique of the conventional approach to population policy-making. The chapter continues with a proposal to substitute an *equal rights* policy for a population (reproductive) policy, a *reproductive rights* policy for a family planning policy, and a *reproductive health* program for a family planning program. Although the issues raised here are most relevant to antinatalist policies and programs in southern countries, they apply to the north as well.

TOWARD MORE RESPONSIVE REPRODUCTIVE POLICIES AND PROGRAMS

An ethical appraisal of a public policy includes two elements: (1) the procedural question of how policies are formulated and implemented, including the participation of those who will be most affected; and (2) the substantive question of the ethics of the policy itself, that is, its implications for freedom, distributive justice, and security/survival (Berelson and Lieberson 1979).

On the *procedural* question, the virtual exclusion of women as a major constituency from the policy-making process in many countries has intensified the antagonism of the women's movement toward many aspects of state reproductive policies and those of international agencies. In many cases this has led to misunderstandings on both sides. Politics is, by and large, a male game. Only 3.5 percent of ministries in 155 countries were headed by women in the late 1980s, and 99 countries had no women ministers at all (Appendix C). Women occupied fewer than 10 percent of legislative seats in 62 of 86 developing countries for which information is available and in 12 of 33 industrialized countries, including Canada, the United States, and the United Kingdom (United Nations 1991:39). The few women who rise to prominence within formal political and bureaucratic structures—as ministers of health and social welfare, for example—rarely express an explicit concern with empowering women. The reasons are understandable. Most successful women have been socialized into the norms of male-dominated professions, while those who appear "too biased" or "too feminist" find their career advancement blocked in all but exceptional circumstances. For these reasons, activists often select themselves out of establishment channels into positions permitting a more critical stance, such as academia or the organized women's movement. As discussed in chapter 4, women leaders and organizations are insisting on having their voices heard in the policy arena. They argue that because reproductive policies and programs affect women most deeply, women must be key actors in the policy-making process. Ensuring the full participation of women's groups, particularly those representing the concerns of exploited classes in both rural and urban areas, becomes a defining element of an ethical policy.

The *substantive* question relates to policy and program content. To be effective, policy approaches must be tailored to the unique circumstances of each country as well as to the diversity of needs within each country. Speaking generally, however, let us consider the proposition that a responsive reproductive policy could create conditions favorable to lower fertility while expanding the exercise of human rights through three major avenues: (1) rights-oriented socioeconomic development; (2) equal rights for women; and (3) the promotion of reproductive health and rights. Following this logic, the previously separated streams of thought combine to create three new equations:

human rights =	development policies
equal rights for women =	population (reproductive) policies
reproductive rights and health =	family planning policies and programs

Ideally, a population policy is part of an overarching *development policy* designed to advance human welfare through such means as employment and income generation, land reform, education, health services, social security, and the reduction of socioeconomic inequalities across countries, regions, and social classes. The intent is to extend to all persons an adequate standard of living together with other basic freedoms and entitlements. In this sense, *a development policy is a human rights policy.* Based on the principles of the Universal Declaration of Human Rights, it promotes social and economic rights; it broadens people's opportunities for survival, security, and mobility; it advocates distributional justice. Ideally, a development policy is a human rights policy in another sense as well: it advances individual freedoms by promoting civil and political rights.

Governments differ in the absolute and relative weights they place on social and economic rights as compared with civil and political rights. Some emphasize both (e.g., models of democratic socialism); some emphasize entitlements over freedoms (e.g., communist regimes); some emphasize freedoms over entitlements (e.g., democratic capitalism); some recognize neither (e.g., authoritarian regimes that enrich the elite and impoverish the masses). An antinatalist (or pronatalist) population policy enacted in the absence of a strategy to expand basic freedoms or entitlements is bound to be considered illegitimate by those who are its objects.

A second avenue of intervention is to promote the equal rights of women and men. In this formulation, *a population policy is an equal rights policy.* It advances women's economic and social rights and women's civil and political rights; it works toward the elimination of all forms of discrimination against girls and women; it undermines pronatalist patriarchal relations in the family, community, and nation. Fertility reduction is not a primary goal, however; rather, it is a secondary outcome of an equal rights policy.

A third avenue of intervention targets specific areas of reproductive health and freedom within the larger framework of a human rights/equal rights policy. "Family planning" undergoes a metamorphosis: it transcends its conventional definition as a system for delivering contraceptive services to embrace a broader range of freedoms and entitlements. *A family planning policy is a reproductive rights policy* designed to ensure that women and men exercise the full range of reproductive rights to which they are, in principle, entitled. It protects individuals against infringements of their rights by both pro- and anti-family planning forces. Similarly, *a family planning program is a reproductive health program* designed to deliver a full range of high-quality sexual and reproductive health services to all who want and need them. The population control element of family planning vanishes with this transformation along with its targets of "contraceptive acceptors" and "births averted." Both are replaced by goals and targets linked directly to the achievement of gender equality and reproductive rights, that is, to the improvement of human welfare. As will be argued below, the "new look" should have a major demographic impact despite (or because of) the reformulation of policy goals.

WHAT IS WRONG WITH THE CONVENTIONAL POPULATION POLICY APPROACH?

A population policy is a deliberate effort by a national government to influence aggregate levels of fertility, mortality, and migration. As noted in chapter 1, it typically includes a reproductive policy, a health policy, and a policy relating to migration and population distribution. A typical policy statement begins with a *rationale* of why there is a population problem. For example, current or projected population growth rates may be said to pose serious obstacles to the achievement of a country's social and economic objectives (for country-specific examples, see Isaacs and Irvin 1991). Second, a statement includes a set of general *goals* and specific *objectives,* such as achieving a better balance of population and resources or improving overall standards of living by altering demographic behavior in specified ways. In some cases, timetables and targets are set for their achievement (e.g., to "achieve birth spacing practice of a minimum of three years by at least 50 percent of mothers by the year 2000," as in India; ibid. p. 13). Third, a policy statement sets forth specific measures for *implementation,* such as improving health and nutrition through community campaigns, slowing cityward migration by investing in rural infrastructures, strengthening family planning services, educating students and the general public on the country's population problems, improving the status of women through changes in their legal status, promoting research and evaluation, and so on (ibid.). Specific government ministries or other organizations are identified as the responsible agents for policy and program implementation.

The process by which population policies emerge in developing countries has drawn criticism from both supporters and detractors of the need for such policies. At the risk of oversimplification, let us consider a typical scenario (Godwin 1975; Roberts 1990; Thomas and Grindle 1990). In this model, demographers working with bilateral or multilateral donor agencies, research organizations, or consulting firms develop sophisticated statistical analyses of the impact of projected population growth rates and characteristics on the development prospects of a particular country. They highlight the difficulties of providing universal schooling and health care, raising per capita incomes, sustaining adequate food production and consumption, and conserving natural resources and the environment, among other issues. With these analyses in hand, experts working for donor organizations such as USAID, UNFPA, or the World Bank form alliances with like-minded local government officials, in-country researchers, or leaders of key NGOs such as family planning associations to propose policy solutions to recipient governments. A donor agency may appoint a population advisor to work with government planners to formulate and implement an "official" demographic policy. Political leaders are urged to make public statements in support of such a policy, with emphasis on the need to reduce birth rates through the promotion of family planning programs.

The process as described is technocratic, externally motivated, and apolitical. Consider, for example, the comments of USAID population experts on their early approach to policy-making in developing countries (Sinding and Hemmer 1975): "(1) [planners] *must be convinced* that some of the values they seek to maximize are unlikely to be advanced under existing demographic conditions; (2) *they must be convinced* that it is possible to affect the demographic variables, especially fertility, through the instruments of public policy; and (3) *they must be convinced* that specific policy measures have a good chance of producing the desired result" (emphases added). A less directive version describes a model of "linkage politics" in which networks of private and official international donors provide assistance to local groups working to establish a political environment conducive to the development of a national policy (Merrick 1990). More attention is paid here to mobilizing local support. National counterpart organizations and individuals who could be recruited for the cause include population researchers, private family planning associations, medical and family welfare associations, legislators, government officials in health and statistical units, and high-level public officials at the presidential and ministerial levels and in the military.

What is wrong with this picture? To the extent that it reflects reality, the model neglects the political constraints on decision makers such as scarce resources, competing demands, uncertain tenure, and political opposition. Defining planners as concerned with promoting the common good and finding optimal solutions based on a "neutral" analysis of "scientific" evidence (Dye 1972), it ignores the fact that governments are often more preoccupied with eliminating political opposition than with meeting the basic human needs of their people. The model implies that governments are incapable of initiating their own programs based on their own analyses and rationales. Conversely, it treats all governments as though they have the legitimacy, political will, and capacity to carry out their policy agendas, ignoring the possibility that new or weak states may have to bargain and compromise with powerful local leaders.

Most important, the scenario reflects a top-down process that relies on experts rather than on consultations with groups who will be most affected by policy decisions. Yet, as noted in chapter 1, people are likely to resist the imposition of state population policies and birth control programs that threaten their strategies for survival and security. Local leaders will intervene to protect their constituents, "in the process usurping the social control of the state and snuffing out compliance with its policies" (Greenhalgh 1990:10). Moreover, by perpetuating the false equation of family planning with population control, the technocratic approach distorts the purposes of both and fuels the fires of anti-family planning sentiment among potential clients and among critics from the right and the left. As a political scientist observes in her analysis of antinatalist policies in sub-Saharan Africa, "Religious officials, traditional sector leaders, minority ethnic groups, and nationalists can sense disadvantage and political ill will in the antinatalist choice. But it is rare that these variables figure, even marginally, in economic and demographic analysis" (Anglim 1975:174).

If the purpose of a demographic policy is to promote sustainable long-term development and improve the quality of life for all people, then the regulation of birth rates is a *means to an end* and not an end in itself. Measuring changes in fertility levels per se tells us little about the achievement of these broader goals. Similarly, if the purpose of reducing infant mortality and expanding people's opportunities for schooling, employment, better health and housing, old-age security, and other benefits is to improve human welfare, then these are *ends in themselves* and not a means to an end such as lower birth rates. Finally, if the purpose of providing family planning services is to enable couples and individuals to regulate their fertility in a safe, effective, and acceptable manner, then this too is an *end in itself* and not a means to an end. Family planning is a social good and a right; it needs no other justification. Program achievements need to be measured in their own terms—as measures of client empowerment, knowledge, satisfaction, and welfare—and not in terms of a population control agenda.

FROM POPULATION CONTROL TO EQUAL RIGHTS

In what sense is an equal rights policy an antinatalist population policy? Its intent is to challenge explicitly those ideological and structural elements of "coercive pronatalism" that deny women genuine reproductive choice. These include early arranged marriage, female seclusion, sexual exploitation in the domestic and public realms, and gender-based discrimination in rights of property, family affairs, education, employment, and political life. Affecting women differentially by economic and social class but universally as a sexual class, patterns of female subordination are embedded, in various forms and degrees, in patriarchal family systems, in social, religious, economic, political, and legal systems, and in state policies in both developing and industrialized countries.

A woman's capacity to make independent choices about marriage, divorce, and childbearing is tied to her capacity for economic and social self-sufficiency. For this reason, a policy of *selective* investment in female schooling, vocational training, employment, and community organizing, which is widely recognized as an appropriate mechanism for accelerating de facto equality, may have a far greater impact on reproductive behavior (as well as on children's health and well being) than so-called gender-neutral investments that almost always favor males (Dixon 1978; Cochrane 1979; Caldwell 1986; Dwyer and Bruce 1988). Moving beyond equality of opportunity, a gender-focused policy would seek equality of results. Acquiring full legal rights is essential, but women need social and economic resources in order to activate them. As discussed in chapter 5, strategies for empowering girls and women include acquiring knowledge and skills, earning independent incomes, and mobilizing grass-roots and national organizations to advance their rights and protect their interests. The *substance* of an equal rights policy, then, is to devise means of promoting women's freedom and security/survival directly, which sets the stage for reproductive rights policies and programs. In contrast, a conventional population policy uses interventions such as socioeconomic investments and family planning programs as the means of reducing birth rates without close consideration of their implications for women's lives in particular contexts.

An equal rights policy, like a population policy, represents a commitment by a national government to institute specific changes. It includes a rationale (e.g., why discrimination against girls and women constitutes a denial of human rights and an obstacle to development), goals and objectives, targets and timetables, and a plan for implementation. The U.N. Convention on the Elimination of All Forms of Discrimination Against Women offers a useful framework for a national equal rights policy. Ratified or acceded to by over 100 countries (Appendix D), the convention calls for governmental intervention to ensure that women enjoy on a basis of equality with men a full range of human rights and fundamental freedoms. In particular, it calls for states parties to institute laws and policies that will (1) eliminate customary practices and prejudices that discriminate against girls and women; (2) ensure women equal rights with men in political and public life and nationality; (3) ensure equal rights in all aspects of education; (4) eliminate discrimination against women in matters of employment, working conditions, benefits, and earnings, including protection against dismissal due to marriage or maternity; (5) accord women equality with men before the law, including full and independent legal status; (6) accord women equal rights at the time of marriage, during marriage, and at its dissolution; and (7) recognize the special problems faced by rural women and their need to participate in development planning, training and education, community organization, credit and land reform schemes, and other development efforts (Appendix A).

Reinforcing and adding to women's rights that have been spelled out in over a dozen international charters and conventions, the convention represents both an equal rights policy and a "women in development" policy. Its power has been weakened, however, by inadequate enforcement mechanisms and by numerous reservations filed by states parties that are intended to avoid confict with religious or customary laws (Cook 1990; Holt 1990). Because the abolition of customary laws and practices that discriminate against women is one of the jewels in the crown of the convention, such reservations render ratification almost meaningless. They are not surprising, however, for the document's preamble and substantive articles are intended to challenge the very foundations of patriarchy. This challenge is bound to elicit resistance from religious elites (in this case, most frequently the protectors of Islamic law) and from defenders of customary practices and laws in traditional non-Islamic societies (e.g., in sub-Saharan Africa). Religious personal status laws and unwritten customary laws almost invariably perpetuate male privilege and control over women in matters of sexuality, marriage, divorce, child custody, and inheritance. They also serve as powerful symbols of cultural identity and anti-Western sentiment (Freedman 1991; Kandiyoti 1991). Thus, Third World governments indebted to or captured by conservative religious or ethnic groups or nationalist movements are likely to protect the status of such laws even where civil codes guarantee equal rights for all citizens in the public sphere.

Ratification obliges states to bring their laws and policies into conformity with the convention's provisions and report periodically to a U.N. monitoring committee (International Women's Rights Action Watch 1988). Many countries have incorporated equal rights provisions in their constitutions (Appendix D), some of which precede the convention by many years. In addition, most governments and international aid agencies have adopted "official" feminist rhetoric by committing themselves—at least on paper, and with limited success—to policies promoting the integration or "mainstreaming" of women in all sectors of development and decision making (Staudt 1985, 1990; Carloni 1987; Duncan and Habib 1988). In conformity with the Forward-Looking Strategies of the U.N. Decade for Women, most governments have established national commissions on the status of women, women's divisions or ministries, and other agencies for monitoring progress and effecting change. The success of these endeavors depends on many factors, of course, and the outcome has been mixed.

An equal rights policy shares with a population control policy a number of problems. Even where the political will exists and the majority of citizens support the principle of equality, the wheels of legislative and policy reform turn slowly. Much depends on the structural and cultural characteristics of the legal system (Freedman 1991). States with powerful ruling families or strong governments may simply impose a policy of female emancipation in order to undermine patriarchal kin groups and communities or regional, ethnic, or religious influence, extend state control, and mobilize women's labor power and political support. Examples include Soviet control of central Asia (Massel 1974), the Democratic People's Republic of Yemen, Iran under Reza Shah, Egypt under Nasser, Iraq under the Ba'th party, and Turkey under Attaturk (Kandiyoti 1991). Weak states will have to bargain with opponents of women's rights; policy statements may reflect little more than accommodation to international political pressures with no intent to implement.

Ideally, however, an equal rights policy will involve a different *process* than the externally driven, top down, and technocratic approach described earlier. First, although policies and programs of equal rights and "women in development" are already in place in most countries, women's organizations in each country can articulate specific principles of most relevance to them and work for their implementation. The goal is to enable women in each country to understand how current laws and policies inhibit their participation in social and economic life and to determine ways in which women might use the political and legal system most effectively to secure their rights. The model is one of change from within. "The call for the granting of basic rights of choice to women and the methods used to secure them must come from within—from within the country itself,

and from within the terms that define that country's cultural reality"
(Freedman 1991:28–29).

Second, whereas women's organizations in the south and the north
have been wary of population control policies and critical of family planning program abuses, they are natural allies of measures designed to
promote women's freedom and welfare. This is not to suggest that wom-
en's groups will see eye-to-eye on all issues, for the case studies in chapter
4 demonstrated that this is not the case. Women's organizations in countries where autonomous groups are permitted cover a spectrum of political, economic, and social orientations. Many are based on class, religious,
regional, or ethnic identities. Yet, despite their many contradictions, organizations representing women's interests are likely to find some common ground on which to articulate their gender-based concerns and
demands for action.

Third, an equal rights policy encourages coalition-building among researchers, government officials, legislators, and activists concerned with
human rights issues, legal reform, family welfare, social justice, and development. Women's organizations and leaders can ally themselves with
like-minded individuals and groups within their own countries while drawing on the support of women's movements in other southern countries,
in the north, and in international agencies. State ratification of the convention offers a useful organizing tool and focus. NGOs can play a central
role in monitoring governmental action or inaction in compliance with its
terms, at the same time organizing grass-roots activities to mobilize
women of all classes and inform them of their rights. In collaboration with
national commissions or women's ministries, NGOs can produce and
disseminate a culturally specific "girls' and women's bill of rights" to
raise the consciousness of key groups in each country, particularly of
women in marginalized circumstances. Freedoms and entitlements to be
included in such a bill of rights cover not only those items mentioned in
the convention, but also sexual and reproductive rights to be elaborated
in each cultural context.

FROM FAMILY PLANNING TO REPRODUCTIVE RIGHTS

A reproductive rights policy is embedded in a human rights/equal rights
policy. It sets the legal and structural framework within which women
and men are able to exercise their right to sexual and reproductive self-
determination and obtain the information and services they need.

Governments may support a conventional family planning policy on
demographic or health grounds, on grounds of human rights or women's
status, or for reasons of social justice and human welfare. In essence, the
mission of a family planning policy is to support the provision of birth

control information and services through public and private sector initiatives. A widely cited scheme for assessing the strength of national family planning program efforts cites eight "policy and stage-setting activities" (Mauldin and Lapham 1987). Five involve the mobilization of governmental support for family planning through official policy rationales, supportive statements from leaders, high-level bureaucratic location of national program leadership, integration of other ministries and government agencies, and budgetary support. China's policy and stage-setting score far exceeds that of other developing countries in this scheme, followed by India, Indonesia, the Republic of Korea, and Mexico as the next strongest (ibid.:564). The implication is that a strong demographic mandate contributes to a strong family planning program.

This implication, however, lies at the heart of the confusion about (and political resistance to) the purpose of family planning. As Judith Bruce points out, "tension [is] created when family planning services are caught between two potentially conflicting mandates: promoting the achievement of demographic objectives and meeting individual health and welfare needs" (Bruce 1990:63) If family planning programs could be unhooked from their demographic mandate, they could focus more clearly on meeting individual needs and providing a range of sexual and reproductive health care. At the same time, a *reproductive rights policy* could provide a framework for ensuring that women and men are protected from infringements on their freedom by *both* antinatalist and pronatalist forces. No one could be denied their right to use a contraceptive method, for example, or to terminate an unwanted pregnancy. At the same time, no one could be forced to use a method (e.g., compulsory sterilization), or persuaded to do so under false pretenses (e.g., by withholding information about side effects), or prevented from stopping a method (e.g., by refusing to remove a contraceptive implant). Any of these actions would involve a violation of basic rights. This formulation is consistent with the 1989 Health Law of Vietnam, for example, which stresses that all individuals must be free to choose the family planning method they wish and declares that "all acts of preventing or forcing the implementation of family planning are prohibited" (Allman et al. 1991:314).

A reproductive rights policy would lay the groundwork for freedom of choice in marriage and divorce, in sexual relations more generally, and in the use of birth control methods. *Marriage laws* and policies backed up by public information campaigns could prohibit the betrothal of young girls; set a minimum age at marriage of at least 18 years for both sexes and require their free and full consent; regulate the size of brideprice and dowry payments which reinforce kinship controls over the bride; ensure that a husband in a polygynous marriage can take a second wife only with the first wife's agreement in court; ensure that a wife can initiate and obtain a divorce on the same grounds as her husband; eliminate divorce by unilateral repudiation of the wife; and establish a woman's right to the custody of young children and financial support following divorce. A father's obligation to support his children would be enforced. *Laws relating to sexual behavior* would attach criminal penalties to incest and the sexual abuse of children; rape and other forms of physical violence; sexual intercourse with under-age females; and recruitment for and profiting from prostitution and sexual slavery. At the same time, homosexual relations between consenting adults and heterosexual relations between consenting unmarried adults would be decriminalized. *Laws on contraceptives* would legalize the importation, manufacture, distribution, and advertising of contraceptives while maintaining appropriate standards of quality control (Isaacs and Cook 1984). They would facilitate the provision of services and supplies by trained non-physicians such as midwives, nurses, and pharmacists. Restrictions on sexual and birth control information and services for adolescents or unmarried people would be repealed (Roemer and Paxman 1985) along with requirements of spousal or parental consent (Cook and Maine 1987). *Voluntary sterilization and abortion* would be legalized on request while maintaining appropriate medical standards and ensuring fully informed consent. Special incentive payments to providers of family planning methods such as IUDs or sterilization, "motivators," and "acceptors" would be eliminated in order to reduce the potential for program abuses. Independent commissions would be established to investigate complaints of coercive, negligent, or other harmful practices of family planning researchers or providers in the public and private sectors and assist clients in protecting their rights.

These are examples of what might be included in a reproductive rights policy. Coalitions of women's groups, human rights advocates, and family planners in each country could draw up a set of principles to guide reproductive laws and policies. The purpose of such a policy is to provide a "shelter" of rights within which people's sexual and reproductive health needs can be fully addressed.

REPRODUCTIVE HEALTH AS A CORE PROGRAM

The concept of reproductive health has gained currency in the 1980s as a symbol of a fresh perspective on women's rights and family planning (e.g., Germain 1987; Germain and Ordway 1989). It incorporates elements of conventional approaches to health and family planning service delivery while broadening their scope and deepening their impact. The concept of reproductive health is premised on the feminist principle that every woman has the right to control her own sexuality and reproduction without discrimination as to age, marital status, income, or other considerations. Ensuring the highest possible standards of reproductive health care for girls and women is fundamental to the exercise of their reproductive rights and freedoms, and to the exercise of the broad array of other human rights to which girls and women are entitled.

Reproductive health refers to a woman's ability (1) to understand and enjoy her own sexuality by gaining knowledge of her own body, her sexual capacities, and her sexual rights; (2) to regulate her fertility safely and effectively by conceiving only when desired, by terminating unwanted pregnancies, and by carrying wanted pregnancies to term; (3) to remain free of disease, disability, or death associated with her sexuality and reproduction; and (4) to bear and raise healthy children (adapted from Germain and Ordway 1989). By laying out these principles, we can see that a reproductive health program involves much more than the delivery of maternal and child health (MCH) or family planning services as conventionally defined.

Reproductive health incorporates a clear feminist and human rights focus for its full realization. It moves birth control out from under the umbrella of "family planning" and "planned parenthood," with their patriarchal connotations, into the realm of individual rights to sexual and reproductive health. It links and transforms existing services in a manner that places women's physical and emotional security at the center. It broadens the concepts of "user's perspective" (or client's perspective) and "quality of care" (Bruce 1980, 1990; Ainsworth 1985)—both of which represent significant advances over earlier thinking—to encompass an agenda for social transformation. It recognizes that reproductive autonomy cannot be obtained by means of birth control alone, even when delivered in a comprehensive and caring way.

The reproductive health framework also helps to move family planners away from their preoccupation with contraceptive acceptance rates and births averted, a preoccupation that has led to charges that singling out "excess fertility" as the most urgent problem represents a cynical disregard for the multiplicity of women's needs (Karkal and Pandey 1989). At the same time, it can move health workers away from their sometimes narrow conception of *maternal* morbidity and mortality to consider a broader range of social and health issues (Sai and Nassim 1989). As noted in chapter 6, reproductive health is consistent with the concepts of *reproductive* mortality and morbidity which involve calculations of the health risks and benefits of sexual behavior and of attempts to prevent pregnancy as well as of pregnancy and childbirth. Perhaps most important, a reproductive health framework elicits positive connotations of health and reproduction rather than negative connotations of fertility control.

A comprehensive program of reproductive health and rights based on feminist principles would (1) build on and learn from women's experience; (2) empower women to overcome their oppression; (3) offer an appropriate array of reproductive health services; (4) ensure fully informed choice of birth control methods, including abortion; (5) offer a choice among delivery systems and providers; (6) provide individual and group counseling and educational programs; (7) reach into the community to change discriminatory attitudes and practices; (8) build linkages with related programs and providers; (9) institute staff training in accountability and philosophy of care; and (10) draw on a sustained commitment from governments, NGOs, and bilateral and multilateral funding agencies. Each of these points is elaborated briefly below.

1. *Building on women's experiences*

Building on and learning from women's experiences is an essential first step in creating a woman-centered reproductive health program. In essence, this means that clinic- or community-based programs would be designed, in large part, *by* women *for* women. Men would not be excluded from sharing the responsibility for practicing birth control or from providing or receiving services; far from it. Culturally sensitive educational and service programs designed by men for men are essential (Gallen 1986). Rather, programs intended primarily for female clients would be planned, implemented, and evaluated with the full participation of women at all levels and stages of decision making. (For a useful analysis of concepts and measures of client participation, see Cohen and Uphoff 1977.)

Involving representatives of client populations in the design and assessment of decentralized community services will ensure that reproductive health programs are informed by women's perceptions of their own needs and priorities in each setting. Women can draw on their experiences with health care and family planning providers such as herbalists, pharmacists, traditional midwives, and physicians and paramedics in the public and private sectors. In a woman-centered program, what the *client* knows about her personal history, health and family planning needs, and about the attitudes of her family and community is just as important as what the *provider* knows about technical topics such as the relative risks of different contraceptives or how a method works (Bruce 1983:51; see also Lipton, Dixon-Mueller and Brindis 1987). Program clients would participate directly in the evaluation of the services they receive through informal group consultations, serving as community advisors, and other means.

Reproductive health programs would be adapted to the specific needs of the women they serve, derived from a fundamental understanding of women's lives in diverse economic and cultural circumstances. Recognizing the centrality of childbearing to women's security and self-esteem, service providers would treat clients' concerns with overcoming infertility with as much care as clients' concerns with avoiding unwanted or closely spaced births. Providers would also recognize that in conditions of economic crisis, women's perceived need for family planning may rank below other needs. In an income-generating and consciousness-raising association of about 7,000 destitute rural women organized in 400 groups in Bangladesh, for example, women who were asked about their objectives in joining the groups generally ranked "to receive family planning" below other goals such as "obtain redress from moneylenders," "stop the dowry system," "send children to schools," "get correct and fair wages," "encourage group savings," and "rescue from torture of husbands" (Banchte Shekha 1986).

Childbearing and fertility regulation among vulnerable groups occur within an environment of social and economic risk and uncertainty (e.g., Schnaiberg and Reed 1974; Cain 1981). Service providers must be acutely aware of the risks as well as the benefits to women of spacing or limiting births or of using a contraceptive method (see chapter 6). Women may fear divorce, abandonment, physical abuse, or social rejection if their contraceptive practice is known, for example, or experience anxiety about method side effects that could alter menstrual patterns or cause subsequent fertility impairments. The more rigid is the patriarchal system enforcing female economic dependency, the greater is the risk to women of restricting their childbearing or of going against their husband's or elders' wishes. The risk is especially severe where labor markets that might otherwise provide some independent economic security for women are most discriminatory.

2. *Empowering women to overcome their oppression*

A reproductive health program forms one component of a comprehensive effort to transform power relations in the family, the community, and the society. It challenges female subordination in the sexual and reproductive spheres as well as in other spheres of women's lives. Reproductive health is related both ideologically and programmatically to these broader human rights goals; indeed, it is subsumed by them.

The essence of a feminist reproductive health program is empowering clients as individuals and in groups, however poor, *to make demands* of themselves, their families, and their communities. In many cases the first step is the most difficult: to encourage women to "break their silence" about their sexual and reproductive problems and their experience with health systems. In Nigeria, for example, sociologist Mere Kisekka (1989c:2) points out that women have "internalised the ethic of 'nobility in suffering' such that pain and discomforts emanating from their reproductive and sexual roles are accepted as the very essence of womanhood. ... [S]ocial stigma, and hence the culture of silence, [is] attached to sexual and reproductive problems, the geneses of which are invariably perceived to be women." The culture of silence characteristic of many societies translates into a reluctance among some women to press for their personal rights even in clinic settings. "Their desire to have their human rights observed is not expressed as an 'entitlement,' " writes one observer, "but rather as a wish for dignified and fair treatment" (Bruce 1987:378).

A feminist reproductive health program means empowering clients to make demands on public and private agencies and individual providers for the type of care they want. It means empowering clients to make demands on their sexual partners for respect and cooperation in sexual relations, fertility regulation, and childbearing and rearing. It also means creating conditions by which women can act unilaterally to control their own fertility, if they wish, through the use of non-detectable contraceptive methods and of tubal ligation or abortion on an outpatient basis. In the words of British historians J. A. and Olive Banks cited earlier in this book (1964:125), a feminist agenda "involves a campaign waged in the face of opposition—a struggle of the underprivileged female against the dominant, privileged male." It may also involve race, caste, and class struggle, with particular emphasis on empowering women in oppressed groups to act on their own behalf.

3. *Offering an appropriate array of reproductive health services*

Designed to meet the needs of girls and women of all ages and economic conditions, the reproductive health concept incorporates a holistic approach to prevention and treatment that centers on the person rather than on a particular part or function of the physical body.

Ideally, a reproductive health program would include (1) education and counseling on sexuality, contraception, abortion, childbearing, hygiene, infection, and disease; (2) screening and treatment of reproductive tract infections (including sexually transmitted diseases), cervical cancer, and other gynecological problems; (3) informed choice of contraceptive methods, with systematic attention to contraceptive safety; (4) safe early abortion for contraceptive failure or non-use; (5) prevention and treatment of infertility; (6) prenatal care, supervised delivery, and post-partum care; and (7) infant and child health services (Germain and Ordway 1989). Services can be offered directly or through referrals, in both public and private sectors. Offering an array of services in one center or community outreach program can encourage followup and continuity of care. In addition, each new service, such as prenatal care or child immunization, pulls in additional clients who then return for other services, such as contraception.

Service priorities will depend on the perceived needs of client populations and on organizational capacity. The Bangladesh Women's Health Coalition, for example, began in 1980 as a single-purpose clinic offering safe, legal menstrual regulation for low-income women (Kay, Germain and Bangser 1991). It added contraceptive services and counseling almost immediately. As the organizational capacity and number of clinics grew, the coalition responded to clients' demands for additional services by adding primary maternal and child health care such as immunization, nutrition education, and referrals for high-risk pregnancy, and a birthing center in one clinic. In the late 1980s the coalition initiated (on a small scale) diagnosis and treatment of common reproductive tract infections which contribute to infertility and other disabilities. Other groups have other concerns. Latin American feminist health collectives have placed a high priority on sexuality and rape counseling, safe abortion services or referrals, dealing with violence against women, and ensuring contraceptive safety and choice, including protection from unsafe biomedical experimentation. A group of Nigerian health activists has identified infertility as a major focus of its immediate concerns (chapter 4), which encompasses the prevention and treatment of infections and other damage caused by unsafe abortion, unsafe delivery, unsafe sexual practices, and customs such as female circumcision. An appropriate constellation of reproductive health services would be responsive to the specific concerns and requirements of diverse populations. Each of the elements of reproductive health is phrased as a social entitlement which forms the foundation of reproductive choice and freedom.

4. *Ensuring informed choice of birth control methods*

A feminist perspective on reproductive health values a broad range of method choice in fertility regulation, including a woman's right to use a less effective method, to use a method only sporadically, to switch freely from one method to another, or to refuse any or all services or products. These options follow logically from the principles of informed choice and self-determination. Every woman will weigh differently from every other woman the relative risks and benefits of each method of birth control and of childbearing at different points in her life (e.g., see Hass 1976; Bruce 1987). Once she is made fully aware of the available options in contraception, sterilization, and abortion through intensive counseling on the risks and benefits of each method—whether male and female methods, natural or artificial—the individual woman is in the best position to know what is right for her.

Unlike the conventional family planning program that urges adoption of long-acting methods such as the IUD, implants, or male or female sterilization, a feminist program would support trial use and method switching. It would also place more reliance on barrier methods such as condoms, diaphragms, cervical caps, sponges, or spermicides, some of which help prevent sexually transmitted diseases. Providers could offer instruction in coitus interruptus (withdrawal), "natural family planning" (periodic abstinence), and breastfeeding as spacing mechanisms for women who are willing to accept a higher risk of pregnancy, or where safe abortion is readily available in cases of method failure.

Concerns about contraceptive choice and safety have posed a dilemma for feminists, just as they have for governments, researchers, program administrators, service providers, and clients themselves. Should a woman be offered methods that may produce or exacerbate other health problems or even cause death, no matter how small the probability? How does one balance the principles of individual freedom and social entitlement in this case? The vehement opposition of some feminist health advocates to the use of hormonal injectables and implants under any conditions is one example of such controversy. Yet, others contend that women should have access to the full range of available methods under conditions of fully informed consent, careful screening for contraindications, and adequate medical followup. These preconditions are, of course, very difficult to meet. Counseling, screening, and followup are inadequate in most developing countries, especially in rural areas, and among some subpopulations in industrialized countries as well.

The challenge of a reproductive health program is to ensure that adequate monitoring is possible within the context of individual choice. There is probably no drug or device or medical procedure without risk. In this sense, the need for client education about possible side effects and informed consent is not unique to family planning. Women should have the freedom to choose, but they are also entitled to protective legislation that regulates the conditions under which drugs, devices, or medical procedures can be tested or marketed and to participate in this legislative process so that their own views are heard.

The right to safe and low-cost or free abortion on request lies at the heart of method choice. Abortion represents a woman's ultimate veto power over an unwanted or mistimed pregnancy—that is, over coerced childbearing—as well as an essential reproductive health service. Abortion will always be necessary as a backup for contraceptive failure or nonuse where women or couples are determined to prevent an unwanted birth. In addition, many women prefer abortion to contraception because it meets their particular needs at a given time better than contraception does. Where abortion is properly performed within the first 12 weeks of pregnancy, the resulting mortality rate is lower than for other family planning methods such as the IUD, tubal ligation, or hormonal pills. The availability of safe, supportive abortion services as a basic component of women's comprehensive reproductive health care is thus neither an unfortunate fact nor a necessary evil, but, like all family planning, is a woman's right, a social entitlement, and a positive social good (Petchesky 1984:387).

5. *Expanding choices among delivery systems and providers*

The concept of choice extends to individual providers and institutional delivery systems. Male and female clients from diverse backgrounds will respond differently to providers of various types, often strongly preferring some over others based on their social values and personal experiences. Systems differ in their ideologies, accessibility, cost, physical and social settings, modes of transaction, type of goods and services, technical competence of providers, and familiarity to the client. Mechanisms of service delivery may determine the acceptability of contraceptive methods and other reproductive health services: "The service delivery experience encapsulates the method, and in the clients' minds, is part of the 'technology.' *Women do not choose simply to use a specific method; they choose to accept interaction with an often complex service apparatus*" (Bruce 1987:36; emphasis added).

Channels of service delivery are so varied that it is not possible to assess the potential advantages and disadvantages of each type (Lapham and Simmons 1987:341–542). A comprehensive reproductive health program would include both clinic-based and community-based delivery systems in the public and private sectors. Clinic-based services include freestanding, mobile, or hospital-based clinics run by governments, NGOs, or private for-profit operators as well as the offices of physicians and other medical or paramedical personnel. Community-based services include pharmacies and other retail outlets in the formal sector, street vendors and traditional health practitioners (e.g., herbalists and midwives) in the informal sector, and field-workers in community programs. The latter offer basic health and family planning information and services house-to-house (usually woman-to-woman) or in specialized settings such as factories and other workplaces, festivals and markets, women's clubs, high schools or adult literacy classes, and cooperatives and credit societies. Community field-workers are often outreach workers for clinic-based programs. Some services and supplies can be offered in the client's home or in other non-clinic settings (e.g., condoms, contraceptive foams and suppositories, resupplies of pills, nutrition supplements, prenatal monitoring, and perhaps immunizations and midwifery), while others are usually referred to clinics (e.g., female and male sterilization, abortion, IUD insertion, gynecological problems, high-risk pregnancies).

Patterns of concentration or diversity in the sources of selected family planning and health services—for example, between public and private sources—can be identified in the Demographic and Health Surveys undertaken in a number of developing countries in the mid 1980s. In Brazil, for example, 93 percent of women using the pill obtained their supplies from a pharmacy and only 4 percent from government health facilities and 1 percent from private physicians or clinics. In contrast, only 3 percent of women in Senegal who used the pill went to pharmacies compared with 43 percent each in government and private health centers. Thai women relied heavily on government facilities (70 percent) and on pharmacies (23 percent) with almost none resorting to private physicians or clinics. Although these comparisons illustrate some apparent distortions in sources of supply, their interpretation requires fuller knowledge of the situation in each country.

By definition, community-based programs are intended to bring essential services closer to clients, especially to low-income and rural households with less access to formal health facilities, and to women. Also by definition, they offer considerably more scope for community participation and entrepreneurial initiative than do clinic-based programs. Community-based services can offer alternatives to formal medical centers, relying instead on more informal contacts between clients and providers, the latter of whom are usually less highly trained and thus socially closer to their clients than are clinical personnel. Moreover, community-based programs in countries with discriminatory labor markets such as Bangladesh have provided important new employment opportunities for thousands of women as health and family planning field-workers (Simmons et al. 1988).

Feminists have supported in principle the diversification of delivery systems as a means of improving access to important reproductive health services among potentially marginalized groups such as teenage girls, ethnic minorities, nonliterate women, or married women who are unable to leave home. Many remain nervous, however, about the implications of distributing contraceptive methods such as the pill in situations where users may not be fully informed about their correct use, contraindications, and possible side effects (International Women's Health Coalition and the Population Council 1986:18; Bruce 1987; Germain 1987). Needed are innovative efforts to educate providers of all types, along with better inserts for contraceptive packaging that can be easily understood by clients with limited reading skills.

6. *Providing counseling and educational programs*

A comprehensive reproductive health program would offer individual and group counseling and educational programs to clinic and community participants on topics such as fertility control and reproductive physiology, male and female sexuality, reproductive health and nutrition, and the elimination of harmful practices such as female circumcision or damaging treatments during pregnancy, childbirth, and the post-partum period.

The need for high quality counseling of individuals and couples in their choice of a birth control method which includes clear information about possible side effects is increasingly recognized as essential to ensuring informed choice and user satisfaction. It has also raised contraceptive acceptance and voluntary continuation rates in a variety of settings (Gallen and Lettenmaier 1987). Training manuals and techniques have been developed to improve providers' communication skills and the accuracy of their technical information, not only for family planning clinic personnel but also for community outreach workers, pharmacists and shopkeepers, and traditional midwives (ibid.). Less has been done in the realm of male and female sexuality, including counseling on how to achieve more pleasurable sexual relations, how to treat sexual dysfunctions, and how to recognize, treat, and prevent reproductive tract infections and sexually transmitted diseases. (AIDs counseling may represent one exception.) The lack of attention paid to female sexuality concerns feminist health advocates in many countries who are confronted in their everyday work with women who in ignorance of their orgasmic capacities feel "used" by their sexual partners.

The key to good counseling is adaptability to the needs and concerns of each client, couple, and group. Feminist women's health collectives in industrialized and some developing countries have experimented with a variety of individual and group counseling methods that share a strong self-help focus and egalitarian ideology (Ruzek 1978). Some of the more radical-feminist self-help clinics in industrialized countries have appealed to a relatively small minority of women, however—usually young and well educated—who share a feminist ideology of alternative health care (Jones, Thoss, and Scottish Health Education Group 1987). Many women in poverty in both industrialized and developing countries, as well as middle-class women, may prefer a more conventional model of counseling and service delivery. For some women this may include a preference for male physicians, for example, and for *more* rather than less social distance between provider and client as a basis for trust and respect. The feminist principle of learning from the experiences and needs of women in diverse circumstances means that both the content and style of counseling and educational programs would be developed through a participatory process.

7. Challenging discriminatory attitudes and behavior in the community

The low status of women has been identified as a root cause of maternal deaths, poor health, and high fertility in many societies (e.g., Starrs 1987). In the light of the broad interpretation of reproductive health and rights proposed here, administrators of family planning and health programs, whether governmental or nongovernmental, would define their missions not only as delivering comprehensive and high quality fertility regulation and other reproductive health services to all social groups, but also as advocating the elimination of those oppressive institutions and practices that impede girls' and women's knowledge of and access to family planning and health services.

A variety of mechanisms could be created to challenge discriminatory attitudes and practices within the community. These can be tailored to the mass media, to political and religious leaders, to the schools, and to community groups of various kinds. Community-based health and family planning field-workers offer a good resource for reaching individuals and households with positive messages. In Bangladesh, for example, female outreach workers in a rural family planning extension project have served as effective change agents in altering the "calculus of choice" that binds women and men to patriarchal attitudes and practices. Workers try to win the support of husbands and other relatives for family planning while encouraging women to make their own decisions, if necessary, which may include surreptitious method use (Simmons et al. 1988). In addition, locally controlled women's income-generation projects, literacy programs, and grass roots community organizing can all change women's (and men's) consciousness and objective options (Rogow 1986:92). Women's organizations are a key resource in this endeavor.

8. *Building linkages with related programs and providers*

The question of whether family planning programs in developing countries should be integrated with health programs or operated as separate administrative entities has elicited a great deal of controversy over the years. Although complete administrative integration might appear to be both effective and efficient and tends to be favored by the medical profession, some family planning advocates fear that integration would dilute the resources and focus of the family planning effort and force a dependency on health ministries and infrastructures which in many countries are relatively weak. Instead, they say, specialized population activities should remain administratively distinct, although linked in some way to health programs (Simmons and Phillips 1987). Such linkages can include adding selected MCH and primary health care services to family planning programs—and vice versa—to create multiple-service packages in clinic or community settings; operating parallel but coordinated health and family planning programs; or establishing a reproductive health referral system at each specialized service delivery point that identifies sources of other specialized services. Similarly, clinic- or community-based workers can remain specialized in their functions or add other reproductive health tasks and referrals to their current "portfolio."

Evidence is mixed on which strategies are more effective in delivering family planning and health services and in attracting clients. Much depends on organizational capacities, worker motivation, and the quality of care provided. Although there is some preference for multiple-service packages in the same location, the bottom line of this debate for women's health advocates is the extent to which girls and women in diverse settings have access to a culturally acceptable and affordable range of services, whatever the mechanism may be.

9. *Training workers in accountability and quality of care*

The successful delivery of reproductive health care requires services that are accessible, acceptable, and of high quality. *Accessible* services are designed with the client's specific needs and abilities in mind with regard to location, mode of delivery, hours of service, costs, and communication skills. *Acceptable* services are those with which clients feel comfortable and satisfied. *High quality* services depend on providers' technical competence, sensitivity to the needs and concerns of each client, continuity of care, and commitment to fully informed personal choice for all women. These guidelines pose a challenge to professional staff and field-workers in southern and northern countries alike. As Judith Bruce (1987:380) concludes in her analysis of users' perspectives on contraceptive technology and delivery systems, "Service delivery systems rarely transcend the structural limitations characteristic of their societies. More frequently, they reflect these limitations or even extend prevailing discriminatory concepts about women's roles and entitlements. But they, too, can be realigned to be conscious in ideology and design of the needs of their clients." "How do we reach these women?" Bruce asks. "How do we protect their interests, their pride, and their privacy? What fears and limits can we help them overcome?" The most effective way to answer these questions is clearly to listen to the women themselves.

Women's health advocates throughout the world have highlighted the need for better training of health and family planning workers in the philosophy and techniques of listening to and empowering their clients. Training is required at all levels, from program managers through professional medical and nonmedical staff through paramedical and support workers. Although training techniques and content need to be tailored to specific situations, elements of quality of care include ensuring technical competence, conveying information accurately and clearly, raising sensitivity to girls' and women's modesty and fears, managing pain, and emphasizing client satisfaction and continuity of care in both clinic-based and community-based programs (Bruce 1990). Good evaluation research, record-keeping, and accountability procedures are also essential. Moreover, every attempt would be made to minimize the hierarchical, top-down approach to service delivery, including those " ... class, race, and other differences that distinguish the interests, experiences, and vulnerability of women with professional training from those of the women whose fertility they are 'managing' " (Jaquette and Staudt 1985:258). Where possible, program staff such as outreach workers, paramedics, and counselors would be recruited and trained from among the ranks of the women they serve. Interpersonal skills would be as important as technical skills in the selection and training of service providers.

10. *Eliciting commitments from governments, NGOs, and bilateral and multilateral funding agencies*

The reproductive health approach does not require massive infusions of additional funding nor does it replace currrent institutionalized delivery systems. Instead, it pulls together elements of major existing programs as building blocks of a more comprehensive approach to women's reproductive health and rights and identifies directions of change (Germain and Ordway 1989:10).

National and international priorities have shifted during the 1970s and 1980s with respect to major initiatives in Family Planning, Maternal and Child Health (MCH), Primary Health Care, Child Survival, and Safe Motherhood. Each of these initiatives incorporates different objectives, program strategies, and client populations. It should be possible to pull the threads together in a manner that identifies current gaps in reproductive health priorities and service delivery at the national and international levels. Family planning programs, for example, whose primary objectives are to promote contraceptive acceptance and reduce fertility, generally focus their attentions on married women of reproductive age who already have two or three children. They are less oriented to younger or unmarried women, women who want to be pregnant or want to terminate a pregnancy, and women with other reproductive health problems (Germain 1987:5). MCH programs serve pregnant and recently delivered women and their young children; safe motherhood initiatives concentrate on pregnant women through delivery; child survival initiatives serve women only indirectly through their emphasis on the mother's role in infant and child health. Missing from all of these client populations are adolescent girls, infertile women, women with reproductive tract infections, women not currently at risk of pregnancy or bearing children, victims of rape and violence, and others who "fall through the cracks" of service delivery— if services are available at all.

A sustained commitment to women's reproductive health and rights would build on current population and health programming as well as on women in development programming in governments; NGOs such as the International Planned Parenthood Federation with its multiple country affiliates; multilateral donor organizations such as the World Bank, World Health Organization, UNICEF, and the United Nations Population Fund

(UNFPA); and bilateral agencies such as the U.S. Agency for International Development. It would involve the critical analysis and coordination of existing efforts in order to define women's reproductive health—and, as a natural byproduct, the health and well-being of children—as a key element of population, health, and development programming.

THE DEMOGRAPHIC SIGNIFICANCE OF GENDER EQUALITY AND REPRODUCTIVE RIGHTS

There is no doubt that the world is faced with an overwhelming problem of sustained population growth at the global level. Although population growth rates have slowed since the 1960s and 1970s almost everywhere except sub-Saharan Africa, the 1990s will see the greatest increase in human numbers of any decade in history: almost one billion people. The demographic momentum engendered by past and current growth rates carries larger and larger waves of human increase in sheer numbers even as the rate of growth declines. Between 1990 and 2010 the world's population is likely to increase by one-third. The populations of southern countries, if they continue growing at 2 percent annually on average, will double in 34 years. The arguments presented in this final chapter are in no way intended to denigrate the seriousness of the population problem or to suggest that nothing need be done. Rather, they are presented as an alternative to conventional calls for "population control" in southern countries and for the intensified recruitment of family planning "acceptors" as its tool.

Analyses of the impact of population trends on economic growth and environmental degradation are clearly important. But the evidence suggests that many top-down approaches to controlling population growth through political campaigns and massive family planning promotions have been relatively ineffective, or have provoked fear and opposition among major population groups and within families, or both (Warwick 1982; Hernandez 1984). Feminist health advocates have been particularly vocal in their criticisms. At the same time, the multiple reproductive health needs of many girls and women remain largely unmet. In India, for example, where massive sterilization campaigns in the 1970s caused a political uproar and where the birth rate has remained stubbornly high, critics contend that the population program has been too focused on statistical objectives and too interested in quick solutions. Needed is a longer-term, more moderated approach centered on a good system of health delivery at the grassroots level together with improvements in literacy, skill development, income generation, physical and emotional security, and respect for human values (Bose 1988). Indian feminists add, "The new strategy should put family planning in the broadest dimension of social change.... It should be ... a people's movement and a community endeavor,'' not an externally imposed program (Karkal and Pandey 1989:106).

The search for a more responsive reproductive policy described in this chapter has considered both policy process and content. Ideally, the process becomes transformed from one that is externally imposed and technocratic to one that is internally motivated and humanistic. Listening to women's voices in the design and implementation of reproductive policies and programs involves a fundamental reorientation of policy-making processes and priorities. Indeed, it constitutes a shift in paradigm: a different world view, requiring different theories and lines of inqury. Turning things upside down, a woman-centered approach begins by trying to understand the concrete material and social conditions of women's lives in different contexts, and the meanings that women attach to their sexual and reproductive experiences. Programs and policies build on and adapt to these experiences.

The policy content becomes transformed as well. In bringing together the previously separated streams of thought about human rights and population processes, four major shifts occur. First, a development policy becomes a human rights policy designed to ensure that all persons have an adequate standard of living together with other basic freedoms and entitlements that are essential to personal security and reproductive choice. Second, a population (reproductive) policy becomes an equal rights policy designed to eliminate discrimination against girls and women in economic, social, political, and cultural life. Its intent is to undermine those gender-based structures and ideologies that curtail girls' and women's control over valued material and social resources and perpetuate patriarchal pronatalist controls. Consider, for example, the Philippines Development Plan for Women created by the National Commission on Women with input from women's organizations and government ministries as an accompaniment to the Medium-Term Philippines Development Plan for 1989–1992 (see chapter 4). The plan for women contained a broad range of sectoral goals and timetables, as well as particular demographic goals that focused on women's and children's well-being.

Third, a family planning policy becomes a reproductive rights policy designed to ensure that women and men are able to exercise genuine sexual and reproductive choice. Standards are set to protect individuals from coercive efforts by both pronatalist and antinatalist forces at the state, community, and family levels. In Brazil, for example, a national Committee on Reproductive Rights worked closely with the National Council for Women's Rights to formulate guidelines on women's sexual and reproductive rights. In the Philippines, a major umbrella organization for women's associations, GABRIELA, formed a Commission on Health and Reproductive Rights to set policy guidelines. Fourth, a family planning program becomes a reproductive health program designed to extend a full range of sexual and reproductive health services to women (and men) of all ages, particularly those who are excluded by reason of economic, social, marital, or pregnancy status from current programs. Again, the feminist-sponsored Integrated Women's Health Program in Brazil together with its associated Policy on Women's Health and Family Planning is an important example of this type. Fertility control forms only one (but a key) element of a reproductive health strategy enabling women to understand and enjoy their own sexuality, to regulate their fertility safely and effectively, to bear and raise healthy children, and to remain free of sexual violence and reproductive disability.

Human rights, women's rights, reproductive health: do they constitute a population policy? Yes and no. Their primary aim is *not* fertility decline, but rather, the expansion of human rights and improvement of human welfare. In this sense, then, the interventions do not—together or separately—constitute a population policy in the limited way we have defined it.

Nevertheless, there is little doubt that such interventions are likely to create conditions favorable to lower fertility if they are designed and implemented through a flexible participatory process to meet the needs of specific population groups within each country. A *rights-oriented development strategy* that improves the distribution of incomes and other resources among population subgroups, for example, can alter the environment of reproductive decision making in fundamental ways. In particular, structural changes combined with rising expectations can reduce the dependence of low-income and landless rural populations on children for their security and survival, reorient their survival/security strategies toward long-term investments in children's health and education, and reverse the inter-generational flow of wealth (e.g., Ridker 1976; Murdoch 1980; Caldwell 1982; Bulatao and Lee 1983). An *equal rights strategy* that explicitly challenges those ideological and structural forces that currently deny girls and women genuine choice can have a demographic impact by altering the circumstances of female dependency, marriage and divorce, schooling and employment, property ownership, inheritance and legal rights, and women's abilities to mobilize politically (United Nations 1975; Cochrane 1979; Bulatao and Lee 1983). A *reproductive rights policy* would remove legal and other impediments to the use of contraception, voluntary sterilization, and abortion, while prohibiting early arranged marriages, encouraging male financial responsibility for the children they father, and facilitating divorce. Each of these interventions is likely to reduce fertility. Finally, each of the ten elements outlined for the *core program in reproductive health* will, arguably, favor lower fertility by altering the conditions of sexual and reproductive decision making and providing services that encourage more sustained contraceptive use (e.g., Jain 1989). These elements consist of designing programs based on women's experiences, empowering women to overcome their oppression, offering an appropriate array of reproductive health services, ensuring informed choice among a range of birth control methods, expanding the channels of service delivery, providing counseling and educational programs, challenging discriminatory attitudes and behavior in the community, building linkages with related reproductive health programs and providers, and eliciting commitments from governments, NGOs, and international funding agencies.

If women are to control their own reproduction safely and effectively, they must also be able to manage their own health and sexuality, to achieve social status and dignity, and to exercise their basic economic and social rights in the family and in society. A population (reproductive) policy cannot be considered apart from an equal rights policy. Redefining the content of a population policy in this way should help to pull together different segments of activists working in northern and southern countries on issues of human rights, women's rights, and reproductive freedom. Most important, ridding family planning of its population control rationale and substituting a broader reproductive rights and health focus should appeal to the population, health, and family planning communities, on the one hand, and to feminist health advocates and human rights activists, on the other. The joining together of these communities in a common endeavor becomes all the more compelling in the context of a global political environment in which threats to women's rights and reproductive freedom are becoming more powerful. Women's rights groups and the population/family planning establishment cannot afford to be divided in their purpose, nor can feminists allow their anti-family planning rhetoric to be coopted by "right-to-life" organizations committed to the abolition of all artificial methods of birth control and to the perpetuation of women's subordination.

APPENDIXES

Appendix A: U.N. Convention on the Elimination of All Forms of Discrimination Against Women

[The Convention was passed by the U.N. General Assembly in 1979 and entered into force as a convention in 1981. The following passages are excerpted from the full document.]

THE STATES PARTIES TO THE PRESENT CONVENTION,

Noting that the Charter of the United Nations reaffirms faith in fundamental human rights, in the dignity and worth of the human person and in the equal rights of men and women,

Noting that the Universal Declaration of Human Rights affirms the principle of the inadmissibility of discrimination and proclaims that all human beings are born free and equal in dignity and rights and that everyone is entitled to all the rights and freedoms set forth therein, without distinction of any kind, including distinction based on sex,

Noting that the States Parties to the International Convenants on Human Rights have the obligation to ensure the equal right of men and women to enjoy all economic, social, cultural, civil and political rights,

Considering the international conventions concluded under the auspices of the United Nations and the specialised agencies promoting equality of rights of men and women,

Noting also the resolutions, declarations and recommendations adopted by the United Nations and the specialised agencies promoting equality of rights of men and women,

Concerned, however, that despite these various instruments extensive discrimination against women continues to exist,

Recalling that discrimination against women violates the principles of equality of rights and respect for human dignity, is an obstacle to the participation of women, on equal terms with men, in the political, social, economic and cultural life of their countries, hampers the growth of the prosperity of society and the family and makes more difficult the full

development of the potentialities of women in the service of their countries and of humanity, . . .
[followed by eight additional points of preamble]
Have agreed on the following:

PART I
ARTICLE 1

For the purposes of the present Convention, the term "Discrimination against women" shall mean any distinction, exclusion or restriction made on the basis of sex which has the effect or purpose of impairing or nullifying the recognition, enjoyment or exercise by women, irrespective of their marital status, on a basis of equality of men and women, of human rights and fundamental freedoms in the political, economic, social, cultural, civil or any other field.

ARTICLE 2

States Parties condemn discrimination against women in all its forms, agree to pursue by all appropriate means and without delay a policy of eliminating discrimination against women and, to this end, undertake:
a) To embody the principle of the equality of men and women in their national constitutions or other appropriate legislation if not yet incorporated therein and to ensure, through law and other appropriate means, the practical realisation of this principle;
b) To adopt appropriate legislative and other measures, including sanctions where appropriate, prohibiting all discrimination against women;
c) To establish legal protection of the rights of women on an equal basis with men and to ensure through competent national tribunals and other public institutions the effective protection of women against any act of discrimination;
d) To refrain from engaging in any act or practice of discrimination against women and to ensure that public authorities and institutions shall act in conformity with this obligation;
e) To take all appropriate measures to eliminate discrimination against women by any person, organisation or enterprise;
f) To take all appropriate measures, including legislation, to modify or abolish existing laws, regulations, customs and practices which constitute discrimination against women;
g) To repeal all national penal provisions which constitute discrimination against women.

ARTICLE 3

States Parties shall take in all fields, in particular in the political, social, economic and cultural fields, all appropriate measures, including legislation, to ensure the full development and advancement of women, for the purpose of guaranteeing them the exercise and enjoyment of human rights and fundamental freedoms on a basis of equality with men.

ARTICLE 4

1. Adoption by States Parties of temporary special measures aimed at accelerating *de facto* equality between men and women shall not be considered discrimination as defined in the present Convention, but shall in no way entail as a consequence the maintenance of unequal or separate standards; these measures shall be discontinued when the objectives of equality of opportunity and treatment have been achieved.
2. Adoption by States Parties of special measures, including those measures contained in the present Convention, aimed at protecting maternity shall not be considered discriminatory.

ARTICLE 5

States Parties shall take all appropriate measures:
a) To modify the social and cultural patterns of conduct of men and women, with a view to achieving the elimination of prejudices and customary and all other practices which are based on the idea of the inferiority or the superiority of either of the sexes or on stereotyped roles for men and women;
b) To ensure that family education includes a proper understanding of maternity as a social function and the recognition of the common responsibility of men and women in the upbringing and development of their children, it being understood that the interest of the children is the primordial consideration in all cases.

ARTICLE 6

States Parties shall take all appropriate measures, including legislation, to suppress all forms of traffic in women and exploitation of prostitution of women.

PART II
ARTICLE 7

States Parties shall take all appropriate measures to eliminate discrimination against women in the political and public life of the country and, in particular, shall ensure to women, on equal terms with men, the right:
a) To vote in all elections and public referenda and to be eligible for election to all publicly elected bodies;
b) To participate in the formulation of government policy and the imple-

mentation thereof and to hold public office and perform all public functions at all levels of government;

c) To participate in nongovernmental organisations and associations concerned with the public and political life of the country.

ARTICLE 8

States Parties shall take all appropriate measures to ensure to women, on equal terms with men and without any discrimination, the opportunity to represent their Governments at the international level and to participate in the work of international organisations.

ARTICLE 9

1. States Parties shall grant women equal rights with men to acquire, change or retain their nationality. They shall ensure in particular that neither marriage to an alien nor change of nationality by the husband during marriage shall automatically change the nationality of the wife, render her stateless or force upon her the nationality of the husband.

2. States Parties shall grant women equal rights with men with respect to the nationality of their children.

PART III
ARTICLE 10

States Parties shall take all appropriate measures to eliminate discrimination against women in order to ensure to them equal rights with men in the field of education and in particular to ensure, on a basis of equality of men and women:

a) The same conditions for career and vocational guidance, for access to studies and for the achievement of diplomas in educational establishments of all categories in rural as well as in urban areas; this equality shall be ensured in pre-school, general, technical, professional and higher tehnical education, as well as in all types of vocational training;

b) Access to the same curricula, the same examinations, teaching staff with qualifications of the same standard and school premises and equipment of the same quality;

c) The elimination of any stereotyped concept of the roles of men and women at all levels and in all forms of education by encouraging coeducation and other types of education which will help to achieve this aim and, in particular, by the revision of textbooks and school programmes and the adaptation of teaching methods;

d) The same opportunities to benefit from scholarships and other study grants;

e) The same opportunities for access to programmes of continuing education, including adult and functional literacy programmes, particularly those aimed at reducing, at the earliest possible time, any gap in education existing between men and women;

f) The reduction of female student drop-out rates and the organisation of programmes for girls and women who have left school prematurely;

g) The same opportunities to participate actively in sports and physical education;

h) Access to specific educational information to help to ensure the health and well-being of families, including information and advice on family planning.

ARTICLE 11

1. States Parties shall take all appropriate measures to eliminate discrimination against women in the field of employment in order to ensure, on a basis of equality of men and women, the same rights, in particular:

a) The right to work as an inalienable right of all human beings;

b) The right to the same employment opportunities, including the application of the same criteria for selection in matters of employment;

c) The right to free choice of profession and employment, the right to promotion, job security and all benefits and conditions of service and the right to receive vocational training and retraining, including apprenticeships, advanced vocational training and recurrent training;

d) The right to equal remuneration, including benefits, and to equal treatment in respect of work of equal value, as well as equality of treatment in the evaluation of the quality of work;

e) The right to social security, particularly in cases of retirement, unemployment, sickness, invalidity and old age and other incapacity to work, as well as the right to paid leave;

f) The right to protection of health and to safety in working conditions, including the safeguarding of the function of reproduction.

2. In order to prevent discrimination against women on the grounds of marriage or maternity and to ensure their effective right to work, States Parties shall take appropriate measures:

a) To prohibit, subject to the imposition of sanctions, dismissal on the grounds of pregnancy or of maternity leave and discrimination in dismissals on the basis of marital status;

b) To introduce maternity leave with pay or with comparable social benefits without loss of former employment, seniority or social allowances;

c) To encourage the provision of the necessary supporting social services to enable parents to combine family obligations with work responsibilities and participation in public life, in particular through promoting the establishment and development of a network of child-care facilities;

d) To provide special protection to women during pregnancy in types of work proved to be harmful to them.
3. Protective legislation relating to matters covered in this article shall be reviewed periodically in the light of scientific and technological knowledge and shall be revised, repealed or extended as necessary.

ARTICLE 12

1. States Parties shall take all appropriate measures to eliminate discrimination against women in the field of health care in order to ensure, on a basis of equality of men and women, access to health care services, including those related to family planning.
2. Notwithstanding the provisions of paragraph 1 of this article, States Parties shall ensure to women appropriate services in connection with pregnancy, confinement and the post-natal period, granting free services where necessary, as well as adequate nutrition during pregnancy and lactation.

ARTICLE 13

States Parties shall take all appropriate measures to eliminate discrimination against women in other areas of economic and social life in order to ensure, on a basis of equality of men and women, the same rights, in particular:
a) The right of family benefits;
b) The right to bank loans, mortgages and other forms of financial credit;
c) The right to participate in recreational activities, sports and all aspects of cultural life.

ARTICLE 14

1. States Parties shall take into account the particular problems faced by rural women and the significant roles which rural women play in the economic survival of their families, including their work in the non-monetized sectors of the economy, and shall take all appropriate measures to ensure the application of the provisions of the present Convention to women in rural areas.
2. States Parties shall take all appropriate measures to eliminate discrimination against women in rural areas in order to ensure, on a basis of equality of men and women, that they participate in and benefit from rural development and, in particular, shall ensure to such women the right:
a) To participate in the elaboration and implementation of development planning at all levels;

b) To have access to adequate health care facilities, including information, counselling and services in family planning;

c) To benefit directly from social security programmes;

d) To obtain all types of training and education, formal and non-formal, including that relating to functional literacy, as well as, *inter alia,* the benefit of all community and extension services, in order to increase their technical proficiency;

e) To organise self-help groups and co-operatives in order to obtain equal access to economic opportunities through employment or self-employment;

f) To particpate in all community activities;

g) To have access to agricultural credit and loans, marketing facilities, appropriate technology and equal treatment in land and agrarian reform as well as in land resettlement schemes;

h) To enjoy adequate living conditions, particularly in relation to housing, sanitation, electricity and water supply, transport and communications.

PART IV
ARTICLE 15

1. States Parties shall accord to women equality with men before the law.

2. States Parties shall accord to women, in civil matters, a legal capacity identical to that of men and the same opportunities to exercise that capacity. In particular, they shall give women equal rights to conclude contracts and to administer property and shall treat them equally in all stages of procedure in courts and tribunals.

3. States Parties agree that all contracts and all other private instruments of any kind with a legal effect which is directed at restricting the legal capacity of women shall be deemed null and void.

4. States Parties shall accord to men and women the same rights with regard to the law relating to the movement of persons and the freedom to choose their residence and domicile.

ARTICLE 16

1. States Parties shall take all appropriate measures to eliminate discrimination against women in all matters relating to marriage and family relations and in particular shall ensure, on a basis of equality of men and women:

a) The same right to enter into marriage;

b) The same right freely to choose a spouse and to enter into marriage only with their free and full consent;

c) The same rights and responsibilities during marriage and at its dissolution;

d) The same rights and responsibilities as parents, irrespective of their marital status, in matters relating to their children; in all cases the interests of the children shall be paramount;

e) The same rights to decide freely and responsibly on the number and spacing of their children and to have access to the information, education and means to enable them to exercise these rights;

f) The same rights and responsibilities with regard to guardianship, wardship, trusteeship and adoption of children, or similar institutions where these concepts exist in national legislation; in all cases the interests of the children shall be paramount;

g) The same personal rights as husband and wife, including the right to choose a family name, a profession and an occupation;

h) The same rights for both spouses in respect of the ownership, acquisition, management, administration, enjoyment and disposition of property, whether free of charge or for a valuable consideration.

2. The betrothal and the marriage of a child shall have no legal effect, and all necessary action, including legislation, shall be taken to specify a minimum age for marriage and to make the registration of marriages in an official registry compulsory.

PART V
ARTICLE 17

1. For the purpose of considering the progress made in the implementation of the present Convention, there shall be established a Committee on the Elimination of Discrimination against Women . . . consisting, at the time of entry into force of the Convention, of eighteen and, after ratification of or accession to the Convention by the thirty-fifth State Party, of twenty-three experts of high moral standing and competence in the field covered by the Convention. The experts shall be elected by States Parties from among their nationals and shall serve in their personal capacity, consideration being given to equitable geographical distribution and to the representation of the different forms of civilisation as well as the principal legal systems. . . .

[The remainder of article 17 describes the functioning of the Committee]

ARTICLE 18

1. States Parties shall undertake to submit to the Secretary-General of the United Nations, for consideration by the Committee, a report on the legislative, judicial, administrative or other measures which they have adopted to give effect to the provisions of the present Convention and on the progress made in this respect. . . .

[The remainder of article 18, and articles 19 through 24, deal with administrative details.]

ARTICLE 25

1. The present Convention shall be open for signature by all States.
2. The Secretary-General of the United Nations is designated as the depositary of the present Convention.
3. The present Convention is subject to ratification. Instruments of ratification shall be deposited with the Secretary-General of the United Nations.
4. The present Convention shall be open to accession by all States. Accession shall be effected by the deposit of an instrument of accession with the Secretary-General of the United Nations. . . .
[Articles 26 through 29 deal with additional administrative details.]

ARTICLE 30

The present Convention, the Arabic, Chinese, English, French, Russian and Spanish texts of which are equally authentic, shall be deposited with the Secretary-General of the United Nations.
IN WITNESS WHEREOF the undersigned, duly authorised, have signed the present Convention.

Appendix B: Selected Demographic Indicators: Countries with Populations of Over One Million Persons, Around 1990

Region and	1990	1990	%Pop	TFR		%Contra	%F15-19	Mat	F life
Country	Pc GNP	pop/mil	Incr	1970	1990	total/mod	married	mort	expec
AFRICA									
Northern Africa									
Algeria	2,170	25.6	2.7	7.5	5.4			140	64
Egypt	630	54.7	2.9	6.6	4.5	38/35	21	318	62
Libya	5,410	4.2	3.1		5.2			80	62
Morocco	900	25.6	2.5	7.1	4.5	36/29	17	300	62
Sudan	420	25.2	2.9	6.7	6.4	9/6		660	51
Tunisia	1,260	8.1	2.2	6.8	4.1	50/40	6	310	66
Unweighted av.	1,798		2.7	6.9	5.0	33/28	15	301	61
Western Africa									
Benin	380	4.7	3.0	6.9	7.1	9/1			48
Burkina Faso	310	9.1	3.3	6.7	7.2		53	810	49
Cote d'Ivoire	790	12.6	3.5	7.4	7.4	3/1	52		54
Ghana	380	15.0	3.2	6.8	6.3	13/5		1000	56
Guinea	430	7.3	2.6	6.4	6.1	1/			44
Guinea-Bissau	180	1.0	2.0	5.2	5.8	1/			47
Liberia	450	2.6	3.2	6.4	6.8	6/6			56
Mali	260	8.1	3.0	6.6	7.1	5/1	49		46
Mauritania	490	2.0	2.8	6.5	6.5	1/	37		48
Niger	290	7.9	3.3	7.1	7.1			420	46
Nigeria	250	118.8	2.8	7.1	6.2	6/4		800	52
Senegal	650	7.4	2.8	6.7	6.5	11/2	33	600	47
Sierra Leone	200	4.2	2.7	6.4	6.5	4/		450	43
Togo	390	3.7	3.7	6.2	7.2	34/3			55

Appendix B (continued)

Region and Country	1990 Pc GNP	1990 pop/mil	%Pop Incr	TFR 1970	TFR 1990	%Contra total/mod	%F15-19 married	Mat mort	F life expec
Unweighted av.	389		3.0	6.6	6.7	8/3	45	680	49
Eastern Africa									
Burundi	220	5.6	3.2	5.8	7.0	9/1	19		51
Ethiopia	120	51.7	2.9	6.7	6.8	2/	53		43
Kenya	380	24.6	3.8	8.1	6.7	27/18		170	60
Madagascar	230	12.0	3.2	6.6	6.6	2/	34	240	55
Malawi	180	9.2	3.4	6.9	7.7	7/1	47	100	48
Mauritius	1,950	1.1	1.4	4.3	2.0	75/45	11	126	72
Mozambique	80	15.7	2.7	6.5	6.3		48		48
Rwanda	310	7.3	3.4	8.0	8.1	10/1	15	210	50
Somalia	170	8.4	2.9	6.6	6.6			1100	47
Tanzania	120	26.0	3.7	6.9	7.1	11/	36	340	55
Uganda	250	18.0	3.5	6.9	7.4	5/3		300	53
Zambia	390	8.1	3.8	6.7	7.2	1/	29	151	54
Zimbabwe	640	9.7	3.1	7.5	5.6	43/36	24	480	60
Unweighted av.	388		3.2	6.7	6.5	18/15	32	322	54
Middle Africa									
Angola	620	8.5	2.8	6.4	6.4	1/			46
Cameroon	1,010	11.1	2.6	5.8	5.8	2/1	44		53
Cen. Af. Rep.	390	2.9	2.6	5.7	5.6		46	600	47
Chad	190	5.0	2.5	6.1	5.8			860	47
Congo	930	2.2	3.0	5.9	5.9		16	1000	50
Gabon	2,770	1.2	2.3	4.2	5.0				53
Zaire	260	36.6	3.1	6.0	6.1	11/			54
Unweighted av.	881		2.7	5.7	5.8	5/1	35	820	50
Southern Africa									
Botswana	940	1.2	2.7	6.9	4.9	33/32	7	250	62
Lesotho	470	1.8	2.9	5.7	5.8	5/2			60

Appendix B (continued)

Region and	1990	1990	%Pop	TFR		%Contra	%F15-19	Mat	F life
Country	Pc GNP	pop/mil	Incr	1970	1990	total/mod	married	mort	expec
Namibia		1.5	3.1	6.1	5.9	48/45			58
South Africa	2,460	39.6	2.7	5.9	4.5	20/17	5	83	64
Unweighted av.	1,290		2.9	6.2	5.3	26/24	6	166	61
ASIA									
Western Asia									
Iraq		18.8	2.7	7.2	6.4	15/13	32		65
Israel	9,750	4.6	1.6	3.8	3.0		6	8	77
Jordan	1,730	4.1	4.1	8.0	7.1	26/21	20		68
Kuwait		2.1	3.0	7.5	4.7		14	4	75
Lebanon		3.3	2.1	6.1	3.6				69
Oman	5,220	1.5	3.8	7.2	7.2				57
Saudi Arabia	6,230	15.0	3.4	7.3	7.2				65
Syria	1,020	12.6	3.8	7.8	6.7	20/15	25	280	67
Turkey	1,360	56.7	2.2	5.6	3.7	77/49	21	210	66
UAE	18,430	1.6	2.7	6.8	4.9		55		73
Yemen	640	9.8	3.5	7.0	7.4	1/			52
Unweighted av.	5,548		3.0	6.8	5.6	28/24	25	126	67
Southern Asia									
Afghanistan		15.9	2.6	7.1	7.1		53	690	42
Bangladesh	180	114.8	2.4	6.9	4.9	33/26	65	600	50
Bhutan	190	1.6	2.0	5.9	5.9			1710	58
India	350	853.4	2.0	5.7	3.9	49/42	44	340	66
Iran		55.6	3.3	7.0	6.2	/22	34		50
Nepal	170	19.1	2.5	6.2	6.1	15/15	50	830	56
Pakistan	370	114.6	3.0	7.0	6.6	8/7	29	500	72
Sri Lanka	430	17.2	1.5	4.7	2.5	62/41	10	60	47
Unweighted av.	282		2.4	6.3	5.4	33/26	41	676	55
Southeast Asia									

Appendix B (continued)

Region and Country	1990 Pc GNP	1990 pop/mil	%Pop Incr	TFR 1970	TFR 1990	%Contra total/mod	%F15-19 married	Mat mort	F life expec
Cambodia		7.0	2.2	6.2	4.5				50
Indonesia	490	189.4	1.7	5.6	3.0	48/44	17	450	57
Laos	170	4.0	2.2	6.2	5.0				50
Malaysia	2,130	17.9	2.5	5.9	3.6	51/30	8	59	72
Myanmar		41.3	1.9	5.7	4.1		16	135	62
Philippines	700	66.1	2.6	6.0	4.1	45/22	14	93	65
Singapore	10,450	2.7	1.3	3.5	1.8	74/59	2	13	76
Thailand	1,170	55.7	1.3	6.1	2.2	66/64	16	81	67
Viet Nam		70.2	2.3	5.9	4.0	53/38		140	64
Unweighted av.	2518		2.0	5.7	3.6	56/43	12	122	62
East Asia									
China	360	1119.9	1.4	6.0	2.3	71/70	4	44	71
Hong Kong	10,320	5.8	0.7	4.0	1.2	81/73	2	3	79
Japan	23,730	123.6	0.3	2.0	1.5	64/60	1	14	81
Korea, North		21.3	1.8	5.7	2.5			41	73
Korea, South	4,400	42.8	0.9	4.5	1.6	77/70	1	14	72
Mongolia		2.2	2.7	5.9	4.8			100	66
Taiwan		20.2	1.1		1.7	78/62			
Unweighted av.	9,702		1.3	4.7	2.3	74/67	2	19	74
NORTH AMERICA									
Canada	19,020	26.6	0.7	2.5	1.7	73/69	5	4	80
United States	21,100	251.4	0.8	2.6	2.1	74/69	5	8	79
Unweighted av.	20,060		0.8	2.6	1.9	74/69	5	6	80
LATIN AMERICA									
Central America									
Costa Rica	1,790	3.0	2.4	5.8	3.3	70/58	15	24	77
El Salvador	1,040	5.3	2.8	6.6	4.6	47/45		70	66
Guatemala	920	9.2	3.0	6.6	5.3	23/19	26	76	64

Appendix B (continued)

Region and Country	1990 Pc GNP	1990 pop/mil	%Pop Incr	TFR 1970	TFR 1990	%Contra total/mod	%F15-19 married	Mat mort	F life expec
Honduras	900	5.1	3.1	7.4	5.3	41/31		50	66
Mexico	1,990	88.6	2.3	6.7	3.8	53/45	20	91	72
Nicaragua	830	3.9	3.4	7.1	5.5	27/23		47	65
Panama	1,780	2.4	2.1	5.6	3.0	58/54	20	57	74
Unweighted av.	1,321		2.7	6.5	4.4	46/39	20	59	69
Caribbean									
Cuba		10.6	1.1	4.3	1.9	65/	27	47	76
Dominican Rep.	790	7.2	2.3	6.7	3.6	50/47		74	68
Haiti	400	6.5	2.9	6.2	6.4	10/9	8	230	56
Jamaica	1,260	2.4	1.9	5.4	2.6	55/51		110	77
Puerto Rico	6,010	3.3	1.1	3.4	2.2	70/62	14	13	78
Trinidad	3,160	1.3	1.6	3.9	2.4	53/44	11	54	73
Unweighted av.	2,324		1.8	5.0	3.2	50/43	12	88	71
South America									
Argentina	2,160	32.3	1.2	3.1	2.7		10	60	74
Bolivia	600	7.3	2.6	6.6	4.9	30/12	16	480	55
Brazil	2,550	150.4	1.9	5.3	3.3	66/56	15	120	68
Chile	1,770	13.2	1.8	4.4	2.7		10	50	75
Colombia	1,190	31.8	2.0	6.0	2.9	65/53		110	67
Ecuador	1,040	10.7	2.4	6.7	3.8	44/36	18	160	68
Paraguay	1,030	4.3	2.8	6.4	4.5	48/35	14	365	69
Peru	1,090	21.9	2.3	6.6	4.0	46/23	14	89	63
Uruguay	2,620	3.0	0.8	2.8	2.4	40/	12	43	74
Venezuela	2,450	19.6	2.3	5.9	3.3	49/	18	59	73
Unweighted av.	1,650		2.0	5.4	3.5	48/36	14	154	69
EUROPE									
Northern Europe									
Denmark	20,510	5.1	0.0	2.2	1.6	63/59	1	4	78

Appendix B (continued)

Region and Country	1990 Pc GNP	1990 pop/mil	%Pop Incr	TFR 1970	TFR 1990	%Contra total/mod	%F15-19 married	Mat mort	F life expec
Finland	22,060	5.0	0.3	2.1	1.7	80/77	1	7	79
Ireland	8,500	3.5	0.6	3.9	2.1	60/	1		77
Norway	21,850	4.2	0.3	2.7	1.9	71/64	1		80
Sweden	21,710	8.5	0.3	2.1	2.1	78/	0		80
United Kingdom	14,750	57.4	0.2	2.5	1.8	83/75	3		78
Unweighted av.	18,230		0.3	2.6	1.9	73/69	1	6	79
Western Europe									
Austria	17,360	7.6	0.1	2.5	1.4	71/56	4	7	78
Belgium	16,390	9.9	0.1	2.3	1.6	81/64	5	9	78
France	17,830	56.4	0.4	2.6	1.8	75/51	1	12	80
Germany	16,200	79.5	0.0	2.3	1.5		2	10	78
Netherlands	16,010	14.9	0.4	2.7	1.6	72/69	1	8	80
Switzerland	30,270	6.7	0.3	2.3	1.6	71/65	1	4	80
Unweighted av.	19,010		0.2	2.4	1.6	74/61	2	8	79
Eastern Europe									
Bulgaria	2,320	8.9	0.1	2.2	2.0	76/8	17	25	75
Czechoslovvakia		15.7	0.2	2.1	2.0	66/25	8	8	75
Hungary	2,560	10.6	-0.2	2.0	1.8	73/62	11	15	74
Poland	1,760	37.8	0.5	2.3	2.1	75/26	4	13	76
Romania		23.3	0.5	3.1	2.3	56/6	14		73
Unweighted av.	2,213		0.2	2.3	2.0	69/25	11	15	75
Southern Europe									
Albania		3.3	1.9	5.1	3.0				74
Greece	5,340	10.1	0.1	2.4	1.5		14	7	78
Italy	15,150	57.7	0.1	2.5	1.3	78/32	5	9	79
Portugal	5,820	10.4	0.2	2.9	1.5	66/33	9	9	77
Spain	9,150	39.4	0.2	2.9	1.3	59/38	5	11	80
Yugoslavia	2,490	23.8	0.5	2.5	1.9	55/12	11	16	75

Appendix B (continued)

Region and Country	1990 Pc GNP	1990 pop/mil	%Pop Incr	TFR 1970	TFR 1990	%Contra total/mod	%F15-19 married	Mat mort	F life expec
Unweighted av.	7,590		0.5	3.0	1.8	64/29	9	10	77
USSR		291.0	0.8	2.4	2.3		9	48	74
OCEANIA									
Australia	14,440	17.1	0.8	2.9	1.8	67/47	4	5	80
New Zealand	11,800	3.3	0.9	3.2	2.1	70/60	2	14	78
Pap. New Guinea	900	4.0	2.3	6.2	5.3	5/	17	900	55
Unweighted av.	9,047		1.3	4.1	3.1	47/54	8	306	71

Source:

Per capita Gross National Product, 1990: Population Reference Bureau 1991.
1990 mid-year population in millions: Population Reference Bureau 1990.
Annual rate of natural increase, 1990: Population Reference Bureau 1991.
Total fertility rate, 1970: United Nations 1991:67–70.
Total fertility rate, 1990: Population Reference Bureau 1991.
Percentage of married women using contraception (total and modern): Population
    Reference Bureau 1991; IPPF 1990; Demographic and Health Survey Data (Ecuador
    and Thailand), 1987.
Percentage of women ages 15–19 currently married: United Nations 1991:26–29.
Maternal morality rate (maternal deaths per 100,000 live births): ibid.: 67–70.
Female life expectancy at birth, in years: ibid.

Appendix C: Selected Indicators of the Status of Women, Around 1990

Region and Country	%F 15-24 illiterate	F/M ratio	%F in Sec School	F/M ratio	%F 15+ ec activ	F as % ec activ	%F Seat par	%F Seat min
AFRICA								
Northern Africa								
Algeria	40	2.61	53	.76	8	9	2.4	3.3
Egypt	62	1.67	58	.68	9	10	3.9	0
Libya					9	9		
Morocco			30	.66	19	20	0	0
Sudan					24	22	0.7	0
Tunisia	37	3.79	38	.74	26	25	5.6	4.2
Unweighted av.	46	2.69	45	.71	16	16	2.5	1.5
Western Africa								
Benin	82	1.50	9	.39	77	48	4.1	0
Burkina Faso	93	1.20	4	.46	77	46		11.5
Cote d'Ivoire			12	.44	48	34	5.7	9.5
Ghana			30	.66	51	40		0
Guinea			4	.31	57	40		0
Guinea-Bissau	82	2.04			57	41	14.7	4.5
Liberia					37	30	6.3	10.5
Mali	86	1.18	4	.42	16	16	3.7	6.3
Mauritania			10	.44	24	22		0
Niger			4	.42	79	47		0
Nigeria			7		46	35		0
Senegal			10	.51	53	39	11.7	12.0
Sierra Leone					38	32		0
Togo	64	2.39	12	.32	47	36	5.2	0
Unweighted av.	81	1.66	10	.44	51	36	7.3	3.9
Eastern Africa								
Burundi			3	.52	78	48	9.2	10.0

Appendix C (continued)

Region and Country	%F 15-24 illiterate	F/M ratio	%F in Sec School	F/M ratio	%F 15+ ec activ	F as % ec activ	%F Seat par	min
Ethiopia			12	.67	52	37		0
Kenya			19	.70	58	40	1.7	0
Madagascar			19	.94	55	39	1.5	4.5
Malawi			3	.60	57	41		0
Mauritius			53	.97	29	27	5.7	4.2
Mozambique	75	2.08	4	.54	79	48	16.0	0
Rwanda	55	1.37	5	.35	79	47	12.9	0
Somalia					53	39	4.0	0
Tanzania	46	2.38	3	.54	77	48		16.0
Uganda			8	.54	62	41		0
Zambia					33	28	2.9	0
Zimbabwe			42	.88	44	34	9.0	4.0
Unweighted av.	59	1.94	16	.66	58	40	7.0	3.0
Middle Africa								
Angola					52	39	14.5	4.8
Cameroon	41	2.00	21	.64	41	33	14.2	6.5
Cen. Af. Rep.	82	1.78	6	.40	68	46		0
Chad			2	.18	23	21		4.2
Congo				.76	51	39	9.8	0
Gabon				.81	47	37	13.4	2.0
Zaire			14		45	35	3.5	0
Unweighted av.	62	1.89	11	.56	47	36	11.1	2.5
Southern Africa								
Botswana	33	1.03	33	1.03	42	36	5.1	0
Lesotho			30	1.53	65	44		3.2
Namibia					24	23		
South Africa					40	36	3.5	0

Appendix C (continued)

Region and Country	%F 15-24 illiterate	F/M ratio	%F in Sec School	F/M ratio	%F 15+ ec activ	F as % ec activ	%F Seat par	%F Seat min
Unweighted av.	33	1.03	32	1.28	43	35	4.3	1.1
ASIA								
Western Asia								
Iraq			37	.63	21	21	13.2	0
Israel	0	1.00	87	1.21	37	34	8.3	3.2
Jordan	24	4.52		.96	9	10	0	0
Kuwait	24	1.28	79	.67	24	14		0
Lebanon					25	27	0	0
Oman			34	.71	9	9		0
Saudi Arabia			35	.66	9	7		0
Syria			47	.70	15	16	9.2	0
Turkey	25	3.86	34	.60	45	34	3.0	0
UAE	44	1.27	68	1.01	18	6	0	0
Yemen					10	12	0	0
Unweighted av.	23	2.39	53	.79	20	17	4.2	0.3
Southern Asia								
Afghanistan	89	1.64			8	9		0
Bangladesh	73	1.31	11	.46	5	7	9.1	2.8
Bhutan			2	.41	43	31	1.3	28.6
India	60	1.77	29	.51	29	25	8.3	0
Iran	58	1.98	44	.68	17	18	1.5	0
Nepal	85	1.55	17		43	32	5.8	0
Pakistan	75	1.38	11	.39	13	12	8.9	0
Sri Lanka	10	1.16	74	1.06	29	27	4.8	5.1
Unweighted av.	64	1.54	27	.58	23	20	5.7	4.6
Southeast Asia								
Cambodia					52	38		
Indonesia	18	1.76	43	.79	37	31		4.9

Appendix C (continued)

Region and Country	%F 15-24 illiterate	F/M ratio	%F in Sec School	F/M ratio	%F 15+ ec activ	F as % ec activ	%F Seat par	%F Seat min
Laos			22	.73	71	44		0
Malaysia	17	1.65	57	1.01	44	35	5.1	0
Myanmar	19	1.63	23		48	36		0
Philippines	8	0.85	71		36	31		10.0
Singapore	4	1.06	70		40	32	3.8	0
Thailand	4	1.58			68	45	3.5	0
Viet Nam	6	1.54			70	47	17.7	0
Unweighted av.	11	8.54	48	.84	52	38	7.5	1.9
East Asia								
China	18	3.73	37	.69	70	43	21.2	0
Hong Kong			76	1.04	48	33		
Japan			96	.99	46	38	1.4	0
Korea, North					64	46	21.1	
Korea, South			84	.87	40	34	2.5	
Mongolia			96	1.07	72	46	24.9	0
Taiwan								
Unweighted av.	18	3.73	78	.93	57	40	14.2	0
NORTH AMERICA								
Canada			106	.95	49	40	9.6	17.1
United States	1	0.86	99		50	41	5.3	5.6
Unweighted av.	1	0.86	102	.95	50	40	7.4	11.4
LATIN AMERICA								
Central America								
Costa Rica	2	0.73	42	1.03	24	22	10.5	0
El Salvador	30	1.09	31	.92	29	25	3.3	0
Guatemala					16	16	7.0	14.3
Honduras					21	20	5.2	0
Mexico	9	1.33	53	.89	30	27	10.8	0

Appendix C (continued)

Region and Country	%F 15-24 illiterate	F/M ratio	%F in Sec School	F/M ratio	%F 15+ ec activ	F as % ec activ	%F Seat par	min
Nicaragua			58	1.68	28	26	13.5	5.0
Panama	7	1.29	63	1.05	30	27	6.0	0
Unweighted av.	12	1.11	49	1.11	25	23	8.0	2.8
Caribbean								
Cuba	1	0.63			36	32	33.9	2.9
Dominican Rep.					15	15	5.0	0
Haiti	49	1.01	19		56	41		0
Jamaica			68		68	46	11.7	0
Puerto Rico	5	0.82			26	29		
Trinidad	1	1.00	85	1.00	34	30	16.7	9.5
Unweighted av.	14	.86	57	1.00	39	32	16.8	2.5
South America								
Argentina	3	0.75	78	1.72	28	28	0	0
Bolivia	24	2.85	35		27	25	3.8	0
Brazil	15	0.85	45		30	28	5.3	1.0
Chile	3	0.74	76	1.06	29	28		0
Colombia			56	.99	22	22		1.0
Ecuador	7	1.40	57	.91	19	19	1.4	0
Paraguay	6	1.02	29	.99	23	21	1.7	0
Peru	10	2.91			25	24	5.6	0
Uruguay	1	0.48			32	31	0	13.3
Venezuela	6	0.81	59	1.19	31	28	3.9	0
Unweighted av.	8	1.31	54	1.14	27	25	2.7	1.5
EUROPE								
Northern Europe								
Denmark			108	1.05	58	45	29.1	13.6
Finland			116	1.12	57	47	31.5	23.5
Ireland			102	1.01	32	29	8.4	5.6

Appendix C (continued)

Region and Country	%F 15-24 illiterate	F/M ratio	%F in Sec School	F/M ratio	%F 15+ ec activ	F as % ec activ	%F Seat par	%F Seat min
Norway			96	1.03	50	41	34.4	33.3
Sweden			92	1.07	55	45	28.5	18.2
United Kingdom			84	.96	46	39	6.3	8.0
Unweighted av.			100	1.04	50	41	23.0	17.0
Western Europe								
Austria			82	.94	44	40	11.5	11.8
Belgium			100	1.03	33	34	7.5	0
France			98	1.08	45	40	6.4	0
Germany			92	.97	*41	*37	*15.4	*11.8
Netherlands			102	1.11	31	31	20.0	6.3
Switzerland				.99	43	37	14.0	12.5
Unweighted av.			95	1.02	40	36	12.5	7.1
Eastern Europe								
Bulgaria			76	1.80	57	46	21.0	5.3
Czechoslovakia			88	1.59	62	47	29.5	0
Hungary	1	1.00	72	1.94	53	45	21.0	4.0
Poland	0	1.00	83	2.62	60	46	20.2	3.4
Romania			80	2.33	60	46	34.4	11.6
Unweighted av.	0	1.00	80	2.06	58	46	25.2	4.9
Southern Europe								
Albania					59	41	28.8	5.6
Greece	1	1.22	93	1.01	25	27	4.3	4.2
Italy	0	1.33	76		30	32	12.9	4.5
Portugal	2	0.78	63	1.14	40	37	7.6	7.1
Spain	1	1.11	111	1.01	22	24	6.4	0
Yugoslavia	2	2.50	79	.94	45	39	18.8	0
Unweighted av.	1	1.39	84	1.02	37	33	13.1	3.6
USSR					60	48	34.5	0

Appendix C (continued)

Region and Country	%F 15-24 illiterate	F/M ratio	%F in Sec School	F/M ratio	%F 15+ ec activ	F as % ec activ	%F Seat par	min
OCEANIA								
Australia			101	.99	46	38	6.1	3.3
New Zealand			88	.98	40	35	14.4	9.4
Pap. New Guinea			9	.60	58	38	0	2.9
Unweighted av.			66	.86	55	37	6.8	5.2

*These figures are for West Germany. The comparable figures for East Germany are: 62%, 45%, 32.2%, 10.3%.

Sources:

Percentage of females 15–24 who are illiterate and ratio of female to male illiteracy rates: United Nations 1991:50–53.

Percentage of females of relevant age enrolled in secondary school and ratio of females to males: World Bank 1991:266–267.

Percentage of females ages 15 and over who are economically active, and females as percentage of total economically active population: United Nations 1991:104–107.

Percentage of seats in parliaments (national legislature) and of ministerial (cabinet) positions occupied by women: ibid.:39–42.

Appendix D: Government Policies Relating to Population and the Status of Women

Region and Country	Govt view of fert	Govt FP	Private Fp	Abortion Grounds	U.N. Equal Rights Conventions					Const
					Disc	Pol	Mar	Educ	Emp	Equal
AFRICA										
Northern Africa										
Algeria	High	govt	IPPF	Narrow	NS			R	R	S
Egypt	High	govt	IPPF	Narrow	RA	R		R	R	G
Libya	Sat	none	NoFPA	Illegal	RA			R	R	
Morocco	High	govt	IPPF	Narrow	NS	R		R	R	G
Sudan	Sat	govt	IPPF	Illegal	NS				R	S
Tunisia	High	govt	IPPF	Broad	RA	R	R	R	R	G
Western Africa										
Benin	Sat	some	IPPF	Illegal	S		R	R	R	G
Burkina Faso	High	govt	IPPF	Illegal	RA					S
Cote d'Ivoire	Sat	some	IPPF	Illegal	S				R	S
Ghana	High	govt	IPPF	Narrow*	RA	R			R	
Guinea	High	govt	IPPF	Narrow	RA	R	R	R	R	N
Guinea Bissau	High	govt	FPA	Narrow	RA					
Liberia	High	govt	IPPF	Narrow*	RA	S		R	R	S
Mali	Sat	govt	IPPF	Illegal	S	R	R		R	
Mauritania	Sat	some	IPPF	Illegal	NS	R			R	N
Niger	High	govt	FPA	Illegal	NS	R	R	R	R	
Nigeria	High	govt	IPPF	Illegal	RA	R		R		
Senegal	High	govt	IPPF	Illegal	RA	R		R	R	S
Sierra Leone	High	govt	IPPF	Narrow	RA	R		R	R	S
Togo	High	govt	IPPF	Broad	RA					S
Eastern Africa										
Burundi	High	govt	NoFPA	Broad	S					S

Appendix D (continued)

Region and Country	Govt view of fert	Govt FP	Private Fp	Abortion Grounds	U.N. Equal Rights Conventions Disc	Pol	Mar	Educ	Emp	Const Equal
Ethiopia	High	govt	IPPF	Narrow	RA	R			R	
Kenya	High	govt	IPPF	Narrow	RA					S
Madagascar	High	some	IPPF	Illegal	RA	R		R	R	S
Malawi	High	govt	NoFPA	Illegal	RA	R			R	
Mauritius	Sat	govt	IPPF	Illegal	RA	R		R		S
Mozambique	Sat	govt	FPA	Illegal	NS				R	S
Rwanda	High	govt	IPPF	Narrow	RA				R	S
Somalia	Sat	some	IPPF	Illegal	NS				R	S
Tanzania	High	govt	IPPF	Narrow	RA	R		R		S
Uganda	High	govt	IPPF	Narrow	RA			R		G
Zambia	High	govt	IPPF	Broad	RA	R			R	S
Zimbabwe	High	govt	FPA	Narrow*	RA					S
Middle Africa										
Angola	High	govt	NoFPA	Illegal	RA				R	
Cameroon	High	govt	FPA	Narrow*	S					S
Cen. Af. Rep.	High	govt	FPA	Illegal	RA	R		R	R	S
Chad	Sat	some		Illegal	NS				R	
Congo	Low	govt	FPA	Narrow	RA	R		R		S
Gabon	Low	none	NoFPA	Illegal	RA	R			R	G
Zaire	High	govt	IPPF	Illegal	RA	R				S
Southern Africa										
Botswana	High	govt	IPPF	Illegal	NS					S
Lesotho	High	govt	IPPF	Narrow	S	R				
Namibia				Narrow*	NS					
South Africa	High	govt	FPA	Narrow*	NS					
ASIA										
Western Asia										
Iraq	Low	none	IPPF	Illegal	RA			R	R	S

Appendix D (continued)

Region and Country	Govt view of fert	Govt FP	Private Fp	Abortion Grounds	U.N. Equal Rights Conventions Disc	Pol	Mar	Educ	Emp	Const Equal
Israel	Low	govt	IPPF	Narrow*	S	R	S	R	R	N
Jordan	High	govt	IPPF	Narrow*	S			R	R	G
Kuwait	Sat	none		Narrow	NS			R	R	
Lebanon	Sat	govt	IPPF	Illegal	NS	R		R	R	G
Oman	Sat	none		Illegal	NS					
Saudi Arabia	Sat	none		Narrow	NS			R	R	
Syria	Sat	govt	IPPF	Illegal	NS				R	G
Turkey	High	govt	IPPF	Broad	RA	R			R	
UAE	Sat	none		Illegal	NS					G
Yemen	High	some	IPPF	Illegal	RA				R	G
Southern Asia										
Afghanistan	High	govt	IPPF	Illegal	S	R			R	S
Bangladesh	High	govt	IPPF	Illegal	RA				R	
Bhutan	Sat	govt	NoFPA		RA					
India	High	govt	IPPF	Broad	S	R			R	S
Iran	High	some		Illegal	NS			R	R	
Nepal	High	govt	IPPF	Narrow	RA	R			R	S
Pakistan	High	govt	IPPF	Illegal	NS	R			R	S
Sri Lanka	High	govt	IPPF	Illegal	RA		S			S
Southeast Asia										
Cambodia	Low	none								
Indonesia	High	govt	IPPF	Illegal	RA	R		R		G
Laos	Sat	none	NoFPA	Illegal	RA	R				
Malaysia		govt	IPPF	Narrow*	NS					G
Myanmar	Sat	some		Illegal	NS	S				S
Philippines	High	govt	IPPF	Illegal	RA	R	R	R	R	
Singapore	Low	govt	IPPF	Broad	NS					G
Thailand	High	govt	IPPF	Narrow*	RA	R				G

Appendix D (continued)

Region and Country	Govt view of fert	Govt FP	Private Fp	Abortion Grounds	U.N. Equal Rights Conventions					Const Equal
					Disc	Pol	Mar	Educ	Emp	
Viet Nam	High	govt	IPPF	Broad	RA				R	G
East Asia										
China	High	govt	IPPF	Broad	RA	R	R	R		S
Hong Kong			IPPF	Narrow*	NS					
Japan	Sat	govt	IPPF	Broad	RA	R				S
Korea, North	Sat	govt		Broad	NS					S
Korea, South	Sat	govt	IPPF	Narrow	NS	R				S
Mongolia	High	none	NoFPA	Narrow	RA	R		R	R	S
Taiwan	Sat		FPA	Broad				R		S
NORTH AMERICA										
Canada	Sat	govt	IPPF	Broad	RA	R			R	S
United States	Sat	govt	IPPF	Broad	S	R	S			G
LATIN AMERICA										
Central America										
Costa Rica	High	govt	IPPF	Narrow	RA	R		R	R	G
El Salvador	High	govt	IPPF	Illegal*	RA	S				G
Guatemala	High	govt	IPPF	Illegal	RA	R	R	R	R	S
Honduras	High	govt	IPPF	Illegal	RA				R	S
Mexico	High	govt	IPPF	Illegal*	RA	R	R		R	S
Nicaragua	High	govt	IPPF	Illegal	RA	R		R	R	S
Panama	Sat	govt	IPPF	Illegal	RA			R	R	S
Caribbean										
Cuba	Sat	govt	IPPF	Broad	RA	R	R	R	R	S
Dominican Rep.	High	govt	IPPF	Illegal	RA	R	R	R	R	G
Haiti	High	govt	FPA	Illegal	RA	R			R	G
Jamaica	High	govt	IPPF	Narrow	RA	R			R	S
Puerto Rico			IPPF	Broad						
Trinidad	High	govt	IPPF	Narrow	RA	R	R		R	N

Appendix D (continued)

Region and Country	Govt view of fert	Govt FP	Private Fp	Abortion Grounds	U.N. Equal Rights Conventions					Const
					Disc	Pol	Mar	Educ	Emp	Equal
South America										
Argentina	Sat	some	IPPF	Narrow*	NS	R	R	R	R	G
Bolivia	High	none	NoFPA	Narrow*	RA	R			R	S
Brazil	Sat	govt	IPPF	Illegal*	RA	R	R	R	R	S
Chile	Sat	govt	IPPF	Illegal	RA	R	S	R	R	G
Colombia	Sat	govt	IPPF	Illegal	RA				R	
Ecuador	High	govt	IPPF	Illegal*	RA	R		R	R	G
Paraguay	Sat	some	IPPF	Illegal	RA	S			R	N
Peru	High	govt	IPPF	Narrow	RA	R		R	R	S
Uruguay	Low	govt	IPPF	Broad	RA	S				G
Venezuela	Sat	govt	FPA	Illegal	RA			R	R	S
EUROPE										
Northern Europe										
Denmark	Sat	govt	IPPF	Broad	RA	R	R	R	R	
Finland	Sat	govt	IPPF	Broad	RA	R	R	R	R	G
Ireland	Sat	none	IPPF	Illegal	RA	R				G
Norway	Sat	none	IPPF	Broad	RA	R	R	R	R	
Sweden	Sat	govt	IPPF	Broad	RA	R	R	R	R	S
United Kingdom	Sat	govt	IPPF	Broad	RA	R	R	R		S
Western Europe										
Austria	Sat	govt	IPPF	Broad	RA	R	R		R	S
Belgium	Sat	some	IPPF	Broad	RA	R			R	G
France	Low	some	IPPF	Broad	RA	R	S	R	R	G
Germany	Low	govt	IPPF	Broad	RA	R	R	R	R	S
Netherlands	Sat	some	IPPF	Broad	RA	R	R	R	R	S
Switzerland	Low	none	FPA	Narrow	S				R	S
Eastern Europe										
Bulgaria	Low	govt	IPPF	Broad	RA	R		R	R	S

Appendix D (continued)

Region and Country	Govt view of fert	Govt FP	Private Fp	Abortion Grounds	U.N. Equal Rights Conventions Disc	Pol	Mar	Educ	Emp	Const Equal
Czechoslovakia	Sat	govt	FPA	Broad	RA	R	R	R	R	S
Hungary	Low	govt	IPPF	Broad	RA	R	R	R	R	S
Poland	Sat	govt	IPPF	Broad	RA	R	R	R	R	S
Romania	Low	none	FPA	Broad	RA	R	S	R	R	S
Southern Europe										
Albania	Sat	none		Narrow	NS	R		R		S
Greece	Low	some	IPPF	Broad	RA	R	S			S
Italy	Low	govt	IPPF	Broad	RA	R	S	R	R	S
Portugal	Sat	govt	IPPF	Narrow*	RA			R	R	S
Spain	Sat	some	IPPF	Narrow*	RA	R	R	R	R	S
Yugoslavia	Sat	govt	IPPF	Broad	RA	R	R	R	R	S
USSR	Sat	govt	IPPF	Broad	RA	R		R	R	S
OCEANIA										
Australia	Sat	some	IPPF	Broad	RA	R		R	R	
New Zealand	Sat	some	IPPF	Narrow*	RA	R	R	R		N
Pap. New Guinea	High	govt	FPA	Narrow	NS	R				S

Sources:

Government's view of current fertility levels (High = too high; Sat. = satisfactory; Low = too low): Population Refernce Bureau 1991.

Government's policy concerning effective use of modern methods of fertility regulation (govt = government (direct) support; some = some (indirect) suppport; none = no support); United Nations 1989:111–114.

Private family planning associations (IPPff = local FP association is affiliate of International Planned Parenthood Federation; FPA = local FP association not IFFP affiliate; no FPA = no private association): IPPF 1990; 1991.

Abortion law: grounds on which abortion is legal (broad = broad social grounds or on request; narrow = narrower health or medical grounds; illegal = illegal except in some countries to save woman's life; * also rape and/or incest): Henshaw and Morrow 1990:27–31

Government policy on U.N. Convention on the Elimination of All Forms of Discrimination Against Women (RA = ratified or acceded; S = signed; NS = not signed): United Nations General Assembly, 1991.

Other U.N. equal rights conventions (equal political rights, equal marriage rights, equal education, equality in employment): Sivard 1985:30.

Constitutional provisions for equal protection under law (G = general equal protection provisions; S = sexual equality provisions; N = no equality provisions): IPPF 1985.

BIBLIOGRAPHY

Agarwal, Bina, ed. 1988. *Structures of Patriarchy: State, Community and House-hold in Modernising Asia* (London, Zed Books).

Ahmad, Alia. 1991. *Women and Fertility in Bangladesh* (New Delhi, Sage).

Ainsworth, Martha. 1985. *Family Planning Programs: The Clients' Perspective.* World Bank Staff Working Paper no. 676 (Washington, D.C.: The World Bank).

Allman, James, Vu Qui Nhan, Nguyen Minh Thang, Pham Bich San, and Vu Duy Man. 1991. "Fertility and Family Planning in Vietnam," *Studies in Family Planning* vol. 22, no. 5 (Sept./Oct.), pp. 308–317.

Alvarez, Sonia E. 1989. "Politicizing Gender and Engendering Democracy," in Alfred Stepan, ed., *Democratizing Brazil: Problems of Transition and Consolidation* (New York: Oxford University Press), pp. 205–251.

Anglin, Patricia A. 1975. "A View on Antinatalist Policies: the African Case," in R. Kenneth Godwin, ed., *Comparative Policy Analysis: The Study of Population Policy Determinants in Developing Countries* (Lexington: Lexington Books), pp. 173–189.

Anker, Richard, Mayra Buvinic, and Nadia H. Youssef, eds. 1982. *Women's Roles and Population Trends in the Third World* (London: Croom Helm).

Anker, Richard, and Catherine Hein, eds. 1986. *Sex Inequalities in Urban Employment in the Third World* (London: Macmillan).

Aries, Nancy. 1987. "Fragmentation and Reproductive Freedom: Federally Subsidized Family Planning Services, 1960–80," *American Journal of Public Health* vol. 77, no. 11, pp. 1465–1471.

Arnold, Fred, R. A. Bulatao, C. Burkpakdi, B. J. Chung, J. T. Fawcett, T. Iritani, S. J. Lee, and T. S. Wu. 1975. *The Value of Children: Introduction and Comparative Analysis,* vol. 1 (Honolulu: East-West Population Institute).

Bachrach, Peter, and Elihu Bergman. 1973. *Power and Choice: The Formulation of American Population Policy* (Lexington: D.C. Heath).

Banchte Shekha. 1986. Funding proposal and program evaluation (Dhaka, The Ford Foundation).

Banks, J. A. 1954. *Prosperity and Parenthood: A Study of Family Planning Among the Victorian Middle Classes* (London: International Library of Sociology and Social Reconstruction).

Banks, J. A and Olive Banks. 1964. *Feminism and Family Planning in Victorian England* (New York: Schocken).

Barnett, Patricia G. 1985. Status Report on Population Problems and Programs of Brazil (Washington, D.C.: Population Crisis Committee).

Barnett, Rosalind C., Lois Biener, and Grace K. Baruch, eds. 1987. *Gender and Stress* (New York: The Free Press).

Barroso, Carmen. 1989. "Maternal Mortality: A Political Question," paper delivered at the Seminar on Maternal Mortality, August 25–27, 1989 (Rio de Janeiro, National Council on Women's Rights).

———. 1990. "The Women's Movements, The State, and Health Policies in Brazil," in Geertje Nijehold, ed., *Beyond the Decade* (London: Gower Press).

Bassnett, Susan. 1986. *Feminist Experiences: The Women's Movement in Four Cultures* (London: Allen and Unwin).

Baulieu, Etienne-Emile. 1989. "Contragestion and Other Clinical Applications of RU 486, an Antiprogesterone at the Receptor," *Science* vol. 245 (22 Sept.), pp. 1351–1357.

Beckman, Linda J. 1983. "Communication, Power, and the Influence of Social Networks in Couple Decisions on Fertility," in Rodolfo A. Bulatao and Ronald D. Lee, eds., *Determinants of Fertility in Developing Countries,* vol. 2 (New York: Academic Press), pp. 415–443.

Beeson, Diane, Helene L. Lipton, Donald H. Minkler, and Philip R. Lee. 1987. "Client-Provider Transactions in Family Planning Clinics," in Robert J. Lapham and George B. Simmons, eds., *Organizing for Effective Family Planning Programs* (Washington, D.C.: National Academy Press), pp. 435–456.

Begum, Syeda Firoza, Haidary Kamal, and G. M. Kamal. 1987. *Evaluation of MR Services in Bangladesh* (Dhaka, Bangladesh Association for the Prevention of Septic Abortion).

Belle, Deborah E., and Ruth F. Tebbets. 1982. "Poverty, Work, and Mental Health: The Experience of Low-Income Mothers," in Anne Hoiberg, ed., *Women and the World of Work* (New York: Plenum), pp. 179–188.

Benería, Lourdes, ed. 1982. *Women and Development: The Sexual Division of Labor in Rural Societies* (New York: Praeger).

Benería, Lourdes, and Martha Roldán. 1987. *The Crossroads of Class and Gender: Industrial Homework, Subcontracting, and Household Dynamics in Mexico City* (Chicago: University of Chicago Press).

Benshoof, Janet. 1987. "The Establishment Clause and Government-funded Natural Family Planning Programs: Is the Constitution Dancing to a New Rhythm?" *Journal of International Law and Politics* vol. 20, no. 1 (Fall), pp. 1–33.

Berelson, Bernard. 1969. "Beyond Family Planning," *Studies in Family Planning* no. 38 (Feb.), pp. 1–16.

Berelson, Bernard, and Jonathan Lieberson. 1979. "Government Efforts to Influence Fertility: The Ethical Issues," *Population and Development Review* vol. 5, no. 4 (Dec.), pp. 581–608.

Berkman, Joyce Avrech. 1979. "Historical Styles of Contraceptive Advocacy," in Helen B. Holmes, Betty B. Hoskins, and Michael Gross, eds., *Birth Control and Controlling Birth: Women-Centered Perspectives* (Clifton: Humana Press), pp. 27–36.

Binkin, Nancy J., Nadine N. Burton, Attaher H. Touré, M. Lamine Traoré, and Roger W. Rochat. 1984. "Women Hospitalized for Abortion Complications in Mali," *International Family Planning Perspectives* vol. 10, no. 1 (March), pp. 8–12.

Birdsall, Nancy, and Lauren A. Chester. 1987. "Contraception and the Status of Women: What is the Link?" *Family Planning Perspectives* vol. 19, no. 1 (Jan./Feb.), pp. 14–18.

Black, Maggie. 1987. *Better Health for Women and Children through Family Planning: Report on an International Conference Held in Nairobi, Kenya, October 1987* (New York: The Population Council).

Blake, Judith. 1961. *Family Structure in Jamaica: The Social Context of Reproduction* (New York: Free Press).

———. 1969. "Population Policy for Americans: Is the Government Being Misled?" *Science* vol. 164 (May 2), pp. 522–529.

———. 1972. "Coercive Pronatalism and American Population Policy," in U.S. Commission on Population Growth and the American Future, *Aspects of Population Growth Policy,* vol. 6 (Washington, D.C.: U.S. Government Printing Office).

Blay, Eva Alterman. 1985. "Social Movements and Women's Participation in Brazil," *International Political Science Review* vol. 6, no. 3, pp. 297–305.

Bledsoe, Caroline H. 1980. *Women and Marriage in Kpelle Society* (Stanford: Stanford University Press).

Bogue, Donald J. 1983. "Normative and Psychic Costs of Contraception," in Rodolfo A. Bulatao and Ronald D. Lee, eds., *Determinants of Fertility in Developing Countries,* vol. 2 (New York: Academic Press), pp. 151–192.

Bongaarts, John. 1991. "The GAP-Gap and the Unmet Need for Contraception," *Population and Development Review* vol. 17, no. 2 (June), pp. 293–314.

Bongaarts, John, W. Parker Mauldin, and James F. Phillips. 1990. "The Demographic Impact of Family Planning Programs," *Studies in Family Planning* vol. 21, no. 6 (Nov./Dec.), pp. 299–310.

Bose, Ashish. 1988. "New Issues in Population Control," National Workshop on New Issues in Population, February 10–11, New Delhi, cited in Malini Karkal and Divya Pandey, *Studies on Women and Population: A Critique* (Bombay: Himalaya Publishing House) p. 80.

Boserup, Ester. 1970. *Woman's Role in Economic Development* (New York: St. Martin's Press).

Boston Women's Health Book Collective. 1973. *Our Bodies, Ourselves: A Book By and For Women* (New York: Simon and Schuster).

———. 1984. *The New Our Bodies, Ourselves* (New York: Simon and Schuster).

Boulding, Elise, Shirley A. Nuss, Dorothy Lee Carson, and Michael A. Green-stein. 1976. *Handbook of International Data on Women* (New York: Halsted).

Boulier, Bryan L. 1985. *Evaluating Unmet Need for Contraception: Estimates for Thirty-Six Developing Countries,* World Bank Staff Working Paper no. 678 (Washington, D.C.: The World Bank).

"Brazil 1986: Results from the Demographic and Health Survey 1988," *Studies in Family Planning* vol. 19, no. 1 (Jan./Feb.), pp. 61–65.

Brody, Eugene B. 1981. *Sex, Contraception, and Motherhood in Jamaica* (Cambridge: Harvard University Press).

Brown, Lester R., et al. 1991. *State of the World 1991: A Worldwatch Institute Report on Progress Toward a Sustainable Society* (New York: W. W. Norton).

Browner, Carole. 1979. "Abortion Decision Making: Some Findings from Colombia," *Studies in Family Planning* vol. 10, no. 3 (March), pp. 96–106.

Bruce, Judith. 1980. "Implementing the User Perspective," *Studies in Family Planning* vol. 11, no. 2 (Jan.), pp. 29–33.

———. 1983. "Users' Perspective on Family Planning: Some Operational and Research Issues" (New York: The Population Council).

———. 1987. "Users' Perspectives on Contraceptive Technology and Delivery Systems: Highlighting Some Feminist Issues," *Technology and Society* vol. 9, no. 3/4, pp. 359–383.

———. 1990. "Fundamental Elements of the Quality of Care: A Simple Framework," *Studies in Family Planning* vol. 21, no. 2 (March/April), pp. 61–91.

Bruce, Judith, and S. Bruce Schearer. 1979. *Contraception and Common Sense: Conventional Methods Reconsidered* (New York: The Population Council).

Bulatao, Rodolfo A., and Ronald D. Lee, eds. 1983. *Determinants of Fertility Decline in Developing Countries* (New York: Academic Press).

Burch, Thomas K. 1983. "The Impact of Forms of Families and Sexual Unions and Dissolution of Unions on Fertility," in Rodolfo A. Bulatao and Ronald D. Lee, eds., *Determinants of Fertility in Developing Countries,* vol. 2 (New York: Academic Press), pp. 532–561.

Buvinic, Mayra, and Nadia H. Youssef. 1978. *Women-Headed Households: The Ignored Factor in Development Planning* (Washington, D.C.: International Center for Research on Women).

Cabrera, Gustavo. 1990. "Fertility Change in Mexico as Related to Population Policies," paper delivered at conference on the Politics of Induced Fertility Change in Developing Countries, Feb. 19–23, 1990, Bellagio, Italy.

Cain, Mead. 1978. "The Household Life Cycle and Economic Mobility in Rural Bangladesh," *Population and Development Review* vol. 4, no. 3 (Sept.), pp. 421–438.

———. 1981. "Risk and Insurance: Perspectives on Fertility and Agrarian Change in India and Bangladesh," *Population and Development Review* vol. 7, no. 3 (Sept.), pp. 435–474.

———. 1984. *Women's Status and Fertility in Developing Countries: Son Preference and Economic Security,* World Bank Staff Working Paper no. 682 (Washington, D.C.: The World Bank).

———. 1986. "The Consequences of Reproductive Failure: Dependence, Mobility, and Mortality Among the Elderly of Rural South Asia,'' *Population Studies* vol. 40, no. 3 (Nov.), pp. 375–388.

Caldwell, John C. 1982. *Theory of Fertility Decline* (London: Academic Press).

———. 1983. ''Direct Economic Costs and Benefits of Children,'' in Rodolfo A. Bulatao and Ronald D. Lee, eds., *Determinants of Fertility in Developing Countries,* vol. 1 (New York: Academic Press), pp. 458–493.

———. 1986. ''Routes to Low Mortality in Poor Countries,'' *Population and Development Review* vol. 12, no. 2 (June), pp. 171–220.

Caldwell, John C., P. H. Reddy, and Pat Caldwell. 1983. ''The Cause of Marriage Change in South India,'' *Population Studies* vol. 37, no. 3 (Nov.), pp. 343–362.

Callahan, Daniel. 1981. ''Population Policy, Universal Rights and National Sovereignty,'' in Daniel Callahan and Phillip G. Clark, eds., *Ethical Issues of Population Aid: Culture, Economics and International Assistance* (New York: Irvington), pp. 315–332.

Camp, Sharon L. 1987. ''The Impact of the Mexico City Policy on Women and Health Care in Developing Countries,'' *Journal of International Law and Politics* vol. 20, no. 1 (Fall), pp. 35–51.

Camp, Sharon L., and Craig R. Lasher. 1989. ''International Family Planning Policy: A Chronicle of the Reagan Years,'' unpublished paper (Washington, D.C.: Population Crisis Committee).

Carloni, Alice Stewart. 1987. *Women in Development: A.I.D.'s Experience, 1973–1985,* A.I.D. Program Evaluation Report No. 18 (Washington, D.C.: U.S. Agency for International Development).

Chamie, Mary. 1977. ''Sexuality and Birth Control Decisions among Lebanese Couples,'' *Signs: Journal of Women in Culture and Society* vol. 3, no. 1, pp. 294–312.

Chaturachinda, Kamheang, Somsak Tangtrakul, Sompol Pongthai, Winit Phuapradit, Areena Phanusopone, Vilai Benchakan, and J. Jarrett Clinton. 1981. ''Abortion: An Epidemiologic Study at Ramathibodi Hospital, Bangkok,'' *Studies in Family Planning* vol. 12, no. 6/7 (June/July), pp. 257–262.

Clark, Adele, and Alice Wolfson. 1984. ''Socialist-feminism and Reproductive Rights: Movement Work and its Contradictions,'' *Socialist Review* vol. 14, no. 6 (Nov./Dec.), pp. 110–120.

Cleland, John, and Germán Rodríguez. 1988. ''The Effect of Parental Education on Marital Fertility in Developing Countries,'' *Population Studies* vol. 42, no. 3 (Nov.), pp. 419–442.

Clinton, R., ed. 1973. *Population and Politics* (Lexington: Lexington Books).

Cochrane, Susan H. 1979. *Fertility and Education: What Do We Really Know?* (Baltimore: Johns Hopkins University Press for The World Bank).

Cohen, John M., and Norman T. Uphoff. 1977. *Rural Development Participation: Concepts and Measures for Project Design, Implementation and Evaluation.* Rural Development Monograph no. 2 (Ithaca: Rural Development Committee, Center for International Studies, Cornell University).

Cohen, Sheldon, and S. Leonard Syme. 1985. *Social Support and Health* (Orlando: Academic Press).

Coleman, Samuel. 1981. ''The Cultural Context of Condom Use in Japan,'' *Studies in Family Planning* vol. 12, no. 1 (Jan.), pp. 28–39.

Committee on the Status of Women in India. 1974. *Towards Equality* (New Delhi: Government of India, Department of Social Welfare).

Cook, Rebecca J. 1989a. "Abortion Laws and Policies: Challenges and Opportunities," *International Journal of Gynecology and Obstetrics,* Supplement 3, pp. 61–88.

———. 1989b. "Antiprogestin Drugs: Medical and Legal Issues," *Family Planning Perspectives* vol. 21, no. 6 (Nov./Dec.), pp. 267–272.

———. 1989c. "Bibliography: The International Right to Nondiscrimination on the Basis of Sex," *Yale Journal of International Law* vol. 14, pp. 161–181.

———. 1990. "Reservations to the Convention on the Elimination of All Forms of Discrimination Against Women," *Virginia Journal of International Law* vol. 30, no. 3, pp. 643–709.

Cook, Rebecca, and Deborah Maine. 1987. "Spousal Veto Over Family Planning Services," *American Journal of Public Health* vol. 77, no. 3, pp. 399–444.

Cook, Rebecca, and Pramilla Senanayake, eds. 1978. *The Human Problem of Abortion: Medical and Legal Dimensions* (London: International Planned Parenthood Federation).

Cornia, Giovanni Andrea, Richard Jolly, and Frances Stewart. 1987. *Adjustment with a Human Face,* vol. 1 (Oxford: Clarendon Press).

Corrêa, Sonia. 1989. "The Reproductive Rights in the Context of Brazilian Demographic Transition," paper presented at the annual meetings of the Population Association of America, Baltimore (March).

Crane, Barbara B. 1990. "The Transnational Politics of Abortion," paper delivered at conference on the Politics of Induced Fertility Change in Developing Countries, Feb. 19–23, 1990, Bellagio, Italy.

Crane, Barbara B., and Jason L. Finkle. 1989. "The United States, China, and the United Nations Population Fund: Dynamics of US Policymaking," *Population and Development Review* vol. 15, no. 1 (March), pp. 23–59.

Cross, Harry. 1988. "A.I.D.'s Population Assistance and the Policy Development Process: Twenty Years of Progress," paper delivered at the annual meetings of the Population Association of America, New Orleans (April).

David, Henry P. 1983. "Abortion: Its Prevalence, Correlates, and Costs," in Rodolfo A. Bulatao and Ronald D. Lee, eds., *Determinants of Fertility in Developing Countries,* vol. 2 (New York: Academic Press), pp. 193–244.

———. 1987. "Incentives and Disincentives in Family Planning Programs," in Robert J. Lapham and George B. Simmons, eds., *Organizing for Effective Family Planning Programs* (Washington, D.C.: National Academy Press), pp. 521–542.

Davis, Angela. 1981. *Women, Race and Class* (New York: Random House).

Davis, Kingsley. 1967. "Population Policy: Will Current Programs Succeed?" *Science* vol. 158 (Nov. 10), pp. 730–739.

Davis, Kingsley, and Judith Blake. 1956. "Social Structure and Fertility: An Analytic Framework," *Economic Development and Cultural Change* vol. 4, no. 3 (April), pp. 211–235.

Davis, Kingsley, and Pietronella van den Oever. 1982. "Demographic Foundations of New Sex Roles," *Population and Development Review* vol. 8, no. 3 (Sept.), pp. 495–511.

Day, Lincoln, and Alice Day. 1964. *Too Many Americans* (Boston: Houghton Mifflin).

Degler, Carl N. 1980. *At Odds: Women and the Family in America from the Revolution to the Present* (Oxford: Oxford University Press).

Demeny, Paul. 1985. "Bucharest, Mexico City, and Beyond," *Population and Development Review* vol. 11, no. 1 (March), pp. 99–106.

———. 1986. "Pronatalist Policies in Low-Fertility Countries: Patterns, Performance, and Prospects," in Kingsley Davis, Mikhail S. Bernstam, and Rita Ricardo-Campbell, eds., *Below-Replacement Fertility in Industrial Societies: Causes, Consequences, Policies,* Supplement to vol. 12 of *Population and Development Review,* pp. 335–358.

Demographic and Health Surveys. Reports for various years, various countries (Columbia, Md.: Institute for Resource Development/Macro Systems Inc.).

Dennis, Carolyne. 1987. "Women and the State in Nigeria: The Case of the Federal Military Government 1984–85," in Haleh Afshar, ed., *Women, State, and Ideology: Studies from Africa and Asia* (New York: State University of New York Press), pp. 13–27.

Devereux, George. 1976. *Abortion in Primitive Society* (New York: International Universities Press).

Dixon, Ruth B. 1976. "Measuring Equality Between the Sexes," *Journal of Social Issues* vol. 32, no. 3, pp. 19–32.

———. 1978. *Rural Women at Work: Strategies for Development in South Asia* (Baltimore: The Johns Hopkins University Press for Resources for the Future).

———. 1982. "Women in Agriculture: Counting the Labor Force in Developing Countries," *Population and Development Review* vol. 8, no. 3 (Sept.), pp. 539–566.

Dixon-Mueller, Ruth. 1988. "Innovations in Reproductive Health Care: Menstrual Regulation Policies and Programs in Bangladesh," *Studies in Family Planning* vol. 19, no. 3 (May/June), pp. 129–140.

———. 1989. "Patriarchy, Fertility, and Women's Work in Rural Societies," in International Union for the Scientific Study of Population, *International Population Conference, New Delhi 1989,* vol. 2 (Liege, Belgium: IUSSP), pp. 291–304.

———, and Judith Wasserheit. 1991. "The Culture of Silence: Reproductive Tract Infections among Women in the Third World" (New York: International Women's Health Coalition).

Donaldson, Peter J. 1990. *Nature Against Us: The United States and the World Population Crisis, 1965–1980* (Chapel Hill: The University of North Carolina Press).

Donovan, Patricia. 1984. "The Adolescent Family Life Act and the Promotion of Religious Doctrine," *Family Planning Perspectives* vol. 16, no. 5 (Sept./Oct.), pp. 222–226.

Duchen, Claire. 1986. *Feminism in France From May '68 to Mitterrand* (London: Routledge and Kegan Paul).

Duncan, Ann, and Masooma Habib. 1988. *Women in Development: A Review of Selected Economic and Sector Reports, 1980–1987* (Washington, D.C.: Women in Development Division, The World Bank).

Duncan, M. Elizabeth, Gerard Tibaux, Andrée Pelzer, Karin Reimann, John F. Peutherer, Peter Simmonds, Hugh Young, Ysamin Jamil, and Sohrab Daroughar. 1990. "First Coitus Before Menarche and Risk of Sexually Transmitted Disease," *The Lancet* vol. 335 (Feb. 10), pp. 338–340.

Dwyer, Daisy, and Judith Bruce, eds. 1988. *A Home Divided: Women and Income in the Third World* (Stanford: Stanford University Press).

Dye, Thomas R. 1972. *Understanding Public Policy* (Englewood Cliffs: Prentice-Hall).

Easterlin, Richard A., ed. 1980. *Population and Economic Change in Developing Countries* (Chicago: University of Chicago Press).

Ehrenreich, Barbara, Mark Dowie, and Stephen Minkin. 1979. "The Charge: Gynocide; The Accused: The U.S. Government," *Mother Jones* vol. 4, no. 9 (Nov.), pp. 26–37.

Ehrlich, Paul R., 1968. *The Population Bomb* (New York: Ballantine).

Ehrlich, Paul R., and Anne H. Ehrlich. 1990. *The Population Explosion* (New York: Simon and Schuster).

Eisenstein, Zillah R. 1986. *The Radical Future of Liberal Feminism* (Boston: Northeastern University Press).

Enabulele, Arlene Bene. 1985. "The Role of Women's Associations in Nigeria's Development: Social Welfare Perspective," in Editorial Committee, Women in Nigeria, *Women in Nigeria Today* (London: Zed Books), pp. 187–194.

Faux, Marian. 1988. *Roe v. Wade: The Untold Story of the Landmark Supreme Court Decision that Made Abortion Legal* (New York: Macmillan).

Fawcett, James T. 1983. "Perceptions of the Value of Children: Satisfaction and Costs," in Rodolfo A. Bulatao and Ronald D. Lee, eds., *Determinants of Fertility in Developing Countries,* vol. 1 (New York: Academic Press), pp. 429–457.

Federal Republic of Nigeria. 1988. National Policy on Population for Development, Unity, Progress and Self-Reliance.

Ferrero, Raúl. 1986. *The New International Economic Order and the Promotion of Human Rights* (New York: United Nations).

Feyistan, Bamikale, and Anne R. Pebley. 1989. "Premarital Sexuality in Urban Nigeria," *Studies in Family Planning* vol. 20, no 6 (Part 1)(Nov./Dec.), pp. 343–355.

Field, Marilyn Jane. 1983. *The Comparative Politics of Birth Control: Determinants of Policy Variation and Change in the Developed Nations* (New York: Praeger).

Fineman, Ruthbeth D. 1988. "The Price of Power: Gender Roles and Stress-Induced Depression in Andean Ecuador," in Patricia Whelehan, ed., *Women and Health: Cross-Cultural Perspectives* (Granby, Bergin and Garvey), pp. 153–169.

Finkle, Jason L., and Barbara B. Crane. 1975. "The Politics of Bucharest: Population, Development, and the New International Economic Order," *Population and Development Review* vol. 1, no. 1 (Sept.), pp. 87–114.

———— 1985. "Ideology and Politics at Mexico City: The United States at the 1984 International Conference on Population," *Population and Development Review* vol. 11, no. 1 (March), pp. 1–28.

Flavier, Juan M., and Charles H. C. Chen. 1980. "Induced Abortion in Rural Villages of Cavite, the Philippines: Knowledge, Attitudes, and Practice," *Studies in Family Planning* vol. 11, no. 2 (Feb.), pp. 65–71.

Folbre, Nancy. 1983. "Of Patriarchy Born: The Political Economy of Fertility Decisions," *Feminist Studies* vol. 9, no. 2 (Summer), pp. 261–284.

Folch-Lyon, Evelyn, Luis de la Macorra, and S. Bruce Schearer. 1981. "Focus Group and Survey Research on Family Planning in Mexico," *Studies in Family Planning* vol. 12, no. 12 (Dec.), pp. 409–432.

Ford, C. S. 1964. *A Comparative Study of Human Reproduction,* 2nd ed. (New Haven: Human Relations Area Files Press).

Fox, Gregory H. 1986. "American Population Policy Abroad: The Mexico City Abortion Funding Restrictions," *Journal of International Law and Politics* vol. 18, no. 2 (Winter), pp. 609–662.

Frankfort, Ellen. 1972. *Vaginal Politics* (New York: Bantam).

Fraser, Arvonne S. 1987. *The U.N. Decade for Women: Documents and Dialogue* (Boulder and London: Westview Press).

Freedman, Lynn P. 1991. "Women and the Law in Asia and the Near East" (New York: Development Law and Policy Program, Columbia University).

Frejka, Tomas. 1973. *The Future of Population Growth: Alternative Paths to Equilibrium* (New York: Wiley).

Frenzen, Paul D., and Dennis P. Hogan. 1982. "The Impact of Class, Education, and Health Care on Infant Mortality in a Developing Society: the Case of Rural Thailand," *Demography* vol.19, no. 3, pp. 391–408.

Fried, Marlene Gerber, ed. 1990. *From Abortion to Reproductive Freedom: Transforming a Movement* (Boston: South End Press).

Fryer, Peter. 1965. *The Birth Controllers* (London: Secker and Warburg).

Gallen, Moira. 1986. "Men: New Focus for Family Planning Programs," *Population Reports, Series J,* no. 3 (Nov-Dec.), pp. 889–919.

Gallen, Moira, and Cheryl Lettenmaier. 1987. "Counseling Makes a Difference," *Population Reports, Series J,* no. 3 (Nov.), pp. 1–31.

Germain, Adrienne. 1975. "The Status and Roles of Women as Factors in Fertility Behavior: A Policy Analysis," *Studies in Family Planning* vol. 6, no. 7 (July), pp. 192–200.

———. 1987. "Reproductive Health and Dignity: Choices by Third World Women," paper prepared for the International Conference on Better Health for Women and Children Through Family Planning, Nairobi, Kenya, October 1987 (New York: International Women's Health Coalition).

Germain, Adrienne, and Peggy Antrobus. 1989. "New Partnerships in Reproductive Health Care," *Populi* vol. 6, no. 4 (Dec.), pp. 18–29.

Germain, Adrienne, and Jane Ordway. 1989. "Population Control and Women's Health: Balancing the Scales" (New York: International Women's Health Coalition).

Gillespie, Duff G., and Judith R. Seltzer. 1990. "The Population Assistance Program of the U.S. Agency for International Development," in Helen M. Wallace and Kanti Giri, eds., *Health Care of Women and Children in Developing Countries* (Oakland: Third Party Publishing), pp. 562–569.

Glass, David V. 1940. *Population Policies and Movements in Europe* (Oxford: Clarendon Press).

Glassheim, E., C. Cargille, and C. Hoffman, eds. 1978. *Key Issues in Population Policy* (Washington, D.C.: University Press of America).

Godwin, R. Kenneth, ed. 1975. *Comparative Policy Analysis: The Study of Population Policy Determinants in Developing Countries* (Lexington: Lexington Books).

Goldman, Emma. 1916. "The Social Aspects of Birth Control," *Mother Earth* vol. 11, no. 12 (April), pp. 468–475.

Goldschmidt-Clermont, Louisella. 1987. *Economic Evaluations of Unpaid Household Work: Africa, Asia, Latin America and Oceania*. Women, Work and Development no. 14 (Geneva: International Labour Office).

Gordon, Linda. 1976. *Woman's Body, Woman's Right: A Social History of Birth Control in America* (New York: Grossman).

Gray, Vivian. 1974. "Women: Victims or Beneficiaries of U.S. Population Policy?" in V. Gray and E. Bergman, eds., *Political Issues in U.S. Population Policy* (Lexington: Lexington Books), pp. 167–187.

Greenhalgh, Susan. 1985. "Sexual Stratification: The Other Side of 'Growth with Equity' in East Asia," *Population and Development Review* vol. 11, no. 2 (June), pp. 265–314.

———. 1990. "State-Society Links: Political Dimensions of Population Policies and Programs, with Special Reference to China," Research Division, Working Papers No. 18 (New York: The Population Council).

Hardee-Cleaveland, Karen, and Judith Banister. 1988. "Fertility Policy and Implementation in China, 1986–88," *Population and Development Review* vol. 14, no. 2 (June), pp. 245–286.

Harrison, Polly Fortier. 1983. To Bear a Child: Meanings and Strategies in Rural El Salvador. Unpublished PhD dissertation (Washington, D.C.: Catholic University of America).

Hartmann, Betsy. 1987. *Reproductive Rights and Wrongs: The Global Politics of Population Control and Contraceptive Choice* (New York: Harper and Row).

Hass, Paula Hollerbach. 1974. "Wanted and Unwanted Pregnancies: A Fertility Decision-Making Model," *Journal of Social Issues* vol. 30, no. 4, pp. 125–164.

———. 1976. "Contraceptive Choices for Latin American Women," *Populi* vol. 3, no. 4, pp. 14–24.

Hatcher, Robert A., Deborah Kowal, Felicia Guest, James Trussell, Felicia Stewart, Gary K. Stewart, Sylvia Bowen, and Willard Cates, eds. 1989. *Contraceptive Technology: International Edition* (Atlanta: Printed Matter).

Heise, Lori. 1992. "Violence Against Women: The Missing Agenda," in M. A. Koblinsky, Judith Timyan, and Jill Gay, eds., *Women's Health: A Global Perspective* (Boulder: Westview).

Helzner, Judith, and Bonnie Shepard. 1990. "The Feminist Agenda in Population VOs," in Kathleen Staudt, ed., *Women, International Development, and Politics: The Bureaucratic Mire* (Philadelphia: Temple University Press), pp. 145–160.

Henry, Alice, and Phyllis T. Piotrow. 1979. "Age at Marriage and Fertility," *Population Reports, Series M,* no. 4 (Nov.), pp. 106–159.

Henshaw, Stanley K., and Evelyn Morrow. 1990. "Induced Abortion: A World

Review, 1990," *Family Planning Perspectives* vol. 22, no. 2 (March/April), pp. 76–89.

Hernandez, Donald J. 1984. *Success or Failure? Family Planning Programs in the Third World* (Westport: Greenwood Press).

Herz, Barbara K. 1984. *Official Development Assistance for Population Activities: A Review.* World Bank Staff Working Papers no. 688, Population and Development Series no. 13 (Washington, D.C.: The World Bank).

————, and Anthony R. Measham. 1987. *The Safe Motherhood Initiative: Proposals for Action* (Washington, D.C.: The World Bank).

Himes, Norman E. [1936] 1970. *The Medical History of Contraception* (New York: Schocken Books).

Hodgson, Dennis. 1991. "Ideological Origins of the Population Association of America," *Population and Development Review* vol. 17, no. 1 (March), pp. 1–34.

Hole, Judith, and Ellen Levine. 1971. *Rebirth of Feminism* (New York: Quadrangle).

Hollerbach, Paula E. 1980. "Power in Families, Communication, and Fertility Decision Making," *Population and Environment* vol. 3, pp. 146–173.

————. 1983. "Fertility Decision-Making Processes: A Critical Essay," in Rodolfo A. Bulatao and Ronald D. Lee, eds., *Determinants of Fertility in Developing Countries,* vol. 2 (New York: Academic Press), pp. 340–380.

Holmes, Helen B. 1979. "Reproductive Technologies: The Birth of a Women-Centered Analysis," in Helen B. Holmes, Betty B. Hoskins, and Michael Gross, eds., *Birth Control and Controlling Birth: Women-Centered Perspectives* (Clifton: Humana Press), pp. 3–20.

Holt, Renée. 1989a. *Abortion: Law, Practice, and Project Possibilities in Kenya, Sierra Leone, Brazil, Mexico, and Indonesia* (New York: Development Law and Policy Program, Columbia University).

————. 1989b. "Abortion in Thailand: Law, Practice, and Reform Possibilities" (New York: Development Law and Policy Program, Columbia University).

————. 1990. "Women's Rights: An International Perspective," in Carol Lefcourt, ed., *Women and the Law* (New York: Clark Boardman).

Hong, Sung-bong, and Christopher Tietze. 1979. "Survey of Abortion Providers in Seoul, Korea," *Studies in Family Planning* vol. 10, no. 5 (May), pp. 161–163.

Hull, Terence H. 1983. "Cultural Influences on Fertility Decision Styles," in Rodolfo A. Bulatao and Ronald D. Lee, eds., *Determinants of Fertility in Developing Countries,* vol. 2 (New York: Academic Press), pp. 381–414.

Hull, Valerie J. 1979. "Women, Doctors, and Family Health Care: Some Lessons from Rural Java," *Studies in Family Planning* vol. 10, no. 11/12 (Nov./Dec.), pp. 315–325.

Hunte, Pamela A. 1985. "Indigenous Methods of Fertility Regulation in Afghanistan," in Lucile F. Newman, ed., *Women's Medicine: A Cross-Cultural Study of Indigenous Fertility Regulation* (New Brunswick: Rutgers University Press).

Huston, Perdita. 1978. *Message from the Village* (New York: Epoch B Foundation).

————. 1979. *Third World Women Speak Out: Interviews in Six Countries on Change, Development, and Basic Needs* (New York: Praeger).

IMPACT. 1988. "Contraceptive Safety: Rumours and Realities" (Washington, D.C.: Population Reference Bureau).

Instituto de Ação Cultural, Organizado pela Equipe do Projeto-Mulher. 1981. *As Mulheres em Movimento* (Rio de Janeiro: Editora Marco Zero).

International Planned Parenthood Federation (IPPF). 1990. "Reproductive Rights Wallchart," *People* vol. 17, no. 4 (Oct.).

————. 1991. "World List of Family Planning Addresses" (London: IPPF).

International Women's Health Coalition (IWHC). 1989. "Statement of the Christopher Tietze International Symposium on Women's Health in the Third World: The Impact of Unwanted Pregnancy," *International Journal of Gynecology and Obstetrics, Supplement 3*, p. 175.

————, and The Population Council. 1986. The Contraceptive Development Process and Quality of Care in Reproductive Health Services: Report of a Meeting Held in New York City, Oct. 8–9, 1986 (New York: IWHC and The Population Council).

International Women's Rights Action Watch. 1988. *Assessing the Status of Women: A Guide to Reporting Using the Convention on the Elimination of Discrimination Against Women* (New York: Development Law and Policy Program, Columbia University).

Isaacs, Stephen L., and Rebecca J. Cook. 1984. "Laws and Policies Affecting Fertility: A Decade of Change," *Population Reports, Series E*, no. 7 (Nov.), pp. 105–151.

Isaacs, Stephen L., Renée Holt, and Kathleen Hill. 1990. *Report on Abortion Law and Practice in 14 Countries* (New York: Development Law and Policy Program, Columbia University).

Isaacs, Stephen L., and Andrea Irvin. 1991. *Population Policy: A Manual for Policymakers and Planners,* 2nd. ed. (New York: Development Law and Policy Program, Columbia University).

Jacobson, Jodi L. 1990. *The Global Politics of Abortion.* Worldwatch Paper 97 (Washington, D.C.: Worldwatch Institute).

Jaffe, Frederick. 1981. *Abortion Politics: Private Morality and Public Policy* (New York: McGraw-Hill).

Jain, Anrudh K. 1989. "Fertility Reduction and the Quality of Family Planning Services," *Studies in Family Planning* vol. 20, no. 1 (Jan./Feb.), pp. 1–16.

Jaquette, Jane S., ed. 1989. *The Women's Movement in Latin America: Feminism and the Transition to Democracy* (Boston: Unwin Hyman).

Jaquette, Jane S., and Kathleen A. Staudt. 1985. "Women as 'At Risk' Reproducers: Biology, Science, and Population in U.S. Foreign Policy," in Virginia Sapiro, ed., *Women, Biology, and Public Policy* (Beverly Hills: Sage Publications), pp. 235–268.

Jayawardena, Kumari. 1986. *Feminism and Nationalism in the Third World* (London: Zed Books).

Jensen, Joan M. 1981. "The Evolution of Margaret Sanger's Family Limitation Pamphlet, 1914–1921," *Signs: Journal of Women in Culture and Society* vol. 6, no. 3 (Spring), pp. 548–567.

Jöchle, Wolfgang. 1974. "Menses-inducing Drugs: Their Role in Antique, Medieval, and Renaissance Gynecology and Birth Control,'' *Contraception* vol. 10, no. 4, pp. 428–436.

Joffe, Carole. 1986. *The Regulation of Sexuality: Experiences of Family Planning Workers* (Philadelphia: Temple University Press).

Johnson, D. Gale, and Ronald D. Lee, eds. 1987. *Population Growth and Economic Development: Issues and Evidence* (Madison: University of Wisconsin Press).

Johnson, Jeanette H., and Julie Reich. 1986. "The New Politics of Natural Family Planning," *Family Planning Perspectives* vol. 18, no. 6 (Nov./Dec.), pp. 277–280.

Johnson, M. Glen. 1988. "Human Rights in Divergent Conceptual Settings: How Do Ideas Influence Policy Choices?'' in David Louis Cingranelli, ed., *Human Rights: Theory and Measurement* (London: Macmillan), pp. 41–59.

Johnson, P. Stanley. 1987. *World Population and the United Nations: Challenge and Response* (New York: Cambridge University Press).

Jones, Maggie, Elke Thoss, and Scottish Health Education Group, 1987. *Alternative Approaches to the Development of Family Planning Programmes: Report on a WHO Study* (Copenhagen: World Health Organization, Regional Office for Europe).

Kabir, Sandra M. 1989. "Causes and Consequences of Unwanted Pregnancy from Asian Women's Perspectives,'' *International Journal of Gynecology and Obstetrics Supplement* 3, pp. 9–14.

Kandiyoti, Deniz, ed. 1991. *Women, Islam and the State* (Philadelphia: Temple University Press).

Karkal, Malini, and Divya Pandey. 1989. *Studies on Women and Population: A Critique* (Bombay: Himalaya Publishing House).

Kay, Bonnie J., Adrienne Germain, and Maggie Bangser. 1991. "The Bangladesh Women's Health Coalition,'' *Quality/Calidad/Qualité* no. 3 (New York: The Population Council).

Kay, Bonnie J., and Sandra M. Kabir. 1988. "A Study of Costs and Behavioral Outcomes of Menstrual Regulation Services in Bangladesh,'' *Social Science and Medicine* vol. 26, no. 6, pp. 597–604.

Kennedy, David M. 1970. *Birth Control in America: The Career of Margaret Sanger* (New Haven: Yale University Press).

Khan, Atiqur Rahman, Roger W. Rochat, Farida Akhter Jahan, and Syeda Feroza Begum. 1986. "Induced Abortion in a Rural Area of Bangladesh,'' *Studies in Family Planning* vol. 17, no. 2 (March/April), pp. 95–99.

Kimball, Linda Amy, and Shawna Craig. 1988. "Women and Stress in Brunei,'' in Patricia Whelehan, ed., *Women and Health: Cross-Cultural Perspectives* (Granby, Bergin and Garvey), pp. 170–182.

King, Timothy, ed. 1974. *Population Policies and Economic Development: A World Bank Staff Report* (Baltimore: The Johns Hopkins University Press).

Kisekka, Mere N. 1989a. "Population Policy and Women's Associations in Nigeria,'' paper presented at the annual meetings of the Population Association of America, Baltimore (March).

———. 1989b. "Mapping Exercise of Women's Associations in Jos, Kano, Mubi, and Zaria,'' unpublished paper (New York: International Women's Health Coalition).

———. 1989c. "Reproductive Health Research and Advocacy: Challenges to Women's Associations in Nigeria," paper presented at the conference of the Society of Obstetrics and Gynaecology of Nigeria, Calabar (September).

Knodel, John, and Malinee Wongsith. 1991. "Family Size and Children's Education in Thailand," *Demography* vol. 28, no. 1 (Feb.), pp. 119–131.

Kocher, James. E. 1973. *Rural Development, Income Distribution, and Fertility Decline* (New York: The Population Council).

Kokole, Omari, and Ali Mazrui. 1990. "The Political Culture of Fertility in Africa: The Tensions of Procreation," paper delivered at conference on the Politics of Induced Fertility Change in Developing Countries, Feb. 19–23, 1990, Bellagio, Italy.

Koso-Thomas, Olayinka. 1987. *The Circumcision of Women: A Strategy for Eradication* (London: Zed Books).

Kritz, Mary M., and Douglas T. Gurak. 1989. "Women's Status, Education, and Family Formation in Sub-Saharan Africa," *International Family Planning Perspectives* vol. 15, no. 3 (Sept.), pp. 100–105.

Kupinsky, Stanley, ed. 1977. *The Fertility of Working Women: A Synthesis of International Research* (New York: Praeger).

Ladipo, Oladipo A. 1989. "Preventing and Managing Complications of Induced Abortion in Third World Countries," *International Journal of Gynecology and Obstetrics, Supplement 3*, pp. 21–28.

Laing, John E. 1984. "Natural Family Planning in the Philippines," *Studies in Family Planning* vol. 15, no. 2 (June), pp. 49–61.

Lee, Luke T., and John M. Paxman. 1977. "Legal Aspects of Menstrual Regulation," *Studies in Family Planning* vol. 8, no. 10 (Oct.), pp. 273–278.

Lee, Nancy C., Herbert B. Peterson, and Susan Y. Chu. 1989. "Health Effects of Contraception," in Allan M. Parnell, ed., *Contraceptive Use and Controlled Fertility: Health Issues for Women and Children* (Washington, D.C.: National Academy Press).

Lesthaeghe, Ron. 1980. "On the Social Control of Human Reproduction," *Population and Development Review* vol. 6, no. 4 (Dec.), pp. 527–548.

LeVine, Robert, Sarah E. LeVine, Amy Richman, F. Medardo Tapia Uribe, Clara Correa, and Patrice M. Miller. 1991. "Women's Schooling and Child Care in the Demographic Transition: A Mexican Case Study," *Population and Development Review* vol. 17, no. 3 (Sept.), pp. 459–496.

Lipton, Helene L., Ruth Dixon-Mueller, and Claire D. Brindis. 1987. "Transactions with Clients: Suggestions for Research, Training, and Action," in Robert J. Lapham and George B. Simmons, eds., *Organizing for Effective Family Planning Programs* (Washington, D.C.: National Academy Press), pp. 499–520.

Liskin, Laurie S. 1980. "Complications of Abortion in Developing Countries," *Population Reports, Series F,* no. 7 (July), pp. 105–155.

Littlewood, T. B. 1977. *The Politics of Population Control* (Notre Dame: University of Notre Dame Press).

Lloyd, Cynthia B. 1991. "The Contribution of the World Fertility Surveys to an Understanding of the Relationship Between Women's Work and Fertility," *Studies in Family Planning* vol. 22, no. 3 (May/June), pp. 144–161.

Lodoño E., and Maria Ladi. 1988. "Towards a New Dimension for Abortion," paper presented at The Christopher Tietze International Symposium, Rio de Janeiro, Brazil, 29–30 October (New York: International Women's Health Coalition).

Luker, Kristin. 1975. *Taking Chances: Abortion and the Decision Not to Contracept* (Berkeley: University of California Press).

———. 1984. *Abortion and the Politics of Motherhood* (Berkeley: University of California Press).

Macklin, Ruth. 1989. "Liberty, Utility, and Justice: An Ethical Approach to Unwanted Pregnancy," *International Journal of Gynecology and Obstetrics, Supplement 3*, pp. 37–50.

Maine, Deborah. 1981. *Family Planning: Its Impact on the Health of Women and Children* (New York: Center for Population and Family Health, Columbia University).

Malthus, Thomas R. [1817] 1963. *An Essay on the Principle of Population*, 5th ed. (Homewood: Richard Irwin).

Mandelbaum, David G. 1988. *Women's Seclusion and Men's Honor: Sex Roles in North India, Bangladesh, and Pakistan* (Tucson: University of Arizona Press).

Marcelo, Alexandrina B. 1989. "Reproductive Rights and Challenges in the Philippines," paper presented at the annual meetings of the Population Association of America, Baltimore (March).

MARHIA. *Medium for the Advancement and Achievement of Reproductive Rights, Health Information and Advocacy.* A Quarterly Publication of the Institute for Social Studies and Action (Quezon City, Philippines, ISSA).

Mashalaba, Nolwandle Nozipo. 1989. "Commentary on the Causes and Consequences of Unwanted Pregnancy from an African Perspective," *International Journal of Gynecology and Obstetrics, Supplement 3*, pp. 15–19.

Mason, Karen Oppenheim. 1986. "The Status of Women: Conceptual and Methodological Issues in Demographic Studies," *Sociological Forum* vol. 1, no. 2, pp. 284–300.

———. 1987. "The Impact of Women's Social Position on Fertility in Developing Countries," *Sociological Forum* vol. 2, no. 4, pp. 718–747.

Mason, Karen Oppenheim, and V. T. Palan. 1981. "Female Employment and Fertility in Peninsular Malaysia: The Maternal Role Incompatibility Hypothesis Reconsidered," *Demography* vol. 18, no. 4 (Nov.), pp. 549–575.

Mason, Karen Oppenheim, and Anju M. Taj. 1987. "Differences Between Women's and Men's Reproductive Goals in Developing Countries," *Population and Development Review* vol. 13, no. 4 (Dec.), pp. 611–638.

Massell, Gregory J. 1974. *The Surrogate Proletariat: Moslem Women and Revolutionary Strategies in Soviet Central Asia, 1919–1929* (Princeton: Princeton University Press).

Mauldin, W. Parker, and Bernard Berelson. 1978. "Conditions of Fertility Decline in Developing Countries," *Studies in Family Planning* vol. 9, no. 5 (May), pp. 89–147.

Mauldin, W. Parker, Nazli Choucri, Frank W. Notestein, and Michael Teitelbaum. 1974. "A Report on Bucharest: The World Population Conference and the Population Tribune, August 1974," *Studies in Family Planning* vol. 5, no. 12 (Dec.).

Mauldin, W. Parker, and Robert J. Lapham. 1987. "The Measurement of Family Planning Inputs," in Robert J. Lapham and George B. Simmons, eds., *Organizing for Effective Family Planning Programs* (Washington, D.C.: National Academy Press), pp. 545–582.

Mba, Nina Emma. 1982. *Nigerian Women Mobilized: Women's Political Activity in Southern Nigeria, 1900–1965* (Berkeley: Institute of International Studies, University of California, Berkeley).

McCabe, James L., and Mark R. Rosenzweig. 1976. "Female Employment Creation and Family Size," in Ronald Ridker, ed., *Population and Development: The Search for Selective Interventions* (Baltimore: Johns Hopkins University Press for Resources for the Future), pp. 322–355.

McPherson, M. Peter. 1985. "International Family Planning: The Reasons for the Program," speech delivered to the American Enterprise Institute, Washington, D.C., Nov. 25, 1985.

Meadows, Donella H. et al. 1972. *The Limits to Growth: A Report for the Club of Rome's Project on the Predicament of Mankind* (Washington, D.C.: Universe Books).

Measham, Anthony R., Michael J. Rosenberg, Atiqur R. Khan, M. Obaidullah, Roger W. Rochat, and Suraiya Jabeen. 1981. "Complications from Induced Abortion in Bangladesh Related to Types of Practitioner and Methods, and Impact on Mortality," *The Lancet* (24 Jan.), pp. 199–202.

Menken, Jane, ed. 1986. *World Population and U.S. Policy: The Choices Ahead* (New York: Norton).

Mernissi, Fatima. 1975. "Obstacles to Family Planning Practice in Urban Morocco," *Studies in Family Planning* vol. 6, no. 12 (Dec.), pp. 418–425.

Merrick, Thomas W. 1990. "The Evolution and Impact of Policies on Fertility and Family Planning: Brazil, Colombia, and Mexico," in Godfrey Roberts, ed., *Population Policy: Contemporary Issues* (New York: Praeger), pp. 147–166.

Merrick, Thomas W., and Douglas H. Graham. 1979. *Population and Economic Development in Brazil: 1800 to the Present* (Baltimore: The Johns Hopkins University Press).

Michele, Andrée. 1960. "La Femme dans la Famille Française," *Cahiers Internationaux* vol. 12 (March-April), pp. 61–76.

Mies, Maria. 1982. *The Lacemakers of Narsapur: Indian Housewives Produce for the Worldmarket* (London: Zed Books).

———. 1986. *Patriarchy and Accumulation on a World Scale* (London: Zed Books).

Monat, Alan, and Richard S. Lazarus, eds. 1977. *Stress and Coping: An Anthology* (New York: Columbia University Press).

Morgan, Robin, ed. 1984. *Sisterhood is Global: The International Women's Movement Anthology* (New York: Doubleday).

Murdoch, William W. 1980. *The Poverty of Nations: The Political Economy of Hunger and Population* (Baltimore: The Johns Hopkins University Press).

Musallam, B. F. 1983. *Sex and Society in Islam: Birth Control Before the Nineteenth Century* (Cambridge: Cambridge University Press).

NARAL Foundation. 1991. *Who Decides: A State-by-State Review of Abortion Rights 1991* (Washington, D.C.: National Abortion Rights Action League).

Narkavonnakit, Tongplaew. 1979. "Abortion in Rural Thailand: A Survey of Practitioners," *Studies in Family Planning* vol. 10, no. 8/9 (Aug./Sept.), pp. 223–229.

National Academy of Sciences. 1971. *Rapid Population Growth: Consequences and Policy Implications* (Baltimore: The Johns Hopkins University Press).

National Research Council, Working Group on Population Growth and Economic Development. 1986. *Population Growth and Economic Development: Policy Questions* (Washington, D.C.: National Academy Press).

——, Working Group on the Health Consequences of Contraceptive Use and Controlled Fertility. 1989. *Contraception and Reproduction: Health Consequences for Women and Children in the Developing World* (Washington, D.C.: National Academy Press).

Newman, Lucile F., ed. 1985. *Women's Medicine: A Cross-Cultural Study of Indigenous Fertility Regulation* (New Brunswick, N.J.: Rutgers University Press).

Ngin, Chor-Swang. 1985. "Indigenous Fertility Regulating Methods among Two Chinese Communities in Malaysia," in Lucile F. Newman, ed., *Women's Medicine: A Cross-Cultural Study of Indigenous Fertility Regulation* (New Brunswick, N.J.: Rutgers University Press).

Nichols, Douglas, O. A. Ladipo, John M. Paxman, and E. O. Otolorin. 1986. "Sexual Behavior, Contraceptive Practice, and Reproductive Health Among Nigerian Adolescents," *Studies in Family Planning* vol. 17, no. 2 (March/April), pp. 100–106.

Nortman, Dorothy. 1975. "Population and Family Planning Programs: A Factbook," *Reports on Population/Family Planning* no. 2 (New York: The Population Council).

Ogunsheye, F. Adetowun, Catherine Di Domenico, Carolyne Dennis, Keziah Awosika, and Olu Akinkoye, eds. 1988. *Nigerian Women and Development* (Ibadan: Ibadan University Press).

Okagbue, Isabella. 1990. "Pregnancy Termination and the Law in Nigeria," *Studies in Family Planning* vol. 21, no. 4 (July/Aug.), pp. 197–208.

Okonjo, Kamene. 1983. "Sex Roles in Nigerian Politics," in Christine Oppong, ed., *Female and Male in West Africa* (London: George Allen and Unwin), pp. 211–222.

Oppong, Christine. 1983. "Women's Roles, Opportunity Costs, and Fertility," in Rodolfo A. Bulatao and Ronald D. Lee, eds., *Determinants of Fertility in Developing Countries,* vol. 1 (New York: Academic Press), pp. 547–589.

Oppong, Christine, and Katharine Abu. 1987. *Seven Roles of Women: Impact of Education, Migration and Employment on Ghanaian Mothers.* Women, Work and Development no. 13 (Geneva: International Labour Office).

Orubuloye, E. I. 1983. "Toward National Policy on Population," in I. O. Orubuloye and O. Y. Oyeneye, eds., *Population and Development in Nigeria* (Ibadan: Nigerian Institute of Social and Economic Research), pp. 170–178.

Overall, Christine. 1987. *Ethics and Human Reproduction: A Feminist Analysis* (Boston: Allen and Unwin).

Overholt, Catherine, Mary B. Anderson, Kathleen Cloud, and James E. Austin, eds. 1984. *Gender Roles in Development Projects: A Case Book* (West Hartford: Kumarian Press).

Paddock, William, and Paul Paddock. 1967. *Famine—1975!* (Boston: Little Brown).

Paige, Karen Ericksen, and Jeffery M. Paige. 1981. *The Politics of Reproductive Ritual* (Berkeley: University of California Press).

Panandiker, V. A. Pai, and P. K. Umashankar. 1990. "The Politics of Population Control in a Diverse, Federal, Democratic Polity: The Case of India," paper delivered at conference on the Politics of Induced Fertility Change in Developing Countries, Feb. 19–23, 1990, Bellagio, Italy.

Papanek, Hanna. 1990. "To Each Less Than She Needs, From Each More Than She Can Do: Allocations, Entitlements, and Value," in Irene Tinker, ed., *Persistent Inequalities: Women and World Development* (New York: Oxford University Press), pp. 162–181.

Papanek, Hanna, and Gail Minault, eds. 1982. *Separate Worlds: Studies of Purdah in South Asia* (Columbia: South Asia Books).

Pariani, Siti, David M. Heer, and Maurice D. Van Arsdol, Jr. 1991. "Does Choice Make a Difference to Contraceptive Use? Evidence from East Java," *Studies in Family Planning* vol. 22, no. 6 (Nov./Dec.), pp. 384–390.

Patai, Daphne. 1988. *Brazilian Women Speak: Contemporary Life Stories* (New Brunswick, N.J.: Rutgers University Press).

Peralta, Ana Maria Rotos, and Marlene C. Ligan. 1975. *Philippine Population: Implications, Program and Policies* (Manila: University of the East Press).

Petchesky, Rosalind Pollack. 1984. *Abortion and Woman's Choice: The State, Sexuality, and Reproductive Freedom* (New York: Longman).

Petchesky, Rosalind, and Jennifer A. Weiner. 1990. Global Feminist Perspectives on Reproductive Rights and Reproductive Health: A Report on the Special Sessions Held at the Fourth International Interdisciplinary Congress on Women, Hunter College, New York City, June 3–7, 1990 (New York: Women's Studies Program, Hunter College).

Petersen, William. 1989. "Marxism and the Population Question: Theory and Practice," in Michael S. Teitelbaum and Jay M. Winter, eds., *Population and Resources in Western Intellectual Traditions* (Cambridge: Cambridge University Press), pp. 77–101.

Piepmeier, K. B., and T. S. Adkins. 1973. "The Status of Women and Fertility," *Journal of Biosocial Science* vol. 5, no. 4 (Oct.), pp. 507–520.

Pierpoint, Raymond, ed. 1922. *Report of the Fifth International Neo-Malthusian and Birth Control Conference, Kingsway Hall, London* (London: William Heinemann).

Pinotti, J. A., and A. Faúndes. 1989. "Unwanted Pregnancy: Challenges for Health Policy," *International Journal of Gynecology and Obstetrics, Supplement 3*, pp. 97–102.

Piotrow, Phyllis Tilson. 1973. *World Population Crisis: The United States Response* (New York: Praeger).

———. 1980. *World Population: The Present and Future Crisis.* Headline Series 251 (Washington, D.C.: Foreign Policy Association).

Population Crisis Committee. 1988. "Country Rankings of the Status of Women: Poor, Powerless and Pregnant," Population Briefing Paper no. 20 (June).

Population Reference Bureau. 1980. World's Women Data Sheet (Washington, D.C.: Population Reference Bureau).

———. 1990. 1990 World Population Data Sheet (Washington, D.C.: Population Reference Bureau).

———. 1991. 1991 World Population Data Sheet (Washington, D.C.: Population Reference Bureau).

Portugal, Ana Marie, ed. 1989. *Mujeres e Iglesia: Sexualidad y Aborto en America Latina* (Washington, D.C.: Catholics for a Free Choice, and Distribuciones Fontamara, S.A.).

———, and Amparo Claro. 1988. "Virgin and Martyr," *Conscience: A Newsjournal of Prochoice Catholic Opinion* vol. 9, no. 4 (July/Aug.), pp. 14–18.

"Priority Statement on Population," 1991. Unpublished statement (available from Zero Population Growth, Washington, D.C.).

Quataert, Jean H. 1979. *Reluctant Feminists in German Social Democracy, 1885–1917* (Princeton: Princeton University Press).

Rainwater, Lee. 1965. *Family Design: Marital Sexuality, Family Size, and Contraception* (Chicago: Aldine).

———. 1960. *And the Poor Get Children* (Chicago: Quadrangle Books).

Rich, William. 1973. *Smaller Families Through Social and Economic Progress.* Monograph no. 7 (Washington, D.C.: Overseas Development Council).

Ridker, Ronald, ed. 1976. *Population and Development: The Search for Selective Interventions* (Baltimore: Johns Hopkins University Press for Resources for the Future).

Riemer, Eleanor S., and John C. Fout. 1980. *European Women: A Documentary History, 1789–1945* (New York: Schocken).

Rinehart, Ward, and Adrienne Kols. 1984. "Healthier Mothers and Children Through Family Planning," *Population Reports, Series J,* no. 27 (May-June), pp. 657–696.

Roberts, Godfrey, ed. 1990. *Population Policy: Contemporary Issues* (New York: Praeger).

Robinson, Caroline Hadley. 1930. *Seventy Birth Control Clinics: A Survey and Analysis Including the General Effects of Control on Size and Quality of Population* (Baltimore: Williams and Wilkins).

Roemer, Ruth, and John M. Paxman. 1985. "Sex Education Laws and Policies," *Studies in Family Planning* vol. 16, no. 4 (July/Aug.), pp. 219–230.

Rogow, Deborah. 1986. "Quality of Care in International Family Planning: A Feminist Contribution," in International Women's Health Coalition and The Population Council, *The Contraceptive Development Process and Quality of Care in Reproductive Health Services: Report of a Meeting Held in New York City, Oct. 8–9, 1986* (New York: IWHC and The Population Council), pp. 72–100.

———. 1990. "From Abortion to Contraception: Getting to the Emerald City," paper prepared for WHO Regional Office for Europe, meeting on "From Abortion to Contraception," Tbilisi, USSR, Oct. 1–13, 1990 (New York: International Women's Health Coalition).

Rosenberg, Alison P. 1986. "A.I.D. Population Policy: The Needs and Rights of Individuals and Families," paper delivered at the annual meeting of the Population Association of America, San Francisco (April).

Rosenberg, M. J., R. W. Rochat, S. Jabeen, A. R. Measham, M. Obaidullah, and
A. R. Khan. 1981. "Attitudes of Rural Bangladesh Physicians Toward
Abortion," *Studies in Family Planning* vol. 12, no. 8/9 (Aug./Sept.),
pp. 318–321.

Rossoff, Jeanie I. 1988. "The Politics of Birth Control," *Family Planning Perspectives* vol. 20, no. 6 (Nov./Dec.), pp. 312–320.

Rosoff, Jeanie I. and Asta M. Kenney. 1984. "Title X and Its Critics," *Family
Planning Perspectives* vol. 16, no. 3 (May/June), pp. 111–119.

Rothman, Barbara Katz. 1982. *In Labor: Women and Power in the Birthplace*
(New York: W. W. Norton).

Rutenberg, Naomi, and Elisabeth A. Ferraz. 1988. "Female Sterilization and Its
Demographic Impact in Brazil," *International Family Planning Perspectives* vol. 14, no. 2 (June), pp. 61–67.

Ruzek, Sheryl Burt. 1978. *The Women's Health Movement: Feminist Alternatives
to Medical Control* (New York: Praeger).

Ryan, Bryce. 1951. "Institutional Factors in Sinhalese Fertility," *Milbank Memorial Fund Quarterly*, vol. 30 (Oct.), pp. 359–381.

Sadik, Nafis, ed. 1984. *Population: The UNFPA Experience* (New York: New
York University Press for the United Nations Fund for Population Activities).

Saffioti, Heleieth. 1969. *A Mulher na Sociedade de Classes: Mito e Realidade*
(São Paulo: Quatro Artes).

Safilios-Rothschild, Constantina. 1969. "Sociopsychological Factors Affecting
Fertility in Urban Greece," *Journal of Marriage and the Family* vol. 31,
no. 3 (Aug.), pp. 595–606.

———. 1982. "Female Power, Autonomy and Demographic Change in the Third
World," in Richard Anker, Mayra Buvinic, and Nadia H. Youssef, eds.,
Women's Roles and Population Trends in the Third World (London: Croom
Helm), pp. 117–132.

Sai, Fred T., and Janet Nassim. 1989. "The Need for a Reproductive Health
Approach," *International Journal of Gynecology and Obstetrics, Supplement 3,* pp. 103–114.

Salaff, Janet. 1981. *Working Daughters of Hong Kong: Filial Piety or Power in
the Family?* (Cambridge: Cambridge University Press).

Sanday, Peggy R. 1974. "Female Status in the Public Domain," in Michelle
Zimbalist Rosaldo and Louise Lamphere, eds., *Woman, Culture and Society* (Stanford: Stanford University Press), pp. 189–206.

Sanger, Margaret. 1920. *Woman and the New Race* (New York: Brentano).

———. 1931. *My Fight for Birth Control* (New York: Farrar-Rinehart).

Sarti, Cynthia. 1989. "The Panorama of Feminism in Brazil," *New Left Review*
no. 17 (Jan./Feb.).

Sayers, Janet. 1982. *Biological Politics: Feminist and Anti-Feminist Perspectives*
(London: Tavistock).

Schmink, Marianne. 1981. "Women in Brazilian Abertura Politics," *Signs: Journal of Women in Culture and Society* vol. 7, no. 1, pp. 115–134.

Schnaiberg, Allan, and David Reed. 1974. "Risk, Uncertainty and Family Formation: The Social Context of Poverty Groups," *Population Studies* vol.
28, no. 3 (Nov.), pp. 513–533.

Schultz, T. Paul. 1990. "Women's Changing Participation in the Labor Force: A World Perspective," *Economic Development and Cultural Change* vol. 38, no. 3 (April), pp. 457–488.

Scrimshaw, Susan C. M. 1976. "Women's Modesty: One Barrier to the Use of Family Planning Clinics in Ecuador," in J. Marshall and S. Polgar, eds., *Culture, Natality, and Family Planning* (Chapel Hill: Carolina Population Center, University of North Carolina), pp. 167–187.

———. 1978. "Infant Mortality and Behavior in the Regulation of Family Size," *Population and Development Review* vol. 4, no. 3 (Sept.), pp. 383–402.

Seaman, Barbara. 1969. *The Doctor's Case Against the Pill* (New York: Avon).

Sen, Gita, and Caren Grown. 1987. *Development, Crises, and Alternative Visions: Third World Women's Perspectives,* 2nd ed. (New York: Monthly Review Press).

Shahani, Leticia Ramos. 1987. "Needed: Urgent Implementation of a Population Policy," Speech before the Philippine Senate, 5 Oct. 1987.

Shearer, S. Bruce. 1983. "Monetary and Health Costs of Contraception," in Rodolfo A. Bulatao and Ronald D. Lee, eds., *Determinants of Fertility in Developing Countries,* vol. 2 (New York: Academic Press), pp. 89–150.

Shedlin, Michele Goldzieher, and Paula E. Hollerbach. 1981. "Modern and Traditional Fertility Regulation in a Mexican Community," *Studies in Family Planning* vol. 12, no. 6/7 (June/July), pp. 278–296.

Sherris, Jacqueline D., and Gordon Fox. 1983. "Infertility and Sexually Transmitted Disease: A Public Health Challenge," *Population Reports, Series L.,* no. 4 (Baltimore: Population Information Program, The Johns Hopkins University).

Shorter, Edward. 1973. "Female Emancipation, Birth Control, and Fertility in European History," *American Historical Review* vol. 78, no. 3 (June), pp. 605–640.

Shrier, Sally, ed. 1988. *Women's Movements of the World: An International Directory and Reference Guide* (London: Longman).

Silvestre, Louise, Catherine Dubois, Maguy Renault, Yvonne Rezvani, Etienne-Emile Baulieu, and André Ulmann. 1990. "Voluntary Interruption of Pregnancy with Mifepristone (RU 486) and a Prostaglandin Analogue," *New England Journal of Medicine* vol. 322, no. 10 (8 March), pp. 645–648.

Simmons, Ruth, Laila Baqee, Michael A. Koenig, and James F. Phillips. 1988. "Beyond Supply: The Importance of Female Family Planning Workers in Rural Bangladesh," *Studies in Family Planning* vol. 19, no. 1 (Jan./Feb.), pp. 29–38.

Simmons, Ruth, Bonnie J. Kay, and Carol Regan. 1984. "Women's Health Groups: Alternatives to the Health Care System," *International Journal of Health Services* vol. 14, no. 4, pp. 619–634.

Simmons, Ruth, and James F. Phillips. 1987. "The Integration of Family Planning with Health and Development," in Robert J. Lapham and George B. Simmons, eds., *Organizing for Effective Family Planning Programs* (Washington, D.C.: National Academy Press), pp. 185–212.

Simon, Julian L. 1981. *The Ultimate Resource* (Princeton: Princeton University Press).

Sinding, Steven W., and Carl J. Hemmer. 1975. "Population Policy Development:

The Application of Theory," in R. Kenneth Godwin, ed., *Comparative Policy Analysis: The Study of Population Policy Determinants in Developing Countries* (Lexington: Lexington Books), pp. 267–282.

Sivard, Ruth Leger. 1985. *Women: A World Survey* (Washington, D.C.: World Priorities).

Smith, Herbert. 1989. "Integrating Theory and Research on the Institutional Determinants of Fertility," *Demography* vol. 26, no. 2, pp. 171–184.

Standing, Guy. 1983. "Women's Work Activity and Fertility," in Rodolfo A. Bulatao and Ronald D. Lee, eds., *Determinants of Fertility in Developing Countries,* vol. 1 (New York: Academic Press), pp. 517–546.

Starrs, Ann. 1987. *Preventing the Tragedy of Maternal Deaths: A Report on the International Safe Motherhood Conference, Nairobi, Kenya, February 1987* (Washington, D.C.: The World Bank).

Staudt, Kathleen A. 1981. "Women's Organizations in Rural Development," in Barbara C. Lewis, ed., *Invisible Farmers: Women and the Crisis in Agriculture* (Washington, D.C.: Office of Women in Development, U.S. Agency for International Development), pp. 329–400.

———. 1985. *Women, Foreign Assistance and Advocacy Administration* (New York: Praeger).

———, ed. 1990. *Women, International Development, and Politics: The Bureaucratic Mire* (Philadelphia: Temple University Press).

Stycos, Joseph M. 1968. *Human Fertility in Latin America* (Ithaca: Cornell University Press).

———. 1977. "Some Minority Opinions on Birth Control," in R. M. Veatch, ed., *Population Policy and Ethics: The American Experience* (New York: Irvington Publishers/Halstead Press).

Stycos, Joseph M., and Robert N. Weller. 1967. "Female Working Roles and Fertility," *Demography* vol. 4, no. 1, pp. 210–217.

"Summary Report of the National Seminar on Reproductive Rights, Embu-São Paulo, Brazil, Sept. 1987" (New York: International Women's Health Coalition).

Symonds, Richard, and Michael Carder. 1973. *The United Nations and the Population Question, 1956–1970* (New York: McGraw-Hill).

Szalai, Alexander, ed. 1972. *The Use of Time: Daily Activities of Urban and Suburban Populations in Twelve Countries* (The Hague: Mouton).

Tadiar, Alfredo Flores. 1989. "Commentary on the Law and Abortion in the Philippines," *International Journal of Gynecology and Obstetrics, Supplement 3,* pp. 89–92.

Tangri, Sandra S. 1976. "A Feminist Perspective on Some Ethical Issues in Population Programs," *Signs: Journal of Women in Culture and Society* vol. 1, no. 4, pp. 895–904.

Thomas, John, and Merillee Grindle. 1990. "National Priorities and Individual Responses: The Political Economy of Population Policy Reform," paper delivered at conference on the Politics of Induced Fertility Change in Developing Countries, Feb. 19–23, 1990, Bellagio, Italy.

Tietze, Christopher, and Stanley K. Henshaw. 1986. *Induced Abortion: A World Review,* 6th ed. (New York: The Alan Guttmacher Institute).

Tinker, Irene, ed. 1990. *Persistent Inequalities: Women and World Development* (New York: Oxford University Press).

———, and Jane Jaquette. 1987. "UN Decade for Women: Its Impact and Legacy," *World Development* vol. 15, no. 3, pp. 419–427.

Trussell, J., and A. R. Pebley. 1984. "The Potential Impact of Changes in Fertility on Infant, Child, and Maternal Mortality," *Studies in Family Planning* vol. 15, no. 6, part 1 (Nov./Dec.), pp. 253–266.

Tulloch, Gail. 1989. *Mill and Sexual Equality* (Hemel Hempstead, England: Harvester Wheatsheaf).

United Nations. 1973a. *Human Rights: A Compilation of International Instruments of the United Nations* (New York: United Nations).

———. 1973b. *The Determinants and Consequences of Population Trends,* vol. 1 (New York: United Nations).

———. 1975. *Status of Women and Family Planning* (New York: United Nations).

United Nations, Department of International Economic and Social Affairs. 1984. *Improving Concepts and Methods for Statistics and Indicators on the Situation of Women* (New York: United Nations).

———. 1985. *Socio-Economic Differentials in Child Mortality in Developing Countries* (New York: United Nations).

———. 1987. *Fertility Behaviour in the Context of Development: Evidence from the World Fertility Survey* (New York: United Nations).

———. 1988a. *Case Studies in Population Policy: Brazil* (New York: United Nations).

———. 1988b. *Case Studies in Population Policy: Nigeria* (New York: United Nations).

———. 1988c. *Compendium of Statistics and Indicators on the Situation of Women, 1986* (New York: United Nations).

———. 1988d. *World Population Trends and Policies* (New York: United Nations).

———. 1989a. *Adolescent Reproductive Behavior: Evidence from Developing Countries,* vol. 2 (New York: United Nations).

———. 1989b. *World Population Monitoring* (New York: United Nations).

———. 1990a. *Patterns of First Marriage: Timing and Prevalence* (New York: United Nations).

———. 1990b. *Population and Human Rights: Proceedings of the Expert Group Meeting on Population and Human Rights, Geneva, 3–6 April 1989* (New York: United Nations).

———. 1991. *The World's Women: Trends and Statistics 1970–1990* (New York: United Nations).

United Nations Fund for Population Activities (UNFPA). 1985. *Population Perspectives: Statements by World Leaders, 2nd ed.* (New York: UNFPA).

———. 1986. *Inventory of Population Projects in Developing Countries Around the World, 1984/85* (New York: UNFPA).

United Nations General Assembly. 1991. "Advancement of Women: Convention on the Elimination of All Forms of Discrimination Against Women, Report of the Secretary-General," A/46/462; 25 Sept. (New York: United Nations).

United Nations Population Fund (UNFPA). 1989a. "Maternal and Child Health and Family Planning," Sectoral Paper, International Forum on Population in the Twenty-first Century, Amsterdam, 6–9 November 1989 (New York: UNFPA).

———. 1989b. *Inventory of Population Projects in Developing Countries Around the World* 1987/88 (New York: UNFPA).

United States. 1974. "Statement by the Honorable Caspar W. Weinberger, Delegation of the United States," United Nations World Population Conference, Bucharest, August 1974.

———. 1984. "Policy Statement of the United States of America at the United Nations International Conference on Population (Second Session, Mexico, D.F., August 6–13, 1984," reprinted in *Population and Development Review* vol. 10, no. 4 (Dec.), pp. 576, 583.

U.S. Agency for International Development, Office of Population. 1974. *Population Program Assistance: United States Aid to Developing Countries* (Washington, D.C.: U.S. Government Printing Office).

———. 1982. "Policy Paper on Population Assistance," reprinted in part as "United States Population Assistance Policy," *Population and Development Review* vol. 9, no. 1 (March, 1983), pp. 185–194.

U.S. Commission on Population Growth and the American Future. 1972. *Population and the American Future* (New York: Signet).

van de Kaa, Dirk J. 1988. "A First Note on the Right to Decide Freely and Responsibly," in B. van Norren and H. A. W. van Vianen, eds., *Profession: Demographer: Ten Population Studies in Honour of F. H. A. G. Zwart* (Groningen, The Netherlands: Geo Pers).

van de Walle, Etienne. 1990. "Seminar on Population Policy in Sub-Saharan Africa: Drawing on International Experience, Kinshasa, Zaire, 27 Feb.–2 March 1989," *IUSSP Newsletter no. 38* (Liege, Belgium: International Union for the Scientific Study of Population), pp. 9–19.

van den Bergh, Pierre L. 1973. *Age and Sex in Human Societies: A Biosocial Perspective* (Belmont: Wadsworth).

van der Vlugt, Theresa, and P. T. Piotrow. 1973. "Menstrual Regulation: What Is It?" *Population Reports, Series F,* no. 2 (April), pp. 9–23.

Veil, Simone. 1978. "Human Rights, Ideologies, and Population Policies," *Population and Development Review* vol. 4, no. 2 (June), pp. 313–321.

Verzosa, Cecilia C., Nora Llamas, and Richard T. Mahoney. 1984. "Attitudes Toward the Rhythm Method in the Philippines," *Studies in Family Planning* vol. 15, no. 2 (March/April), pp. 74–78.

Vieille, Paul. 1978. "Iranian Women in Family Alliance and Sexual Politics," in Nikki Keddie and Lois Beck, eds., *Women in the Muslim World* (Cambridge: Harvard University Press), pp. 451–472.

Villarreal, Jorge. 1989. "Commentary on Unwanted Pregnancy, Induced Abortion, and Professional Ethics: A Concerned Physician's Point of View," *International Journal of Gynecology and Obstetrics, Supplement 3,* pp. 51–56.

Ward, Kathryn B. 1984. *Women in the World-System: Its Impact on Status and Fertility* (New York: Praeger).

Ward, Martha C. 1986. *Poor Women, Powerful Men: America's Great Experiment in Family Planning* (Boulder: Westview).

Ware, Helen. 1977. "Women's Work and Fertility in Africa," in Stanley Kupinsky, ed., *The Fertility of Working Women* (New York: Praeger), pp. 1–34.
———. 1981. *Women, Demography, and Development* (Canberra: Australian Na-
tional University).
Warwick, Donald P. 1982. *Bitter Pills: Population Policies and Their Implemen-
tation in Eight Developing Countries* (Cambridge: Cambridge University
Press).
Wasserheit, Judith N. 1989. "The Significance and Scope of Reproductive Tract
Infections Among Third World Women, *International Journal of Gyne-
cology and Obstetrics, Supplement 3*, pp. 145–168.
Weller, Robert H. 1968. "The Employment of Wives, Role Incompatibility and
Fertility: A Study Among Lower and Middle Class Residents of San Juan,
Puerto Rico," *Milbank Memorial Fund Quarterly* vol. 46, no. 4 (Oct.),
pp. 507–526.
Westoff, Charles F. 1988. "The Potential Demand for Family Planning: A New
Estimate of Unmet Need and Estimates for Five Latin American Coun-
tries," *International Family Planning Perspectives* vol. 14, no. 2 (June),
pp. 45–53.
Whelehan, Patricia, ed. 1988. *Women and Health: Cross-Cultural Perspectives*
(Granby: Bergin and Garvey).
Wieringa, Saskia, ed. 1988. *Women's Struggles and Strategies* (Aldershot, Great
Britain: Gower Press).
Winikoff, Beverly, and Maureen Sullivan. 1987. "Assessing the Role of Family
Planning in Reducing Maternal Mortality," *Studies in Family Planning* vol.
18, no. 3 (March), pp. 128–143.
Winter, Jay M. 1989. "Socialism, Social Democracy, and Population Questions
in Western Europe, 1870–1950," in Michael S. Teitelbaum and Jay M.
Winter, eds., *Population and Resources in Western Intellectual Traditions*
(Cambridge: Cambridge University Press), pp. 122–146.
Wollstonecraft, Mary. [1792] 1982. *Vindication of the Rights of Woman* (London:
Penguin).
WomanHealth. 1987. "In Support of Senate P.S. Resolution No. 39. Joint Statement of WomanHealth, Women's Health Care Foundation, Inc., Institute
for Social Studies and Action" (Manila: WomanHealth).
———. 1988. "WomanHealth Proposed Amendments to Senate Resolution No.
39 Introduced by Senators Shahani, Tanada, Romulo and Mercado" (January, 1988) (Manila: WomanHealth).
Women in Nigeria. 1985. *The WIN Document: Conditions of Women in Nigeria
and Policy Recommendations* (Samaru, Zaria: Women in Nigeria).
World Bank. 1984. *World Development Report 1984* (New York: Oxford University Press).
———. 1987. "Nigeria: First National Population Project," Initiating Project Brief
(Washington, D.C.: World Bank, 26 May).
———. 1991. *1991 World Development Report: The Challenge of Development*
(Washington, D.C.: World Bank).
World Health Organization (WHO). 1985a. *Coverage of Maternity Care: A Tabulation of Available Information* (Geneva: Division of Family Health,
WHO).

————. 1985b. *Women, Health and Development: A Report by the Director-General*, WHO Offset Publication No. 90 (Geneva: WHO).

————. 1986. *Maternal Mortality Rates: A Tabulation of Available Information.* 2nd ed. (Geneva: Division of Family Health, WHO).

————. 1991. *Creating Common Ground: Women's Perspectives on the Selection and Introduction of Fertility Regulation Technologies.* WHO/HRP/ITT/91 (Geneva: WHO).

World Health Organization Task Force on Psychosocial Research in Family Planning. 1981. "A Cross-Cultural Study of Menstruation: Implications for Contraceptive Development and Use," *Studies in Family Planning* vol. 12, no. 1 (Jan.), pp. 3–16.

World Population Conference, Bucharest, 1974. *Report of the Symposium on Population and Human Rights, Amsterdam, 21–29 January 1974* (New York: United Nations).

————. 1975. *The Population Debate: Dimensions and Perspectives. Report of the World Population Conference*, Bucharest, 1974 (New York: United Nations).

Woycke, James. 1988. *Birth Control in Germany 1971–1933* (London: Routledge).

Wulf, Deirdre, and Peter D. Willson. 1984. "Global Politics in Mexico City," *Family Planning Perspectives* vol. 16, no. 5 (Sept./Oct.), pp. 228–232.

Yusuf, Bilkisu. 1985. "Nigerian Women in Politics: Problems and Prospects," in Editorial Committee, Women in Nigeria, *Women in Nigeria Today* (London: Zed Books), pp. 212–216.

Zimicki, Susan. 1989. "The Relation between Fertility and Maternal Mortality," in Allan M. Parnell, ed., *Contraceptive Use and Controlled Fertility: Health Issues for Women and Children* (Washington, D.C.: National Academy Press), pp. 1–47.

INDEX

Index

217; definition and purpose, 5, 15–
17, 195–97; demographic targets,
16, 19, 51–52, 68, 101–2, 104, 195,
202; effectiveness, 22, 56–57, 65,
69; and equal rights, 16, 194–95;
ethical aspects, 18–20, 52, 57, 193–
94; government positions, 17–18,
70, 76; implementation, 16, 21–22,
84, 91, 95–96, 99, 102–3, 195–96;
incentive schemes, 16–17, 19–20,
52, 56; influence of foreign donors,
21, 79, 89, 94, 100, 102–3, 183, 196–
97; influence of interest groups, 5,
21–22, 89, 94, 101, 103–5, 196–97;
and national sovereignty, 7, 19; in
Nigeria, 94–96; participation/
exclusion of women, 20, 33, 53, 78,
83–84, 91–92, 94–95, 100–1, 193–94,
217; in Philippines, 99–103. *See also*
U.S. population policy
Pregnancy: adolescent and
nonmarital, 98, 117–18, 129, 142,
160, 171, 179; unwanted and
mistimed, 87, 114, 164, 167–71. *See
also* Childbirth; Maternal mortality
Pro-choice movement (abortion), 39,
44–47, 65–66, 91
Prostitution, 14, 35, 101, 113
Puerto Rico, 43, 172

Race: discrimination, 6, 8; charges of
genocide, 64–65; and the women's
movement: 47, 65, 85
Reproductive health: array of
services, 207–8; definitions: 97, 143,
160–61, 177, 203–4, 218; funding,
215–16; policies, 195, 201–2, 205–7;
programs, 89–90, 98–99, 104, 204–
16, 218–19; providers, 210–11. *See
also* Maternal mortality
Reproductive rights: and the
Convention, 9, 12; as a feminist
agenda, 5, 12, 14, 47, 82; as
freedoms and entitlements, 12, 113–
14, 192, 201–2; indicators of,
113–15
Resource theory, 131, 149
Right-to-life movement (anti-

abortion), 33, 46, 66–67, 71–72, 76,
91, 101, 184, 219
Risk and uncertainty (social and
economic), 26, 112, 116–17, 206
Roe v. Wade (U.S. Supreme Court
decision on abortion), 46, 66–67,
75
Roles, women's social: in the
community, 157; conjugal relations,
150–53; content and profiles, 148;
domestic work, 157; effects of
fertility regulation on, 148–60;
incompatibility of, 118, 124–25, 148,
155; as individuals, 159–60; kinship
relations, 157; maternal, 155–57;
occupational, 153–55; segregation
of, 131, 150; strain and conflict,
149
Roman Catholic church, 43, 45, 59–
60, 76, 85, 91, 100–101,183–84
Romania, 19, 185
Rural women, 11, 64, 123, 125, 135,
142, 168, 199, 206, 211, 218
Rwanda, 126

Sanger, Margaret, 32, 37–43, 45, 49,
59, 139
Saudi Arabia, 11
Senegal, 97, 184, 211
Sexuality: abstinence, 35–36, 75, 97,
133, 151; and birth control, 32, 35–
37, 40, 43, 46, 101, 152–53;
exploitation, 11, 99, 101, 113, 203,
208; and individual freedom, 14, 42,
46, 113, 128, 203–4; pleasure and
dissatisfaction, 35–36, 131, 149, 151,
212; premarital and nonmarital,
116–17, 164, 169–70
Sexually transmitted diseases, 49, 97–
99, 101, 104, 129, 143–45, 207–8,
212
Singapore, 18–19, 43, 153, 164, 168,
172, 184
Soviet Union, 11, 25, 39, 43, 45,
200
Spain, 45, 186
Sri Lanka, 19, 58, 63, 118, 128–29
Status of women: autonomy and

and the family, 8, 127–28, 130; to political participation, 8–9, 119–20, 136–37, 193; to property and social security, 128, 133–35. *See also* Convention; Education; Employment; Marriage, Family
World Bank, 63, 79, 102, 196, 215
World Fertility Surveys, 77, 97
World Health Organization, 139, 141, 181, 186, 215

World Population Conference, Bucharest (1974), 51, 67–69, 70, 73, 79, 86, 88, 94, 135–36, 182
World Population Plans of Action, 12, 68, 73, 135, 182–83

Yemen, 200

Zaire, 184
Zambia, 184
Zimbabwe, 73, 97

About the Author

RUTH DIXON-MUELLER was Professor of Sociology at the University of California, Davis, until 1988 and Research Associate in Demography at the University of California, Berkeley, until 1992. She now lives and works in Costa Rica. She has served as a consultant for the U.S. Agency for International Development, the U.N. World Food Programme, the International Labor Office, the U.S. International Center for Training and Research on the Advancement of Women (INSTRAW), and the International Women's Health Coalition, among other organizations. Dixon-Mueller is the author of *Rural Women at Work: Strategies for Development in South Asia* and *Women's Work in Third World Agriculture*, and articles on U.S. international population policy, abortion policy and women's health, contraceptive use, and women's rights and fertility.